GENITOURINARY CANCER

CONTEMPORARY ISSUES
IN CLINICAL ONCOLOGY
VOLUME 5

SERIES EDITOR

Peter H. Wiernik, M.D.

Gutman Professor and Chairman
Department of Oncology
Montefiore Medical Center
Chief, Division of Medical Oncology
Albert Einstein College of Medicine
Associate Director for Clinical Research
Albert Einstein Cancer Center
New York, New York

GENITOURINARY CANCER

Edited by

Marc B. Garnick, M.D.

Associate Professor of Medicine
Harvard Medical School
Dana-Farber Cancer Institute
Associate Physician
Brigham and Women's Hospital
Boston, Massachusetts

CHURCHILL LIVINGSTONE   **1985**
NEW YORK, EDINBURGH, LONDON, AND MELBOURNE

Acquisitions editor: *William R. Schmitt*
Copy editor: *Kim Loretucci*
Production editor: *Michiko Davis*
Production supervisor: *Kerry A. O'Rourke*
Compositor: *Kingsport Press*
Printer/Binder: *The Murray Printing Co.*

© Churchill Livingstone Inc. 1985

Distributed in the United Kingdom by Churchill Livingstone,
Robert Stevenson House, 1–3 Baxter's Place, Leith Walk
Edinburgh EH1 3AF and associated companies, branches
and representatives throughout the world.

First published in 1985
Printed in U.S.A.

ISBN 0–443–08350–9
9 8 7 6 5 4 3 2 1

Library of Congress Cataloging in Publication Data
Main entry under title:

Genitourinary cancer.

  (Contemporary issues in clinical oncology; v. 5)
  Includes bibliographies and index.
  1. Generative organs, Male—Cancer. 2. Genito-
urinary organs—Cancer. I. Garnick, Marc B.
II. Series: Contemporary issues in oncology; v. 5.
[DNLM: 1. Urogenital Neoplasms—therapy.
W1 CO769MRF v. 5 / WJ 160 G3303]
RC280.G52G46 1985   616.99'46   84–17620
ISBN 0–443–08350–9

Manufactured in the United States of America

To
Arnold D. Kates

A man of creativity, individuality, and simplicity
whose joy for life is inspirational

Contributors

George J. Bosl, M.D.
Assistant Professor of Medicine
Cornell University Medical College
Assistant Attending Physician
Solid Tumor Service
Director, Continuing Medical Education
Memorial Sloan-Kettering Cancer Center
New York, New York

William DeWolf, M.D.
Associate Professor of Surgery
Harvard Medical School
Division of Cellular Genetics
Charles A. Dana Research Institute
Beth Israel Hospital
Boston, Massachusetts

Lawrence H. Einhorn, M.D.
American Cancer Society Clinical Professor of Oncology
Professor of Medicine
Indiana University School of Medicine
University Hospital
Indianapolis, Indiana

Marc S. Ernstoff, M.D.
Assistant Professor of Medicine
Section of Medical Oncology
Yale University School of Medicine
New Haven, Connecticut

Mehmet F. Fer, M.D.
Visiting Scientist
Biological Response Modifiers Program
National Cancer Institute
Frederick Cancer Research Facility
Frederick, Maryland

L. Michael Glode, M.D.
Associate Professor of Medicine
University of Colorado Health Sciences Center
Denver, Colorado

F. Anthony Greco, M.D.
Professor of Medicine
Director, Division of Oncology
Vanderbilt University Medical Center
Nashville, Tennessee

John D. Hainsworth, M.D.
Assistant Professor of Medicine
Division of Oncology
Vanderbilt University Medical Center
Nashville, Tennessee

Daniel F. Hayes, M.D.
Clinical Fellow in Medicine
Harvard Medical School
Dana-Farber Cancer Institute
Boston, Massachusetts

John M. Kirkwood, M.D.
Associate Professor of Medicine and Dermatology
Yale University School of Medicine
New Haven, Connecticut

Bert L. Lum, Pharm.D.
Assistant Professor of Clinical Pharmacology
School of Pharmacy
University of the Pacific
Coordinator, Clinical Pharmacy
V.A. Medical Center
Palo Alto, California

Clarke F. Millette, Ph.D.
Associate Professor of Anatomy
Laboratory of Human Reproduction and Reproductive Biology
Harvard Medical School
Boston, Massachusetts

Perinchery Narayan, M.D.
Assistant Professor of Urologic Surgery
University of Minnesota Health Sciences Center
Minneapolis, Minnesota

Derek Raghavan, M.B., B.S., Ph.D., F.R.A.C.P.
Oncologist, Department of Clinical Oncology
Research Director
Urological Cancer Research Unit
Royal Prince Alfred Hospital
Honorary Consultant
Ludwig Institute for Cancer Research
Sydney, New South Wales, Australia

Jerome P. Richie, M.D.
Associate Professor of Urologic Surgery
Harvard Medical School
Chief, Urologic Oncology
Brigham and Women's Hospital
Boston, Massachusetts

Mark S. Soloway, M.D.
Professor of Urology
University of Tennessee Center for the Health Sciences
Memphis, Tennessee

Frank M. Torti, M.D.
Clinical Associate Professor of Medicine
Division of Oncology
Stanford University Medical Center
Stanford, California
Staff Physician
V.A. Medical Center
Palo Alto, California

Judith L. Vaitukaitis, M.D.
Professor of Medicine and Physiology
Boston University School of Medicine
Head, Section of Endocrinology and Metabolism
Boston City Hospital
Boston, Massachusetts

Nicholas J. Vogelzang, M.D.
Assistant Professor of Medicine
Section of Hematology/Oncology
The University of Chicago
Division of Biological Sciences and
The Pritzker School of Medicine
Chicago, Illinois

James L. Wade III, M.D.
Fellow
Section of Hematology/Oncology
Department of Medicine
The University of Chicago
Division of Biological Sciences and
The Pritzker School of Medicine
Chicago, Illinois

Stephen D. Williams, M.D.
Associate Professor of Medicine
Indiana University School of Medicine
Chief, Hematology-Oncology Service
Indianapolis Veteran's Administration Medical Center
Indianapolis, Indiana

Preface

The mission of *Contemporary Issues in Clinical Oncology,* as originally conceived by Dr. Wiernik, is to produce a "practical, clear, concise, and useful series that will provide the physician with a state-of-art and science base to design treatment for today's patients. . . . The theme of this series is to provide multidisciplinary approaches to common problems and to justify them with laboratory and clinical data."

Genitourinary Cancer specifically addresses these goals and, I believe, fulfills them admirably. This current volume addresses the major controversial areas in the discipline and, as importantly, provides the framework for changes in therapeutic practice in the 1980's.

The volume has been divided into four sections, each discussing the "leading edge" issues of current treatment. In the testis cancer section, Dr. Vaitukaitis provides an overview of the biology and clinical applications of tumor markers in germ cell neoplasms. Both the clinician and laboratory scientist should study this chapter to appreciate fully the methodology in performing these assays and their appropriate clinical interpretation. Dr. Raghavan explores the possibility of therapy with "orchiectomy alone" for stage I nonseminomatous germ cell tumors. Given the high curability rate of patients with metastatic testicular cancer who undergo combination chemotherapy, the policy of orchiectomy alone for patients with early stage disease, followed by chemotherapy at relapse, deserves further study. Likewise, combination chemotherapy has assumed a primary role in treating patients with advanced forms of seminoma, as described by Drs. Williams and Einhorn, who are leaders in the field. Dr. Bosl presents a well-organized overview of the "VAB" combination chemotherapy program conducted at Memorial Sloan-Kettering Cancer Center and demonstrates the enormous advances that have been made in this disease over the past 25 years.

Clinical acumen and pathologic expertise are required in diagnosing and managing extragonadal germ cell tumors. Accordingly, the experience from Vanderbilt University Hospital and Indiana University is discussed by Drs. Fer, Hainsworth, and Greco. They appropriately emphasize some of the controversies on optimal approaches to these very unusual, but treatable, neoplasms.

The last chapter in the testis cancer section delves into the natural biology of seminomatous germ cell tumors, a subject under intensive investigation by Drs. Narayan, Millette, and DeWolf. The potential and future clinical implications of their research are discussed.

The three issues discussed in the prostate cancer section are all areas of great interest in therapeutic management. Dr. Richie provides a very sober and conservative approach to the potential usefulness of lymph node sampling in the management of patients with prostate cancer. Perhaps one of the most exciting areas in the management of disseminated prostate cancer comes from the basic science work in controlling the normal hypothalamic pituitary gonadal axis and the subsequent development of gonadotropin-releasing hormone analogs. Dr. Glode provides an overview of these new analogs, which will clearly be used in a commonplace fashion in the future. Likewise, Drs. Torti and Lum provide an exhaustive and a critical appraisal of the use of chemotherapy for patients with prostate cancer, with special emphasis on those who have become refractory to hormonal therapy.

The bladder cancer section addresses two specific issues: the use of intravesical chemotherapy in the management of superficial disease and the use of chemotherapy followed by definitive radiation therapy, surgery, or both in the management of muscle invasive cancers. Dr. Soloway's review of intravesical chemotherapy trials provides the reader with the author's seasoned judgment on optimal approaches for various stages of superficial disease. Dr. Raghavan provides exciting data for both local and systemic control of muscle invasive bladder cancer with the use of "upfront" chemotherapy followed by definitive radiation therapy, surgery, or both. Clearly, the therapeutic implications of these two chapters will have a major impact in the management of superficial and invasive disease in the coming years.

The last section describes new agents that are useful in managing a variety of urologic cancers. Etoposide, which was recently released in the United States for refractory testicular carcinoma, may produce antineoplastic activity in other neoplasms as well. Drs. Wade and Vogelzang provide an overview of the use of this podophyllotoxin derivative. Great professional and public interest has accompanied the use of interferons as a potential panacea for ills ranging from the common cold to cancer. Drs. Kirkwood and Ernstoff provide a very critical, yet optimistic, appeal for the use of interferons in urologic cancer, with special emphasis on the most refractory of all urologic cancers—renal adenocarcinoma. They provide the foundation for both the basic science and clinical aspects of these very interesting glycoproteins.

The concluding chapter on special surgical applications by Dr. Hayes critically reviews the enormous body of literature on this commonly asked question: is surgical removal of metastatic deposits beneficial? Dr. Hayes specifically addresses the potential role of pulmonary nodulectomy in selected patients with urologic cancers. He presents a clear and comprehensible discussion that the clinician should find useful in his daily practice.

The design and implementation of this volume have been enjoyable and intellectually satisfying. The readers of this volume should praise the contributors for their timely and critical presentations.

I would like to acknowledge Ms. Robin Gibbs, my editorial assistant in the preparation of this volume, and Ms. Kim Loretucci of Churchill Livingstone whose managerial skills allowed this volume to be published in such a timely fashion.

Marc B. Garnick, M.D.
Boston, Massachusetts

Contents

GENITOURINARY CANCER

1 | Biological Markers in Germ Cell Neoplasms

Judith L. Vaitukaitis

Over the past several years, markedly improved chemotherapy-induced response rates among young men presenting with germinal cell tumors of the testis have been attained.[1] Those advances reflect the development of new combinations of chemotherapeutic agents and the introduction of *cis*-platinum and several other drugs. In general, cure rates correlate with the stage of germinal cell testicular cancer at the time of patient presentation.[1] Moreover, accurate clinical staging of the cancer is imperative so that the clinician can select appropriate therapy. Fortunately, several tumor markers have proved useful for improving accuracy of clinical staging as well as monitoring patient responses to therapy and detecting early tumor recurrences. The most widely used markers are human chorionic gonadotropin (hCG) and alphafetoprotein (AFP). In addition, lactic dehydrogenase (LDH) and carcinoembryonic antigen (CEA) have also been used, along with several other markers that either have not proved useful or have not been extensively studied. Since hCG and AFP have been most valuable for monitoring patients with germinal cell cancers, this presentation will focus on those two markers. Monitoring hCG and AFP levels has proved invaluable for staging, monitoring therapy, and detecting recurrent tumor growth weeks to months prior to that discernable with other diagnostic techniques. A few other markers appear promising, but insufficient data are available to adequately assess their usefulness.

HUMAN CHORIONIC GONADOTROPIN

Structure and Physiology

Human chorionic gonadotropin, a glycoprotein hormone, of approximately 45,000 daltons, is normally synthesized in large quantities by the human placenta. It is comprised of two noncovalently linked, dissimilar subunits, designated alpha

1

and beta, and shares a common quaternary structure with the pituitary glycoprotein hormones—luteinizing hormone (LH), follicle stimulating hormone (FSH), and thyroid stimulating hormone (TSH).[2] The isolated subunits are essentially devoid of significant intrinsic biological activity. All four glycoprotein hormones share a common alpha subunit. The primary amino acid sequence of the alpha subunit is essentially identical among those glycoprotein hormones. However, it is the beta subunit that confers both immunological and biological specificities of the glycoprotein hormone.[2] The biological effects of LH and hCG are indistinguishable, which reflects the extensive structural homology of the beta subunits of these two glycoprotein hormones. At least 70 percent of the amino acids of the beta subunits of LH and hCG are homologous.[3] Since the initial therapy of many men who present with germinal cell tumors of the testis usually requires castration and frequently chemotherapy or radiation, high circulating levels of LH are commonly observed and reflect primary gonadal failure induced by therapy. Disruption of the negative feedback loop between the testis and the hypothalamic–pituitary axis results in high or castrate levels of LH. Since LH concentrations in blood may be high, sensitive, specific assays that selectively measure low hCG levels in the presence of castrate or high levels of LH are imperative.

The synthesis of the hCG subunits is controlled by separate messenger ribonucleic acids (mRNA) translated from genes on chromosomes 10 and 18.[4] In the normal placenta, unbalanced synthesis and secretion of the subunits of hCG is observed so that excess free alpha and no significant free beta is present.[5] Not only does the placenta synthesize and secrete hCG, but other human tissues, including the pituitary, gastrointestinal tract, liver, and possibly even the testis also synthesize hCG at low levels.[6-8] Probably because those tissues synthesize hCG, low levels of hCG are present in normal peripheral blood.[9] Borkowski et al.[9] tested pools obtained from apparently normal individuals for the presence of hCG using a variety of techniques. Less than 1 ng/ml or approximately 5 mIU/ml (second International Standard for hCG) or 9.3 mIU/ml (first International Reference Preparation for hCG) was found. In addition to low levels of hCG, a small amount of free immunoreactive alpha also circulates in normal people.[5,10] The major site of secretion of free alpha is from the pituitary, which, like the placenta, synthesizes excess free alpha along with the intact glycoprotein hormones.[11] The glycoprotein hormones do not dissociate spontaneously in peripheral blood, and consequently, high circulating levels of glycoprotein hormones do not contribute to the free alpha or free beta subunits of hCG and other glycoprotein hormones observed in selected clinical settings.[10] In fact, when hCG or pituitary glycoprotein hormones are synthesized and secreted at high levels, more alpha is synthesized and secreted for reasons not understood. However, unbalanced synthesis and secretion of one or both hCG subunits may be observed among some patients with hCG-secreting tumors.[5]

The subunits of hCG can be dissociated by chemical means and isolated in a highly purified form;[12] they possess negligible intrinsic biologic activity,[2] however. Moreover, the plasma half-life of the free subunits is significantly shorter than that for the parent hormone hCG. In man, the plasma half-life for alpha is approximately 13 minutes, for free hCGβ approximately 41 minutes.[13] The fully glycosylated hCG molecule has a plasma half-life of approximately 24 to 36 hours. Because of the prolonged plasma half-life of fully glycosylated hCG, it is usually impossible to discern small arteriovenous gradients of that hormone across tumors secreting it. However, if altered hCG or free subunits are secreted by a tumor, then a small gradient may be discerned because of the markedly shorter plasma half-lives of incompletely glycosylated hCG and its subunits.

Clinical Signs of Human Chorionic Gonadotropin Secretion

Both hCG and LH bind to the same specific plasma membrane receptors of the Leydig cells of the testis. As a result, young prepubertal boys who have tumors secreting low levels of hCG frequently will present with signs of prococious puberty, reflecting increased testosterone secretion induced by biologically active hCG secreted by their tumors. Those tumors-inducing signs of precocious puberty in boys include intracranial midline tumors.[2,14] Human chorionic gonadotropin does not cross the blood-brain barrier efficiently.[15] Approximately 1 percent of hCG crosses the blood-brain barrier in normal pregnancy. In those cases in which low levels of hCG are present in the peripheral blood of young boys presenting with precocious puberty, differential blood : cerebrospinal fluid (CSF) ratios may help ascertain the site of the tumor. For example, a blood : CSF ratio less than 60 : 1 strongly suggests that the site of the hCG-secreting tumor is within the central nervous system.[15-17] Hepatoblastomas may also secrete hCG and induce precocious puberty in young boys.[17,18]

Men with testicular cancer may present with gynecomastia, since the high level of hCG secreted by many tumors may initially induce synthesis of relatively more estradiol by Leydig cells,[19] to induce gynecomastia. In most cases, however, the gynecomastia is a result of concomitant estradiol synthesis by hCG-secreting tumors.[20]

Specific Human Chorionic Gonadotropin Radioimmunoassay

Because hCG assay specificity and sensitivity are required for valid hCG immunological assays, the assays currently available will be discussed. Specific hCG radioimmunoassays are frequently called "β subunit assays." That term is a misnomer, since one is usually using the assay to selectively measure the intact hormone or hCG rather than simply free hCGβ. The term "β subunit assay" came about because the assay initially developed incorporated an antiserum to the highly purified β subunit of hCG,[21] which recognized conformationally dependent antigenic sites on the hCG molecule.[22] Extensive structural homology exists between LHβ and hCGβ, so that the assay is a relatively specific assay for hCG in serum or plasma samples. Since circulating LH attains a finite concentration physiologically, whether it be in the normal reproductive state in women or in the castrate state of both sexes, that approach was feasible. Unfortunately, many investigators who generate antisera with hCGβ fail to recognize this limitation. As a result, false positive hCG levels may be reported in those settings in which high or castrate levels of LH circulate in men with germinal cell tumors of the testis who have previously undergone castration or received chemotherapy or radiation therapy that induced primary gonadal failure.

Since only a few antisera have sufficient specificity and sensitivity, some antisera selected for "specific" hCG assays cross-react with high physiological levels of LH and induce spuriously high hCG levels. The normal limit for circulating hCG in normal controls with both intact gonadal function and those with primary gonadal failure needs to be established to validate a specific hCG assay. If one suspects that high physiological LH levels are inducing false positive hCG levels, then the patient can be treated with exogenous testosterone to suppress circulating levels of LH and to eliminate cross-reactivity induced by high LH levels in the specific hCG assay.[23] Consequently, in validating a specific hCG assay, it is imperative not only to define the upper limit of normal for hCG concentrations for that assay, but also to ascertain empirically whether there is any significant cross-reactivity among samples containing castrate or high circulating levels of LH. Furthermore, one must carefully determine whether repeated freeze-thaw cycles of serum or plasma samples have induced spuriously high hCG levels. Although an assay may be carefully validated for serum or plasma hCG levels, that same assay may yield spurious levels if urine hCG concentrations are monitored. Metabolites of both hCG and LH are present in urine, and they may have markedly different affinities for the polyclonal or monoclonal antibody incorporated within the specific hCG radioimmunoassay. Finally, urine frequently contains nonspecific substances that interfere with the antigen–antibody reaction and may induce falsely high hCG levels. Extraction procedures, corrected for recoveries, are usually required for valid urinary hCG assays. Even though an assay may be carefully validated, the quality control of the assay may vary such that spuriously high levels of hCG are obtained in assays that are not within quality control. The best way of monitoring hCG assay quality control is simply to carefully monitor the slope of the dose-response line for highly purified hCG and its 20, 50, and 90 percent intercepts in order to ascertain whether there has been a significant shift of that dose-response line to the right, which is usually accompanied by higher hCG levels in unknown or test samples, and to incorporate replicated samples with low, medium, and high hCG levels, which are within the dose–response range of the standard used in the assay. The latter permits calculation within and between assay coefficients of variation that differ with the level of hCG present in the quality control samples.

Moreover, if one is using an immunoradiometric assay (IRMA), one must be certain that at least two different aliquots of the patient's serum are within the linear portion of the hCG standard dose–response line, since there is a marked "hook effect" with IRMAs for those samples with high hormone concentrations. Immunoradiometric assays incorporate labeled antibody instead of labeled hormone in the reaction mixture. If the ligand or hormone is present in marked excess, spuriously low hormone concentrations may be reported, since an insufficient amount of antibody is present in the assay tube and, as a result, a "hook effect" is observed. Spuriously low hormone concentrations will be reported from the assay. One must systematically ascertain whether dilutions of the sample are within the linear portion of the hCG standard dose–response range to obviate that potential effect. Since hCG levels may vary widely among patients, and even within the same patient with an hCG-secreting germinal cell tumor of the testis, IRMA assays are not very practical in routine clinical laboratories when ligand or hormone concentrations exceed the upper range of the linear portion of the standard curve. Several different volumes of the sample should be assayed to assure that concentrations of hCG added to the assay tubes are within the linear portion of the dose-response of that IRMA assay.

Human chorionic gonadotropin levels in plasma or other biological samples are usually reported in terms of milli International Units/ml (mIU/ml) of either the second International Standard for hCG or the first International Reference Preparation for hCG. The second International Standard for hCG has been the most widely used reference preparation, but its supply has been exhausted and, consequently, that preparation is no longer distributed by the World Health Organization (WHO). That relatively crude International Reference Preparation (5,300 IU/mg, bioassay) has been replaced by the more highly purified first International Reference Preparation of hCG, which has an assigned potency of 9,300 IU/mg in terms of both its biological and immunological activities.[24,25] That highly purified reference preparation was previously designated hCG CR119 by the Center for Population Research, National Institute of Child Health and Human Development in Bethesda, Maryland. A large quantity of that hormone was donated by that organization to WHO for international distribution as the first IRP for hCG. Consequently, when standardizing an assay, one should provide a factor for converting units of the second International Standard hCG and the first IRP hCG. This is of extreme importance when a patient is being followed over several months, since a hospital's clinical laboratory may send samples for assay to different reference laboratories using either or both reference preparations for assay dose interpolation. Some laboratories report results in terms of one, but not both preparations. In years to come, that will no longer be a problem, since the purification techniques now available for hCG yield preparations of similar high immuno- and bioactivities.

In some cases, urinary hCG concentrations are determined, since a urine specimen is easier to obtain than blood samples. However, nonspecific factors in urine may interfere with the antigen–antibody complex, so in measuring urinary hCG levels, antisera to the carboxyl terminal peptide of hCG are preferred because of greater absolute specificity for hCG. The beta subunit of hCG contains an additional 25 to 30 amino acids not present on LHβ.[3] That carboxyl terminal portion of hCGβ serves as the immunogen for carboxyl terminal hCG assays.[26] Excellent hCG specificity can be attained, but unfortunately, the sensitivities of hCGβ carboxyl terminal antisera are usually tenfold lower than those using the entire hCGβ subunit as immunogen.[22] To overcome decreased sensitivity, a 24-hour urine collection or an aliquot of a 24-hour urine sample is concentrated and extracted prior to the hCG carboxyl terminal assay.[27] Results should be normalized to 24-hour excretion or to grams of creatinine in the urine. Those assays, although considerably more tedious, may be invaluable adjuncts to monitoring patients with low levels of hCG not detected by conventional, sensitive, specific hCG assays. It is imperative that the upper normal limit of urinary hCG excretion be defined for each assay.

Antisera to hCG may be generated solely in vivo or with a combined in vivo/in vitro technique in which immunoglobulin-secreting cells harvested from a host animal previously immunized with hCGβ are fused with myeloma or other related cell lines in vitro.[28] Antisera generated in vivo are polyclonal, since many immunoglobulin-producing cells recognize different portions of the hCG molecule with varying affinities. Those cells recognize several antigenic portions of the hCGβ molecule that may be common to both LHβ and hCGβ, as well as those that may be unique to hCG. A polyclonal antiserum contains a population of immuno-globulin molecules with varying specificities and affinities for the immunogen, usu-ally hCGβ, for specific hCG assays. In some cases, those immunoglobulin molecules that recognize common antigenic determinants of LHβ and hCGβ may be selec-tively removed by affinity chromatography with LH convalently linked to an insolu-ble matrix. In some cases, the cross-reacting antibody populations may be adsorbed by simply adding LH to the hCGβ antisera. In others, monoclonal antibody gener-ated by the hybridoma technique yields monoclonal antibody with a single immuno-logical recognition site to hCGβ. The advantage of the monoclonal antibody is that it is generated to one unique site on the hCGβ molecule and, even if used in a more concentrated state, will only recognize that portion of the molecule. In contrast, if after having validated a polyclonal antibody for use in a specific hCG assay, an investigator uses it in a more concentrated state, then cross-reacting immunoglobulin molecules that recognize common antigenic portions of LHβ and hCGβ may yield spurious hCG concentrations. Unfortunately, some monoclonal antibodies may not recognize low levels of hCG in some patients who have altered metabolism and/or altered forms of hCG, and the monoclonal antibody may not recognize the altered form of circulating hCG. That difficulty may theoretically be overcome by pooling several different monoclonal antibodies with varying speci-ficities, which increases the probability of detecting altered forms of hCG. Finally, screening clones synthesizing antibody to hCGβ is tedious, since most clones have very low affinity, and consequently, the sensitivity of the antibody is not adequate for clinical application.

Human Chorionic Gonadotropin Secretion Among Germinal Cell Tumors of the Testis

Men with seminomas may have abnormally high circulating levels of hCG approximately 5 to 20 percent of the time.[29] That range reflects assay specificities and sensitivities, for the most part. The hCG secretion is usually limited to giant syncytiotrophoblasts within the seminoma.[30,31] In other cases, hCG may be secreted by small nests of either choriocarcinoma or embryonal cell carcinoma within the tumor, which is predominantly seminoma. Obviously, sampling errors in histologi-cal sectioning may result, since other histological tumor types may comprise only a very small fraction of the entire tumor. It is important to discern whether other histological types of testicular germinal cell cancers are present, since treatment for patients may be altered, assuming the tumors cannot be totally removed by simple orchiectomy.

Table 1-1 summarizes the incidence of abnormally high hCG levels among

Table 1-1. Incidence of Immunoreactive hCG (> 5 mIU/ml)[a] in Sera of Men with Testicular Cancer

Histology	Examined (N)	Positive (N)	Positive (%)
Choriocarcinoma	15	15	100
Embryonal	62	37	60
Seminoma	19	7	37
Teratoma/Mixed	32	21	66
Total	132	80	63

[a] Second International Standard hCG

men with germinal cell tumors of the testis. In short, all men with choriocarcinomas of the testis have increased circulating hCG levels at the time of presentation. Men with embryonal cell carcinomas have abnormally high hCG levels approximately two-thirds of the time prior to therapy,[2] frequencies that have been confirmed in several other studies.[29] Monitoring hCG levels among men has provided an invaluable aid to clinicians to more accurately stage germinal cell cancers.[32-34] Many times, the tumor is thought to be localized to the testis or to the retroperitoneal nodes that are removed at the time of initial surgery. However, a persistently high level of hCG or a transient decrease in hCG concentration different from that calculated from the known plasma half-life of hCG may provide the first indication that tumor persists, either within retroperitoneal nodes or at distant sites. In that setting, most oncologists initiate chemotherapy.[34,35] Although lymphangiograms, urograms, and venograms have been used to stage patients with germinal cell tumors of the testis, errors that simply reflect the relative sensitivities of those approaches still persist.[32-34] Unfortunately, not all germinal cell tumors of the testis secrete hCG. In some cases, alphafetoprotein levels (AFP) or other tumor markers may be secreted (see below). In essence then, if the tumor secretes hCG, then hCG concentrations can be used for adjunctive management of the patient. Moreover, since hCG levels may decrease to the normal range after surgery, one must continue to monitor hCG levels, preferably twice a week initially, to ascertain whether hCG levels remain within the normal range or increase after the initial surgical procedure. Figure 1-1 depicts serum hCG levels before and during chemotherapy. Elevated hCG levels persisted in spite of striking clinical evidence of tumor regression discerned by conventional techniques. The patient died several months later with brain metastases. In my own clinical experience, if hCG levels are low but persistently above the normal range in spite of continued aggressive chemotherapy, gross tumor growth subsequently becomes evident and hCG levels progressively increase.

Figure 1-2 depicts circulating levels of hCG in a patient undergoing chemotherapy for germinal cell tumor of the testis; in addition, urinary excretion of hCG, determined by specific hCG assay, is also presented over the same sampling period. Although plasma levels of hCG decreased to within normal limits (≤ 1 ng/ml or 5 mIU/ml, second International Standard hCG), urinary hCG concentrations were persistently above the normal level of hCG excretion. Subsequently, both plasma and urinary hCG levels became abnormally high. In spite of continued therapy,

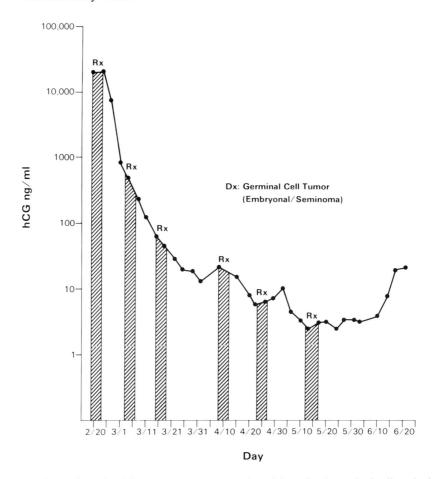

Fig. 1-1. Serum hCG levels in a young man presenting with a mixed germinal cell testicular tumor (embryonal/seminoma). Human chorionic gonadotropin, levels in nanograms per milliliter, can be converted to mIU in terms of the second International Standard hCG by multiplying by a factor of 5 or multiplying the nanograms by a factor of 9.3 to convert to mIU in terms of the 1st International Reference Preparation for hCG. Although not indicated, the patient continued to receive chemotherapy throughout May, and thereafter. In spite of continuous chemotherapy, the patient died with extensive disease, including metasases to the brain. (Vertical hatched bars, times of intensive chemotherapy.)

the patient died. The study underscores the need for sensitive assays for hCG in plasma or serum, since even in the face of those sensitive assays, abnormally high hCG levels may be excreted in urine, reflecting occult tumor. Many commercial assay kits have normal limits of serum hCG levels of 25 or 50 mIU/ml (depending on the reference preparation) simply because of significant cross-reactivity with LH or poor affinity of the antibody for hCG. Normal individuals have less than 5 mIU/ml (second International Standard of hCG) in serum.[9] Even after a patient attains normal levels of hCG after surgery and/or chemotherapy, longitudinal

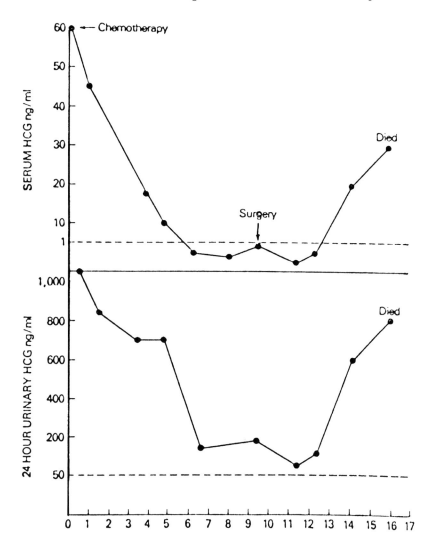

Fig. 1-2. Measurement of simultaneous serum and 24-hour urinary hCG by radioimmu-noassay in a patient with stage III testicular embryonal carcinoma undergoing intensive chemotherapy. Although serum hCG levels attained normal levels after the first five months of chemotherapy, urinary hCG excretion remained abnormally high. Residual tumor was resected between the ninth and tenth month. However, serum hCG levels again became abnormally high in the thirteenth month of follow-up. During the entire course, the patient's 24-hour urine excretion of hCG remained abnormally high. Levels in terms of either the second International Standard hCG or the first International Reference Preparation can be attained by using the conversion factors in Figure 1-1. (Javadpour N, Chen H-C: Improved human chorionic gonadotropin detection with carboxylterminal radioimmunoassay of the β subunit on concentrated 24-hour urine in patients with testicular cancer. J Urol 126:176–178, The Williams & Wilkins Co., 1981.)

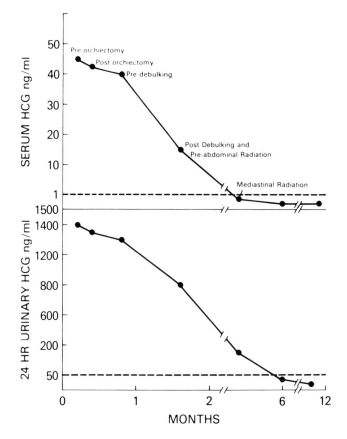

Fig. 1-3. Simultaneous serum and 24-hour urine hCG levels determined by radioimmunoassay in a patient with stage II seminoma. After the patient had undergone surgery and radiotherapy, serum hCG levels finally decreased to within the normal range, but urinary hCG excretion did not decrease to the normal range for another few months. (Javadpour N: Management of seminoma based on tumor markers. Urol Clin North Am 7:773–778, 1980.)

monitoring of the patient with serial blood hCG and AFP levels is mandatory, since a rise in the concentration of either marker usually heralds recurrent tumor.[32-36] Ideally, one would wish to monitor urinary hCG excretion once serum levels are within normal limits. Unfortunately, that technique is quite cumbersome and not available for routine analysis.

Figure 1-3 depicts circulating and excreted hCG levels in a patient with stage II seminoma. The patient was treated with surgery and radiation. Serum hCG levels attained normal levels a few months before urinary hCG concentrations attained the normal range of hCG excretion. The studies in this patient again underscore the need for sensitive specific hCG assays.

ALPHAFETOPROTEIN

Alphafetoprotein was the first oncofetal protein to serve as a tumor marker. Initially it was thought to be uniquely present among patients with tumors. However, with the advent of more sensitive radioimmunoassay techniques, it became apparent that normal individuals had low but significant levels of AFP in peripheral blood.[37,38] Alphafetoprotein is a glycoprotein with a molecular weight of 70,000.[39] It is synthesized by parenchymal cells of the liver, yolk sac, and gastrointestinal tract of the fetus.[40] In the fetus, serum concentrations of AFP may approach 3×10^6 ng/ml between the 12th and 15th week of gestation, but levels subsequently fall to $10-150 \times 10^3$ g/ml at the time of birth. By 1 year of age, AFP levels are equivalent to those found in the normal adult (<40 ng/ml). Alphafetoprotein was initially found in serum of animals with chemically induced hepatomas and in patients with hepatocellular carcinomas.[40] As more sensitive techniques became available, elevated AFP levels were found in patients with germinal cell tumors of the testis, as well as in patients with tumors of endodermal origin.[38,41]

Initially, agar-gel precipitation tests were used to quantitate AFP concentrations. However, that approach has a level of sensitivity of approximately 3,000 ng/ml, which is inadequate for monitoring patients undergoing therapy. Subsequently, more sensitive radioimmunoassays were developed to measure low levels of AFP in the serum of normal individuals, as well as individuals with tumors.[37,38]

Based on immunocytochemical techniques, alphafetoprotein is not secreted by seminomas of the testis. Consequently, if a patient presents with what appears to be a pure seminoma, but with elevated AFP levels, then nonseminomatous disease is considered to be present and appropriate therapy should be undertaken. However, one must carefully ascertain whether the elevated AFP level reflects drug or infection-induced hepatic injury, which is frequently accompanied by increased AFP levels. Up to 75 percent of men with nonseminomatous testicular germ cell tumors may have elevated AFP levels.[38] The upper limit of normal for the AFP radioimmunoassay is 40 ng/ml.[38] When monitoring both AFP and hCG levels among patients with nonseminomatous germ cell tumors of the testis, approximately 90 percent of the patients have elevated levels of either or both markers.[42] The relative frequency of abnormal AFP and hCG levels observed among men with germinal cell testicular tumors of different histological types will vary with the specificity and sensitivity of the assays.

In monitoring some patients, discordant secretion of hCG and AFP may become evident with chemotherapy (Figs. 1-4A and 1-4B). In Figure 1-4A, although both hCG and AFP levels were abnormally high prior to therapy of a man with germinal cell testicular cancer, they returned to within normal limits within several weeks of initiating chemotherapy. On the other hand, hCG concentrations increased significantly between four and six months of chemotherapy and remained abnormally high thereafter even after the chemotherapeutic agents were changed; AFP levels remained within normal limits during the entire course of therapy. Figure 1-4B depicts serial hCG and AFP levels in another patient with advanced testicular germinal cell cancer. With initiation and continuation of chemotherapy hCG con-

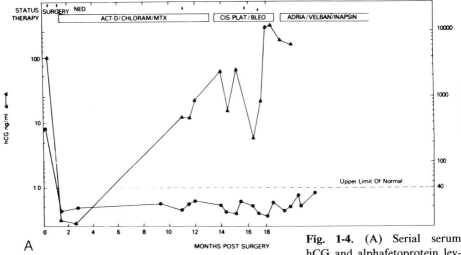

A

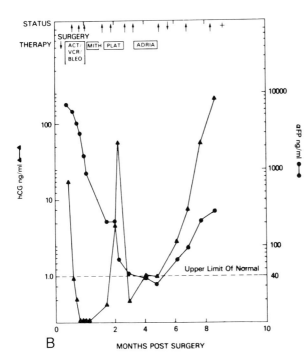

B

Fig. 1-4. (A) Serial serum hCG and alphafetoprotein levels during the course of chemotherapy of a patient with advanced germinal cell testicular cancer. The horizontal dotted line reflects the upper limit of normal for both hCG and alphafetoprotein levels. One nanogram of hCG is equivalent to 5 mIU (second International Standard hCG). (B) Serial hCG and alphafetoprotein levels prior to surgery in a patient who presented with germinal cell testicular cancer. Tumor marker levels were monitored intermittently thereafter during chemotherapy with a variety of drugs. The horizontal line reflects the upper limit of normal for hCG and AFP levels. (Waldmann TA: Tumor markers in the diagnosis and management of patients with testicular germ-cell neoplasms, pp. 374–377, In Anderson T (moderator): Testicular germ-cell neoplasms: Recent advances in diagnosis and therapy. Ann Int Med 90:373–385, 1979.)

centrations remained abnormally high; however, AFP levels decreased to within the normal range for several weeks, but increased markedly two months after surgery. The AFP levels decreased markedly with initiating *cis*-platinum therapy, but increased markedly shortly thereafter. The observations in these two patients underscores the caution with which one should interpret tumor marker concentrations. If the marker is present at abnormally high levels and those levels cannot be attributed to any other intercurrent process, then the abnormal level usually heralds persistent or recurrent tumor. If, on the other hand, the tumor marker levels are within normal limits, tumor growth may persist and should be monitored with other adjunctive clinical techniques.

Localization of Human Chorionic Gonadotropin and Alphafetoprotein

Using immunocytochemical localization of AFP and hCG, small elements of embryonal carcinoma or choriocarcinoma can sometimes be discerned in tissue that otherwise appears to be pure seminoma.[30,31] Alphafetoprotein is present within cells of embryonal cell carcinoma and endodermal sinus tumor. Also hCG, but not AFP may be localized within syncytiotrophoblastic giant cells found in seminomas, embryonal cell carcinomas, and choriocarcinomas.

Since hCG has a relatively long plasma half-life of 24–36 hours, and AFP has a half-life of approximately 7 days, differential arteriovenous (A–V) concentrations of those markers does not usually prove helpful. If an altered form of hCG is secreted by the tumor, however, then one may discern A–V difference across a tumor bed. In those cases, the level of glycosylation must be altered to affect the hCG plasma half-life significantly. Alternatively, free alpha or beta subunits of hCG may be secreted by the tumor. Since alpha and beta subunit half-lives are significantly shorter than those of native hCG, tumor secretion of free subunit may be discerned with selective blood sampling across the tumor bed. In man, the plasma half-life of alpha is approximately 13 minutes, that for hCGβ is approximately 41 minutes.[13] A few cases have been observed in which free alpha subunit was secreted by the tumor, and because A–V differences were readily apparent, tumor could be localized.

LACTIC DEHYDROGENASE

Lactic dehydrogenase is present in human serum in multiple molecular forms.[43] Five different isozyme patterns have been described.[43] In selected clinical settings, the isozymes of LDH may prove helpful, since different LDH isozyme patterns may localize injury to different tissue types. Abnormally high LDH 1 and 2 isozymes result from injury to the heart, kidney, brain, and red cells, whereas LDH isozymes 4 and 5 are increased with injury to the liver, skeletal muscle, and skin.[44] In sera of healthy subjects, LDH isozymes 1 and 2 are predominant.[44] Total LDH levels in sera may be determined biochemically by ascertaining the conversion of pyruvate and reduced nicotinamide adenine dinucleotide (NADH) to lactate and NAD. The normal LDH range will vary from laboratory to laboratory. Since LDH is a ubiquitous intracellular enzyme, serum LDH elevations need not reflect the presence of metastatic germ cell tumors. No histopathological correlations can be made between LDH levels and specific nonseminomatous histopathological cell types.[45] In the study reported by Bosl et al., 65 percent of 351 patients with

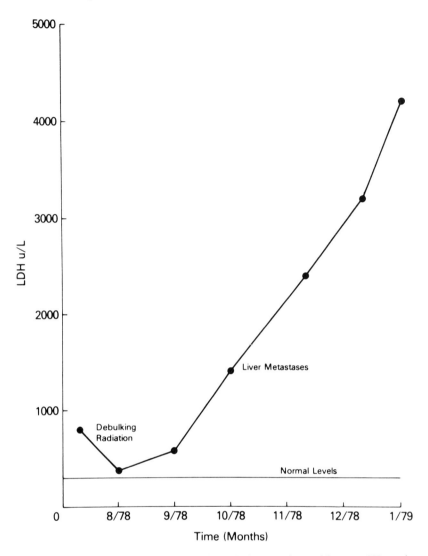

Fig. 1-5. Serial lactic dehydrogenase (LDH) levels in a patient with stage III seminoma before and after surgery. As the tumor mass extended, the LDH levels increased markedly. (Javadpour N: Management of seminoma based on tumor markers. Urol Clin North Am 7:773–781, 1980.)

metastatic germ cell testicular tumors presented with abnormally high LDH levels.[45] In that same report, 60 percent of 245 patients had abnormally high hCG levels and 47 percent of 201 patients had elevated AFP levels. In that study, the upper limit of normal for hCG was 2 ng/ml or approximately 10 mIU/ml in terms of the second International Standard for hCG; the upper limit of normal for AFP was 40 ng/ml. Interestingly, their data analysis suggested an inverse relationship between the initial serum levels of AFP, hCG, and LDH before treatment and the patient's response and survival with treatment for testicular cancer.[45] Other studies have reported abnormal LDH levels among men with advanced testicular cancer.[46] Monitoring LDH levels among men with seminomas may prove clinically useful, since other markers are frequently normal. In the initial studies of abnormal LDH levels among men with seminoma, dysgerminoma, or teratoma, 13 of 15 patients had abnormally elevated LDH isoenzymes 1 and/or 2.[44] However, caution must be exercised, since elevated LDH levels may not reflect tumor, but rather other intercurrent illnesses or forms of cellular injury. The correlation of elevated LDH levels in the face of normal hCG and AFP levels with occult tumor is poorly defined. If no other cause of an elevated LDH level can be discerned, it is not clear whether persistent or recurrent tumor exists, as has been noted when either hCG or AFP levels are abnormally high. Serial assays of LDH may be a useful adjunct to monitoring men with advanced testicular cancers, especially in those settings in which normal hCG and AFP levels are observed. However, more observations need be made to help clarify the clinical importance of elevated LDH levels. Figure 1-5 depicts serial LDH levels in a patient with advanced seminoma, which continued to increase as the seminoma became more widespread. Needless to say, however, the metastatic seminoma was clearly discernible by conventional radiographic and other related techniques.

PREGNANCY-ASSOCIATED PROTEINS

Pregnancy-associated proteins include trophoblastic specific, pregnancy-associated, and fetal proteins.[47] The trophoblast specific proteins include hCG, human placenta lactogen, pregnancy-specific glycoprotein (SP 1), and several other proteins. The fetal-associated proteins include AFP and CEA. The pregnancy-associated proteins include an alpha 2 glycoprotein, sex hormone-binding globulin, and several other placental proteins poorly defined in terms of function.[47] Pregnancy-specific $\beta 1$ glycoprotein (SP 1) was independently described by Tatarinov and Masyukevich, Bohn, and Lin et al.[48-50]

As with hCG, increased SP 1 levels are noted approximately at the same time of implantation during early pregnancy.[51] In contrast to hCG, however, SP 1 levels continue to increase throughout most of pregnancy; and SP 1 appears to have a relatively long half-life of approximately 36 to 48 hours.[51] Low, but significant levels of SP 1 circulate among normal individuals. Unfortunately, not all investigators carefully define the upper limit of normal for SP 1 levels.

Using immunocytochemical techniques, SP 1 was localized to the same cells in which hCG was found.[52] The concordant immunoperoxidase localization of hCG and SP 1 was found in syncytiotrophoblastic cells of choriocarcinoma, in syncytiogiant cells of embryonal carcinomas or teratomas, and in mononuclear embryonal carcinoma cells. However, in some cases only immunoperoxidase staining was evident for hCG and not for SP 1.[51] In that study of 41 patients with advanced testicular cancer, abnormal hCG levels were observed in 61 percent of patients, but only 27 percent had abnormal SP 1 levels. An abnormal SP 1 level was always associated with an abnormal hCG level. Consequently, monitoring SP 1 levels added nothing to patient management. That is in contrast to the study reported by Lange et al.[53] However, in that study, a fivefold lower upper limit of normal of SP 1 levels was used to define abnormal levels, which was probably too low. That undoubtedly contributed to the differences between the two studies.

Another pregnancy protein, termed early pregnancy factor (EPF), has been characterized biologically in preliminary clinical studies.[54] Early pregnancy factor is measured with an in vitro assay.[55] Using that relatively insensitive test, normal healthy males and men with benign testicular tumors or nongerminal cell tumors had no detectable circulating EPF.[56] However, 10 of 11 men with nonseminomatous germ cell tumors and 1 of 10 men with a seminoma had abnormal levels of EPF in serum. Obviously, more studies with a more sensitive technique need to be carried out to ascertain whether EPF can be a useful marker in monitoring men with testicular germ cell cancers.

Placental alkaline phosphatase (PLAP) may be a useful marker for monitoring men with seminomas. PLAP differs from common tissue alkaline phosphatases both immunologically and chemically.[57] PLAP is synthesized by the syncytio-trophoblast of the normal placenta by the twelfth week of gestation, with the level of secretion increasing throughout pregnancy.[58] Limited results of studies are available to assess the clinical utility of monitoring serial PLAP levels in combi-nation with hCG concentrations in men with seminomas. In one study using an enzyme-linked immunoabsorbent assay, PLAP levels were monitored in patients with different stages of seminoma.[59] In 10 men who presented with active stage I seminomatous disease, five had abnormally high circulating PLAP levels (> 1.85 ng/ml); of seven men presenting with stage II, six had abnormally high PLAP levels; only one of five men presenting with stage III active seminoma had an abnormally high PLAP concentration. In contrast, only 2 of 10 men with stage III nonseminomatous germ cell tumor (NSGCT) had abnormally high levels of PLAP, and none of seven men with stage I or II NSGCT had abnormal PLAP levels. Results of that study, which included longitudinal monitoring of both hCG and PLAP levels in men with seminomatous disease, suggest that PLAP may be a useful marker.

It is interesting that PLAP concentrations often mirror the hCG concentrations in men with seminoma. However, discordance between hCG and PLAP levels has been observed and resembles that described above for AFP and hCG levels in men with nonseminomatous cancer undergoing therapy. For reasons not well understood at this time, PLAP levels appear to be more commonly elevated in men with pure seminomas rather than in those with nonseminomatous testicular cancer. Obviously, more studies need be undertaken to validate these preliminary observations to assess better the clinical utility of PLAP in men with seminomas. However, preliminary observations strongly suggest that PLAP may be a useful marker.

CARCINOEMBRYONIC ANTIGEN

Carcinoembryonic antigen was initially isolated from colonic carcinoma by Gold and Freedman.[60] A glycoprotein with a molecular weight of approximately 200,000, CEA is approximately 50 percent carbohydrate. The value of CEA as a tumor marker among men with germinal cell testicular cancers has been assessed in several studies and not proven useful.[45,61] In some studies, fewer than 10 percent of men had abnormally high CEA levels, and those levels do not correlate with disease activity. Moreover, CEA levels apparently are not associated with a specific cell type.[45] Serum CEA levels are usually measured immunologically, but unfortunately, the upper limit of "normal" concentrations is usually not carefully defined. In short, monitoring CEA levels among men with germinal cell testicular cancers is useless.

ACKNOWLEDGMENTS

This work was supported in part by a National Institute of Health Grant RR-533.

REFERENCES

1. Einhorn LH: Testicular cancer as a model for a curable neoplasm. Cancer Res 41:3275, 1981
2. Vaitukaitis JL, Ross GT, Braunstein GD, Rayford PL: Gonadotropins and their subunits: Basic and clinical studies. Recent Prog Hor Res 32:289, 1976
3. Morgan FJ, Birken SJ, Canfield Re: Comparison of chorionic gonadotropin and luteinizing hormone: A note on a proposed structural difference in the beta subunit. FEBS Lett 37:101, 1973
4. Bordelon-Riser ME, Siciliano MJ, Kohler PO: Necessity for human chorionic gonadotropin production in human-mouse hybrids. Somatic Cell Genet 5:597, 1979
5. Vaitukaitis JL: Changing placental concentration of hCG subunits during gestation. J Clin Endocrinol Metab 38:755, 1974
6. Chen HC, Hodgen GD, Matsuura B, Lin JL, Gross E, Reichert LE, Birken S, Canfield RE, Ross GT: Evidence for gonadotropin from non-pregnant subjects that has physical, immunologic, and biologic similarities to human chorionic gonadotropin. Proc Natl Acad Sci USA 72:2885, 1976
7. Yoshimoto Y, Wolfsen AR, Odell WD: Human chorionic gonadotropin-like substance in nonendocrine tissues of normal subjects. Science 197:575, 1977
8. Braunstein ED, Rasor J, Wade ME: Presence in normal testes of a chorionic gonadotropin-like substance distinct from human luteinizing hormone. N Engl J Med 292:1339, 1975
9. Borkowski A, Maquardt C: Human chorionic gonadotropin in the plasma of normal, nonpregnant subjects. N Engl J Med 303:298, 1980
10. Edmonds M, Molitch M, Pierce JG, Odell WD: Secretion of alpha subunits of luteinizing hormone (LH) by the anterior pituitary. J Clin Endocrinol Metab 41:551, 1975
11. Prentice LG, Ryan RJ: LH and its subunits in human pituitary, serum and urine. J Clin Endocrinol Metab 40:303, 1975
12. Morgan FJ, Canfield RE, Vaitukaitis JL, Ross GT: The preparation and characterization of the subunits of human chorionic gonadotropin (hCG). p. 733. In Berson S, Yalow R (eds): Methods in Investigative and Diagnostic Endocrinology. Vol 2B, Part 3. North-Holland Publishers, Amsterdam, 1973

13. Wehman RE, Nisula BC: Metabolic clearance rates of the subunits of human chorionic gonadotropin in man. J Clin Endocrinol Metab 48:753, 1979

14. Sklar CH, Conte FA, Kaplan SL, Grumbach MM: Human chorionic gonadotropin-secreting pineal tumor: Relationship to pathogenesis and sex limitation of sexual precocity. J Clin Endocrinol Metab 53:656, 1981

15. Bagshawe KD, Orr AH, Rushworth AGJ: Relationship between concentrations of human chorionic gonadotropin and plasma and cerebrospinal fluid. Nature (London) 217:950, 1968

16. Bagshawe KD, Harland S: Detection of intracranial tumors with special reference to immunodiagnosis. Proc Roy Soc Med 69:51, 1976

17. Ahmed SR, Shalet SM, Price DA, Pearson D: Human chorionic gonadotropin secreting pineal germinoma and precocious puberty. Arch Dis Childhood 9:743, 1983

18. Hung W, Blizzard RM, Migeon CJ, et al.: Precocious puberty in a boy with hepatoma and circulating gonadotropin. J Pediatr 63:895, 1963

19. Lipsett MB: Physiology and pathology of the Leydig cell. N Engl J Med 303:682, 1980

20. Kirschner MA, Cohen FB, Jespersen D: Estrogen production and its origin in men with gonadotropin producing neoplasms. J Clin Endocrinol Metab 39:112, 1974

21. Vaitukaitis JL, Braunstein GD, Ross GT: A radioimmunoassay which specifically measures human chorionic gonadotropin in the presence of human luteinizing hormone. Am J Obstetr Gynecol 113:751, 1972

22. Chen H-C, Matsuura S, Ohashi M: Limitations and problems of hCG-specific antisera. p. 231. In Segal S (ed): Chorionic Gonadotropin. Plenum Press, New York, 1980

23. Catalona WJ, Vaitukaitis JL, Fair WR: Falsely positive specific hCG assays in patients with testicular tumors. J Urol 122:126, 1979

24. Bangham DR, Grab B: The second international standard for chorionic gonadotropin. Bull WHO 31:111, 1964

25. Storring PL, Gaines-Das RE, Bangham DR: International reference preparation of human chorionic gonadotropin for immunoassay: Potency estimates in various bioassay and protein-binding assay systems and international reference preparations of the alpha and beta subunits of human chorionic gonadotropin for immunoassay. J Endocrinol 84:295, 1980

26. Birken S, Canfield R, Lauer R, Agosto G, Gabel M: Immunochemical determinants unique to human chorionic gonadotropin: Importance of sialic acid for antisera generated to the human chorionic gonadotropin β-subunit COOH-terminal peptide. Endocrinology 106:1659, 1980

27. Ayala AR, Nisula BC, Chen H-C, Hodgen DG, Ross GT: Highly sensitive radioimmunoassay for chorionic gonadotropin in human urine. J Clin Endocrinol Metab 47:767, 1978

28. Khazaeli MB, England BG, Dieterle RC, Nordblom GD, Kabza GA, Bierwaltes WH: Development and characterization of a monoclonal antibody which distinguishes the beta subunit of human chorionic gonadotropin (BhCG) in the presence of hCG. Endocrinology 109:1290, 1981

29. Hussa RO: Human chorionic gonadotropin, a clinical marker: Review of its biosynthesis. Ligand Rev suppl, 2 3:6, 1982

30. Morinaga S, Ojima M, Sasano N: Human chorionic gonadotropin and alpha-fetoprotein in testicular germ cell tumors. Cancer 52:1281, 1983

31. Kurman RJ, Scardino PT, McIntire KR, Waldmann TA, Javadpour N: Cellular localization of alpha-fetoprotein and human chorionic gonadotropin in germ cell tumors of

the testis using an indirect immunoperoxidase technique: A new approach to classification utilizing tumor markers. Cancer 40:2136, 1977

32. Scardino PT, Cox HD, Waldmann TA, McIntire KR, Mittemeyer V, Javadpour N: The value of serum tumor markers in the staging and prognosis of germ cell tumors of the testis. J Urol 118:994, 1977

33. Javadpour N: Improved staging for testicular cancer using biologic tumor markers: A prospective study. J Urol 124:58, 1980

34. Lange PH, Nochomovitz LE, Rosai J, et al: Serum alphafetoprotein and human chorionic gonadotropin in patients with seminoma. J Urol 124:472, 1980

35. Bosl GJ, Lange PH, Nochomovitz LE, et al: Tumor markers in advanced nonseminomatous testicular cancer. Cancer 47:572, 1981

36. Perlin E, Engeler E, Edson M, et al: The value of serial measurement of both human chorionic gonadotropin and alphafetoprotein for monitoring germinal cell tumors. Cancer 27:215, 1976

37. Ruoslahti E, Seppala M: Studies of carcinofetal proteins. III. Development of a radioimmunoassay for alphafetoprotein in serum of healthy human adults. Int J Cancer 8:374, 1971

38. Waldmann TA, McIntire KR: The use of a radioimmunoassay for alphafetoprotein in the diagnosis of malignancy. Cancer 34:1510, 1974

39. Ruoslahti E, Phiko H, Seppala M: Alpha-fetoprotein: Immunochemical purification and chemical purification and chemical properties. Expression in normal state and in malignant and nonmalignant liver disease. Transplant Rev 20:38, 1974

40. Gitlin D, Boesman M: Sites of serum alphafetoprotein synthesis in the human and in the rat. J Clin Invest 46:1010, 1967

41. Abelev GI: Alpha-fetoprotein in oncogenesis and its association with malignant tumors. Adv Cancer Res 14:295, 1971

42. Lange PH, McIntire KR, Waldmann TA, et al: Serum alphafetoprotein and human chorionic gonadotropin in the diagnosis and management of nonseminomatous germ-cell testicular cancer. N Engl J Med 295:1237, 1976

43. Vesell ES, Bearn AG: Localization of lactic acid and dehydrogenase activity in serum fractions. Proc Soc Exptl Biol Med 94:96, 1957

44. Zondag HA, Klein F: Clinical application of lactate dehydrogenase isoenzymes: Alterations in malignancy. Ann NY Acad Sci 151:578, 1968

45. Bosl GJ, Geller NL, Cirrincione C, Nisselbaum D, Vergrin D, Whitmore WK, Golbey RB: Serum tumor markers in patients with metastatic germ cell tumors of the testis. A 10-year experience. Am J Med 75:29, 1983

46. Edler Von Eyben F: Biochemical markers in advanced testicular tumors. Serum lactate dehydrogenase, urinary chorionic gonadotropin and total urinary estrogens. Cancer 41:1826, 1966

47. Horne CHW, Nisbel AD: Pregnancy proteins: A review. Invest Cell Pathol 2:217, 1979

48. Tatarinov YS, Masyukevich VN: Immunological identification of a new, beta-globulin in the blood serum of pregnant women. Byull Eksp Biol Med (Russia) 69:66, 1970

49. Bohn H: Detection and characterization of pregnancy proteins in the human placenta and their quantitative immunochemical determination in sera from pregnant women. Arch Gynaakol 210:440, 1971

50. Lin T-M, Halbert SP, Kiefer D, Spellacy WN: Three pregnancy-associated human plasma proteins: Purification, monospecific antisera and immunological identification. Int Arch Allergy Appl Immunol 47:35, 1974

51. Mandelein M, Rutanen E-M, Heikenheimo M, Jalanko H, Seppala M: Pregnancy-specific

beta-1-glycoprotein and chorionic gonadotropin levels after first-trimester abortions. Obstet Gynecol 52:314, 1978

52. Suurmeijer AJH, DeBruign WHA, Oosterhuis JW, Sleyfer DT, Schraffordt Koops H, Fleuren GJ: Non-seminomatous germ cell tumors of the testis. Immunohistochemical localization and serum levels of human chorionic gonadotropin (hCG) and pregnancy-specific beta-1-glycoprotein (SP 1): Value of SP 1 as a tumor marker. Oncodevelop Biol Med 3:409, 1982

53. Lange PH, Brenner RD, Horne CHW, Vessella RL, Fraley EE: Is SP 1 a marker for testicular cancer? Urology 15:251, 1980

54. Morton H, Rolfe BE, Cavanagh AC: Early pregnancy factor: Biology and clinical significance. p. 391. In Grudzinskas GG (ed): Pregnancy Proteins. Academic Press, Sydney, Australia, 1982

55. Morton H, Rolfe BE, Clunie CJA, Anderson MJ, Morrison J: An early pregnancy factor detected in human serum by the rosette inhibition test. Lancet 1:394, 1977

56. Rolfe BE, Morton H, Cavanagh AC, Gardiner RA: Detection of an early pregnancy factor-like substance in sera of patients with testicular germ cell tumors. Am J Reprod Immunol 3:97, 1983

57. Nathanson L, Fishman WH: New observations of the Regan isoenzyme of alkaline phosphasase in cancer patients. Cancer 27:1388, 1971

58. Stigbrand, T, Millan JL, von Schoultz B: Placental alkaline phosphatase: Clinical significance. pp. 155–164. In Grudzinskas JG, Teisner B, Seppala M (Ed): Pregnancy Proteins, 1982

59. Lange PH, Millan JL, Stigbrand T, Vessella RL, Ruoslahti E, Fishman WH: Placental alkaline phosphatase as a tumor marker for seminoma. Can Res 42:3244, 1982

60. Gold P, Freedman SO: Demonstration of tumor-specific antigens in human chorionic carcinomata by immunological tolerance and absorption techniques. J Exp Med 121:439, 1965

61. Talerman A, van der Rompe WB, Haye WG, Baggerman L, Boekestein-Tjahjadi HM: Alpha-fetoprotein and carcinoembryonic antigen in germ cell neoplasms. Br J Cancer 35:288, 1977

2 | Orchiectomy Alone for Stage I Nonseminomatous Germ Cell Tumors

Derek Raghavan

In recent years, the advances in the treatment of germ cell tumors of the testis have yielded a major increase in the survival of patients with this hitherto lethal disease. The careful use of tumor marker assays has resulted in the earlier detection of occult residual cancer after the completion of radiotherapy, surgery, or chemotherapy, providing a useful warning of recurrence or resistance to treatment.[1]

The improvements in noninvasive diagnostic techniques, such as computerised tomography[2,3] and lymphoscintigraphy,[4] with increased powers of resolution, have further contributed to the management programs by allowing increased accuracy of staging and of ongoing evaluation.

However, the introduction of *cis*-platinum in combination chemotherapy regimens has made the most dramatic contribution to patient survival, particularly in the case of metastatic disease. The five-year survival rates of patients with metastases have increased from less than 20 percent[5] to more than 60 percent.[6-8] Long-term survival figures now approach 100 percent for patients with small volume metastatic disease.[6,7] However, bulky metastatic tumors remain an important management problem (Table 2-1), and considerable effort is being directed toward improving the survival in this patient group[8-11] in whom death rates may still be as high as 40 to 50 percent.[6,8]

Table 2-1. Chemotherapy of Testicular Cancer: Tumor Bulk Versus Complete Response[a]

Protocol	Small Volume Tumor	Large Volume Tumor	Markers Only
VAB IV[50]	9/10	16/31	—
VAB VI[8]	4/6	7/21	6/7
PVB[6]	51/54	60/92	11/11
BEP[10]	13/14	15/19	3/3

[a] Excluding subsequent complete remissions from surgery. Note the variation in the definition of "large volume" in different studies.

As the survival of patients with early stage disease and small volume metastatic cancer is now largely assured, the emphasis is now on reducing the toxicity of the primary treatment of stage I testicular cancer, without loss of overall efficacy.

NATURAL HISTORY AND PATHOLOGY

The treatment regimens for stage I nonseminomatous germ cell tumors (NSGCT) have been based largely on the natural history of the disease. Testicular cancer usually has a stepwise pattern of spread—metastasis initially occurs to the ipsilateral iliac and paraaortic lymph nodes. The afferent channels usually traverse long distances before entering lymph nodes. The lymphatics from the right testis terminate in nodes around the vena cava, whereas the left-sided drainage is to nodes lateral to the aorta from the level of the aortic bifurcation to the left renal hilum and around the origin of the inferior mesenteric artery. Contralateral spread is usually only present in association with large volume retroperitoneal metastases.[12]

Subsequently, metastases may occur in the lung, liver, mediastinum, brain, bone, or supraclavicular nodes. Rarely, distant metastases may be found in the absence of clinically detected retroperitoneal disease.[13-15] Spread from the retroperitoneal lymph nodes probably occurs via the thoracic duct to the left subclavian vein, although there may also be direct lymphatic spread to the mediastinum. Metastases are usually detected within 18 months of diagnosis.

If the major natural barrier to spread, the tunica albuginea, is breached (for example, by transscrotal aspiration or biopsy, or by local tumor infiltration), the pattern of spread is altered as a function of the lymphatic drainage of the epididymis and scrotum—to the external iliac and inguinal nodes. There is then an increased prevalence of scrotal recurrence, of inguinal node metastases, and possibly of distant metastases.[13,16]

Several adverse prognostic features have been identified for stage I NSGCT. It is now generally accepted that local tumor extension (to the rete testis, epididymis, spermatic cord, or scrotal wall—i.e. advanced "T" stage) correlates with an increased prevalence of regional and distant metastases.[14,15,17-20] In a series of 59 patients with clinical stage I tumors treated at the Royal Marsden Hospital between 1973 and 1978, 14 relapsed. Their T stage (Table 2-2) was assessed in 49 patients— the relapse rate of 18 percent for T_1 tumors was significantly different ($p < 0.01$)

Table 2-2. T Staging of Testicular Cancer[a]

T Stage	Description
T_1	Tumor limited to the body of the testicle
T_2	Tumor extending through tunica albuginea
T_3	Tumor extending into rete testis or epididymis
T_{4a}	Invasion of spermatic cord by tumor
T_{4b}	Invasion of scrotal wall by tumor

[a] U.I.C.C. Classification—does not specify intratesticular blood vessel or lymphatic invasion.

from the 60 percent relapse rate in T_2–T_4 tumors.[14] The major limitation of this study was the absence of data from retroperitoneal lymph node dissections, and accordingly, a second study was undertaken at the University of Minnesota.[15] This confirmed the importance of T stage as an independent prognostic variable— among 46 patients with negative lymph node dissections (pathological stage I), 45 had T_1 tumors and only one had locally extensive disease (T_{4a}); this latter patient subsequently developed distant metastases. By contrast, of the 16 patients with T_2–T_4 tumors who underwent lymph node dissection, 15 had regional or distant metastases detected at the time of operation. From a total of 40 patients with T_2–T_4 tumors, including those who did not undergo node dissection, 37 (92 percent) developed metastases during the course of their disease.[15]

Histological evidence of vascular or lymphatic invasion within the testis has been proposed as an adverse prognostic factor, although it is not yet statistically proven.[18-20] It has also been suggested that embryonal carcinoma and choriocarcinoma correlate with an increased metastatic rate,[13,17-19] although this may be a function of their association with advanced T stage.[14,15]

Finally, a prolonged half-life or persistence of the levels of circulating tumor markers after orchiectomy correlates with a high metastatic rate,[14] indicating the presence of residual disease after a potentially curative procedure.

Factors that appear not to influence the prognosis of early stage testicular cancer include the side of the tumor, its size, the absolute blood levels of tumor markers, and the presence of elements of yolk sac tumor.[14,15]

The increased understanding of the biology and natural history of testicular cancer[13,21] has explained, to some extent, the failures of the established treatment programs and may ultimately yield a more rational approach to future patient management.

CONVENTIONAL MANAGEMENT

The optimal management of stage I NSGCT has been controversial for several decades.[7,13,16,22-29] For most of that time, the proponents of radiotherapy and of retroperitoneal lymph node dissection (RPLND) have attempted to demonstrate a difference between the respective survival rates, both of which are in the range of 80 to 95 percent. More recently, adjuvant chemotherapy has been proposed as a solution to the problem posed by stage I NSGCT.[30]

Much of the debate has been characterized by a lack of rational thought and the expression of biased viewpoints. Several factors have made the respective arguments difficult to assess:

1. The patient populations receiving treatment are not identical—for example, "pathological stage" I NSGCT (on the basis of RPLND) is a more clearly defined and select group than is "clinical stage" I, which forms the basis of the radiotherapy data and which represents a mixture of true stage I and occult stage II–IV tumors
2. Historical series are frequently cited for comparison; for example, reports of the efficacy of RPLND may describe outdated radiotherapy series (to indicate the inadequacy of radiotherapy), and vice versa
3. The use of combined modality treatment (for example, the addition of adjuvant chemotherapy)[28] may have obscured the true role of the specific treatment being reported
4. The details of the selection processes for patient accrual, follow-up, and reporting are rarely provided
5. Much of the data regarding the accuracy of "noninvasive" staging antedates the introduction of computerized axial tomography and other sophisticated imaging techniques
6. The skill and experience of the clinicians involved in therapy (particularly in the case of RPLND) is a variable that is difficult to quantify

Despite these problems, the relative merits of RPLND and radiotherapy can be contrasted to some extent.

RADIOTHERAPY

Radiotherapy yields long-term survival rates of 80 to 95 percent (Table 2-3),[7,14,22-25] depending upon the techniques of staging, the extent of local tumor spread,[14,20] and the irradiation techniques employed.[7,22-25]

In addition to the high cure rate, this approach is associated with relatively little acute toxicity, no treatment-related decrease in fertility,[24,31] avoidance of the problems of major surgery, and to some extent, a lesser dependence upon the specific technical expertise of the individual clinician.

However, there are important drawbacks to the use of radiotherapy in this context. These are:

1. Less accurate staging, with the possibility of occult lymph node metastases (which may be resistant to irradiation)
2. Bone marrow suppression, which may prejudice subsequent chemotherapy[6,7,13]

Table 2-3. Radiotherapy for Clinical Stage I Nonseminomatous Germ Cell Tumors of the Testis[a]

Dose (rads)	Patients (N)	Histology	Long-Term Survival (%)	Reference
4,000	30	TC	100	25
4,000	29	TC	97	7
4,000	11	TC	100	51
4,000+	29	TCC + EC	86	52
4,000	20	EC	80	25
4,000	9	EC	90	7
4,000	8	EC	88	51

[a] Results include "salvage" chemotherapy. Note that clinical stage I ≠ pathological stage I.

3. The risk of radiation-induced second malignancies[13,32,33]
4. The potential loss of time from work during a four- to six-week period required for a complete course
5. Acute and chronic gastrointestinal side effects (especially if subsequent abdominal surgery is performed)[13,23]

In addition, the relapse rate after radiotherapy may be as high as 20 percent, and require further treatment.[7,14,24,25]

RETROPERITONEAL LYMPH NODE DISSECTION

The proponents of the surgical approach to clinical stage I NSGCT have reported "cure" rates approaching 100 percent, with a range of 80 to 100 percent (Table 2-4).[13,16,26-29] This approach yields a greater accuracy of staging, at least with respect to the retroperitoneum, and the provision of surgical cure for a proportion of patients with occult stage II disease. However, it should not be forgotten that distant metastases do occur in patients with pathological stage I NSGCT.[15,16]

An important benefit of RPLND is the absence of bone marrow toxicity, in case subsequent chemotherapy is required.

Nevertheless, this treatment option is also associated with problems, as follows:

1. Acute and chronic toxicity of major intraabdominal surgery (including the risk of infection, pulmonary emboli, hemorrhage, chylous ascites, bowel obstruction, and pancreatitis)[13,16,34-36]
2. The risk of a "geographical miss"—especially in the case of prior scrotal violation, with a consequently aberrant pattern of spread (to inguinal nodes, etc.); the chances of actually "missing" retroperitoneal tumor deposits will increase in the hands of an inexperienced surgeon
3. Retrograde ejaculation—this problem is associated with the interruption of the sympathetic nerve supply of the seminal vesicles and ejaculatory ducts during an extensive dissection of the retroperitoneal tissues; however, it should not be forgotten that many patients with germ cell tumors have

Table 2-4. Retroperitoneal Lymph Node Dissection for a Pathological Stage I Nonseminomatous Germ Cell Tumors of the Testis[a]

Patients (N)	Long-Term Survival (%)	References
30	100	26
42	100	28
28	100	27
25	93	29
72	97.5–92.6	34
36	86	53

[a] Includes adjuvant or salvage chemotherapy.

impaired fertility at presentation,[31,33,37,38] and furthermore, the ejaculatory incompetence may reverse after varying periods of time[38]

The relapse rate after RPLND for pathological stage I NSGCT ranges from 5 to 20 percent, although relapse only rarely occurs in the field of dissection.[13,26-29]

THE END RESULTS OF RADIOTHERAPY VERSUS THOSE OF RETROPERITONEAL LYMPH NODE DISSECTION

If one compares the best published results with radiotherapy or RPLND, there is no statistically significant difference between the cure rates achieved (95 versus 99+ percent), particularly if one considers the potential for random variation in relatively small series of patients.

In both instances, salvage chemotherapy is required in up to 15 to 20 percent of patients to achieve these results.[7,13,22-29] In some series, adjuvant chemotherapy has also been used routinely.[28] The statement, "You can't do better than 100 percent" is really not a valid argument in support of RPLND when one considers the highly selected subsets of patients and clinicians involved, and the relatively small number of cases.

On balance, there is less risk with RPLND, in experienced hands, especially with respect to myelosupression and the occurrence of second malignancies. However, in centers where RPLND is not practiced routinely, the hazards of perioperative toxicity or of inadequate dissection (with false negative results) may outweigh the potential limitations of radiotherapy.

Ideally, a randomized clinical trial would be required to resolve the issue. However, to distinguish between 95 and 99 percent cure rates would require a large number of patients and the collaboration of several centers with different philosophies of management, and would thus probably not be feasible.

In fact, it is perhaps of greater importance to consider whether the end results of treatment could be improved by decreasing the toxicity of management programs, rather than by attempting to demonstrate imagined differences between two effective therapeutic options.

A novel approach to reducing the toxicity of treatment of stage I NSGCT was introduced in 1979 by Michael Peckham and his colleagues at the Royal Marsen Hospital: the "surveillance policy."[14,39]

SURVEILLANCE POLICY FOR CLINICAL STAGE I NONSEMINOMATOUS GERM CELL TUMORS

The surveillance policy, a program in which orchiectomy alone is the treatment for carefully selected patients with clinical stage I NSGCT, is currently being evaluated in several centers, including the Royal Marsden Hospital (London),[39] Memorial Sloan-Kettering Cancer Center (New York),[40] The University of Texas (Dallas), National Tumor Institute (Milan), Princess Margaret Hospital (Toronto),[41-42] The Christie Hospital (Manchester),[43] The Cancer Institute (Melbourne), and Royal Prince Alfred Hospital (Sydney).[44] Although the entry criteria vary, most of these studies have the following features in common:

1. Clinical stage I tumor after extensive noninvasive staging
2. T_1 tumors—limited to the body of the testis, without extension to spermatic cord or paratesticular structures
3. Normal circulating levels of alphafetoprotein (AFP) and human chorionic gonadotropin (hCG), or levels that have fallen in accordance with normal half-life values over orchiectomy (5 to 6 days for AFP and 24 to 36 hours for hCG)
4. Carefully selected patients—likely to be cooperative and to attend follow-up visits meticulously
5. No prior history of scrotal interference

The specific entry requirements regarding the tumor itself vary from center to center. For example, patients with tumors that exhibit local vascular or lymphatic invasion are excluded from entry into the Melbourne study, because of the possible prognostic implications of these pathological features.[18,20]

PROTOCOL OF SURVEILLANCE

Patients with clinical stage I disease are considered for entry into the study after orchiectomy. They undergo careful physical examination and extensive staging investigations (including serial tumor marker estimations; CT scans of the chest, abdomen, and pelvis; lymphangiography; routine hematological and biochemical screening; and, occasionally, radionuclide scans). Patients thought to have stage I disease after these investigations are admitted to the study.

Each patient is then seen at monthly intervals for the first year, every other month for the next 6 to 12 months, and then less frequently (usually every 3 months). Tumor markers are assayed at each visit, in addition to an extensive program of investigations (which varies from one center to another)—in general, CT scans of the chest, abdomen, and pelvis are peformed every 2 to 3 months, with regular plain X-rays of the chest and abdomen (to follow residual lymphographic dye).

RATIONALE OF THIS APPROACH

This approach to the management of stage I testicular cancer is feasible and ethical, but it must be approached with considerable care, since

1. Orchiectomy alone cures up to 32 percent of unselected patients with stage I testicular cancer who have undergone only limited staging investigations[45]
2. Patients without adverse prognostic factors in clinical stage I NSGCT have a low risk of recurrence[14] and may thus have a higher chance of cure by orchiectomy
3. However, in view of the limitations of noninvasive staging,[2-4,13,28] approximately 20 percent of these patients can be expected to relapse
4. The cure rates with chemotherapy approach 100 percent for small volume metastatic disease,[6-9] but are lower for patients with large pulmonary or retroperitoneal metastases; intensive monitoring and follow-up are thus essential to facilitate the early use of salvage chemotherapy, if required, to maximize the chance of cure.

PRELIMINARY RESULTS

Royal Marsden Hospital

More than 200 patients have been studied worldwide since 1979 (Table 2-5), with follow-up periods ranging from three months to more than four years. The initial report from the Royal Marsden Hospital[39] documented a series of 53 patients, 9 of whom (17 percent) had relapsed. Most of the relapses occurred within six months of orchiectomy, and all patients were rendered free of disease with chemotherapy. Relapse was most commonly associated with embryonal carcinoma histology. Tumor markers were elevated at the time of relapse in 50 percent of the patients. These data were recently updated at the November 1983 meeting of the American Society of Therapeutic Radiologists (M.J. Peckham, personal communication)—16 relapses have occurred among 84 patients (19 percent); circulating tumor marker levels were raised in 13 cases at relapse; relapses occurred in the retroperitoneum, lungs, and supradiaphragmatic lymph nodes; in three patients, persistently raised tumor marker levels were the only index of recurrence; embryonal carcinoma was the histological element most commonly associated with relapse.

Table 2-5. "Surveillance Policy" for Clinical Stage I Nonseminomatous Germ Cell Tumors of Testis: Preliminary Data

Center	Patients (N)	Number of Relapses (%)	Dominant Site of Relapse	Number Free of Disease
Royal Marsden Hosp.[39][a]	84	16 (19)	Retroperitoneum, lungs	84
Memorial-Sloan-Kettering[40]	45	9 (20)	Retroperitoneum	44
Princess Margaret Hosp.[41]	24	10 (42)	Retroperitoneum	24
U. of Texas[a]	11	3 (27)	Nodes	11
Christie Hosp.[43]	18	3 (17)	Lungs, node, retroperitoneum	18
Royal Prince Alfred Hosp.	12	2 (18)	Node, lung	12
Totals	194	43 (22)		

[a] Personal communication.

Other Centers

The world experience appears to support Peckham's data, with the exception of the results obtained in Canada[41,42] (Table 2-5). In general, relapses occur within nine months of orchiectomy, are associated with embryonal carcinoma histology, and are characterized by the presence of raised circulating levels of AFP and/or hCG at relapse. Metastases are reported most commonly in the retroperitoneum or the lungs.

Memorial Sloan-Kettering Cancer Center

Forty-five patients with T_1 tumors have been followed at Memorial Hospital since 1979.[40] Patients have undergone rigorous staging investigations, as previously outlined. The criteria of exclusion from the study have included T_{2-4} tumors, elements of choriocarcinoma, pure seminoma, and the likelihood of inadequate follow-up. The staging investigations have included a detailed history and examination, biochemical and tumor marker screening, plain X-rays of the chest and abdomen, intravenous pyelography, lymphography, and CT scanning of the abdomen and pelvis. Eighty percent of the patients have remained continuously free of disease. Eight of the nine relapses have occurred within the first eight months, although one patient relapsed two years after orchiectomy. Relapses were documented in lymph nodes and in the lung, with an increased prevalence in patients with embryonal carcinoma.

The Christie Hospital and Holt Radium Institute

A similar study was initiated in 1979 in Manchester.[43] Thirty-eight patients were staged after orchiectomy, of whom 18 were eligible for a surveillance policy. After a median follow-up period of nine months, three relapses were documented

(17 percent)—in the lung, retroperitoneum, and an inguinal lymph node. The three relapsed patients have achieved long-term complete remissions with chemotherapy.

Royal Prince Alfred Hospital

Since 1981, 12 patients have been followed according to the principles outlined above. The series includes two patients who refused to undergo lymph node dissection or radiotherapy, although they were not considered suitable candidates for a surveillance policy. One of these patients was thought to be "unreliable"; the other had evidence of spermatic cord involvement. To date, two relapses have occurred—one in the lungs and another in a lymph node; circulating markers were elevated at relapse in one patient and normal in the other.

Four patients with prior scrotal interference (Table 2-6) have been included in the study because of the uncertainty regarding the likely pattern of spread of the tumors and to avoid unnecessary scrotal irradiation or chemotherapy.

Princess Margaret Hospital

Since 1981, 24 patients have been followed, including 9 with embryonal carcinoma and 15 with teratocarcinoma. To date, 10 patients (42 percent) have relapsed—the sites of relapse have included lung and retroperitoneal nodes; in one patient, the relapse was signaled by elevation of tumor markers with no demonstrable masses. The relapses occurred between two and nine months after orchiectomy and were seen more commonly in patients with teratocarcinoma (as distinct from the other series described above).

CRITICISMS OF THE SURVEILLANCE POLICY

The major drawback to this policy is its potential lack of safety. It has been suggested that AFP and hCG are not reliable tumor markers for stage I NSGCT because their levels are elevated in less than 10 percent of patients.[28] However, in two series of patients reported from Royal Marsden Hospital,[14,39] between 42 and 75 percent had raised levels of tumor markers in the blood at presentation; similar results were reported from the University of Minnesota.[1] This discrepancy may be explained by different blood sampling schedules after orchiectomy.

The results of the "watch policy" at the Princess Margaret Hospital, Toronto, have caused considerable concern, with a relapse rate of 42 percent in a series of 24 cases. The reasons for this discrepancy, compared with the other reported series (Table 2-5), are not clear. Nevertheless, this study indicates quite clearly that the role of this treatment program is not yet proven and requires further evaluation. As the cure rates for metastatic disease have not yet reached 100 percent, a relapse rate of 40 percent from a "surveillance policy" would constitute a major hazard to the survival of patients with this curable disease.

Furthermore, data regarding the prevalence of second malignancies induced

Table 2-6. Royal Prince Alfred Hospital Surveillance Policy[a]

Patient	Age	Entry	Histology	Tumor Stage	Side	Orchidectomy	Initial AFP ($\mu g/l$)	Initial hCG ($\mu g/l$)	Antecedent History (months)	Time of Relapse (months)	Site of Relapse	Treatment	Outcome
1	35	11/81	EC/Y/TD/S	T_1	R	Ing[b]	1390	<1	2	9	Node	PVB	CR
2	24	2/82	EC/Y/TD/S	T_1	L	Ing	1000	15	2	4	Lung	PVB	CR
3	25	5/82	EC/Y	T_1	R	Ing-Scrot[b]	<5	<5	2	—	—	—	—
4	23	5/82	EC	T_1	R	Ing	<5	<5	1	—	—	—	—
5	25	8/82	TC/Y/ST	T_1	R	Ing	36	<5	1.5	—	—	—	—
6	21	12/82	EC	T_1	L	Ing	<5	<5	2	—	—	—	—
7	24	12/82	TC	T_1	R	Ing	270	150	1	—	—	—	—
8	28	1/83	EC	T_1	L	Scot[b]	29	23	1	—	—	—	—
9	24	3/83	EC	T_4	L	Ing	<5	<5	1	—	—	—	—
10	35	3/83	EC/TD	T_1	R	Ing	11	<5	1	—	—	—	—
11	35	7/83	EC	T_1	L	Ing[b]	181	15	2	—	—	—	—
12	30	8/83	EC/Y	T_1	R	Ing	<5	<5	1	—	—	—	—

[a] EC, embryonal carcinoma; TC, teratocarcinoma; Y, yolk sac tumor (endodermal sinus tumor); ST, syncytiotrophoblastic cells; CR, complete remission; Ing, inguinal; Scrot, scrotal; TD, differentiated teratoma; PVB, cis-platinum–vinblastine–bleomycin.
[b] Scrotal interference.

by *cis*-platinum–containing combination chemotherapy have not yet been collected. There have only been sporadic reports of leukemias and an isolated case report of a solid tumor occurring in patients treated with the combination of *cis*-platinum, bleomycin, and vinblastine.[33,46] However, the increasing incidence of second malignancy in patients treated with chemotherapy for Hodgkin's disease is an alarming precedent.

FUTURE DIRECTIONS

The preliminary data from more than 200 patients suggest that a surveillance policy is a feasible option for the management of patients with clinical stage I testicular cancer, although its safety remains in doubt. This approach to management should be tested carefully and not merely be used as an easy option for the patient or the clinician. All patients entered on such programs must be monitored closely in referral centers, by experienced clinicians, with excellent diagnostic facilities. It is pertinent to note that in most of the centers currently evaluating these programs, including our own, the patients are followed personally by the senior clinician directing the study (M.J. Peckham, P. Peters, T. Sandeman, personal communications).

Several issues remain to be clarified:

Optimal Criteria for Inclusion in a Surveillance Study. It is not yet known with certainty whether histological evidence of vascular or lymphatic invasion within the testis constitutes an adverse prognostic factor in the context of a surveillance policy and whether this adverse prognosis (if present) is of sufficient importance to require adjuvant chemotherapy. Similarly, the duration of the antecedent history has been shown to correlate with the extent of spread of the tumor and with ultimate prognosis;[47,48] it is possible that this variable should also be taken into consideration into the selection of patients for these studies.

Furthermore, the most appropriate management of patients with T_{2-4} tumors has not been defined. Such patients have been excluded from surveillance studies because of the high likelihood of relapse; in some centers, these patients are treated by RPLND, whereas others receive chemotherapy. As has been shown, RPLND may not be sufficient treatment to achieve cure outside the field of node dissection.[13,15,16] However, not all patients with T_{2-4} tumors will relapse,[14,15,18] and a case could be made for including all such patients in a carefully monitored surveillance program, thus avoiding unnecessary chemotherapy for some of them. Nevertheless, such an approach could increase the risk of death—for example, after rapid progression and metastasis or in the presence of cerebral metastases.

Another factor that should be considered is the significance of prior scrotal violation (aspiration, biopsy) or antecedent testicular surgery (orchipexy, herniorrhaphy).

When is a Patient Cured? Although more than 90 percent of the relapses to date have occurred within the first nine months after orichiectomy, the report of a late relapse at two years[40] mandates caution in long-term follow-up and counseling of patients with respect to prognosis.

Diagnosis of Relapse.   At present, persistently raised levels of AFP of hCG in the blood are equated with relapse in all the studies in progress. However, the methods and criteria for the diagnosis of relapse in the absence of raised levels of tumor markers vary: For example, should a "new" mass on an abdominal CT scan be biopsied or merely followed serially? It is our practice to obtain a tissue diagnosis whenever possible, to avoid the risk of a falsely positive scan and to avoid the delay associated in following serial CT scans.

Treatment of Relapse.   The protocols for the management of relapse after a period of surveillance differ in each center—for example, combination chemotherapy is employed by Peckham's group, whereas retroperitoneal metastases may be irradiated by others.[41] In fact, the optimal treatment for small volume metastatic NSGCT is not yet known with any certainty, and is the subject of several ongoing randomized trials.

What are the Psychological Implications of the Surveillance Policy?   The emotional stresses associated with cancer have been extensively studied.[49] In the surveillance study, which is universally applied with fully informed patient consent, patients know that they may be at risk of receiving chemotherapy (and of possible death) in order to avoid unnecessary toxicity associated with radiotherapy or node dissection. As yet, there are no published data regarding an increase of psychological trauma due to the 12- to 24-month period of active surveillance, especially with respect to patients who "fail" and require further treatment.

The potential benefits from this program of management for stage I testicular cancer are great. Nevertheless, there is also the possibility of increasing morbidity, particularly if the relapse rate eventually proves to be substantially greater than 20 percent (with the associated requirement for chemotherapy); the psychological effects of such an approach will also need to be studied. Furthermore, the cost-effectiveness of a protocol that requires intensive and repeated investigations will have to be addressed.

However, of greatest importance, the possibility that there will be a sudden increase in the mortality rate of patients with a curable cancer must not be forgotten—a particular risk as the study is being evaluated concurrently in several centers without a mechanism for regular and rapid communication of toxicity. We must continue to be very careful and to improve the system for registering patients and transmitting appropriate data between participating centers.

REFERENCES

1. Lange, PH, Raghavan D: Clinical applications of tumor markers in testicular cancer. p. 111. In Donohue JP (ed): Testis Tumors. Williams & Wilkins, Baltimore, 1983
2. Husband JR, Peckham MJ, MacDonald JS, Hendry WF: The role of computed tomography in the management of testicular teratoma. Clin Radiol 30:243, 1979
3. Husband JE, Barrett A, Peckham MJ: Evaluation of computed tomography in the management of testicular teratoma. Br J Urol 53:179, 1981
4. Kaplan WD: Iliopelvic lymphoscintigraphy. Sem Nuc Med 13:42, 1983
5. Li MC, Whitmore WF, Golbey R, Grabstald H: Effect of combined drug therapy on metastatic cancer of the testis. JAMA 174:145, 1960

6. Einhorn LH: Testicular cancer as a model for a curable neoplasm: The Richard and Hinda Rosenthal Foundation Award Lecture. Cancer Res 41:3275, 1981

7. Peckham MJ, Barrett A, McElwain TJ, Hendry WF, Raghavan D: Non-seminoma germ cell tumours (malignant teratoma) of the testis: Results of treatment and an analysis of prognostic factors. Br J Urol 53:162, 1981

8. Vugrin D, Whitmore WF, Jr, Golbey RB: VAB-6 combination chemotherapy without maintenance in treatment of disseminated cancer of the testis. Cancer 51:211, 1983

9. Ozols RF, Deisseroth AB, Javadpour N, et al: Treatment of poor prognosis nonseminomatous testicular cancer with a "high-dose" platinum combination chemotherapy regimen. Cancer 51:1803, 1983

10. Peckham MJ, Barrett A, Liew KH, et al: The treatment of metastatic germ cell testicular tumours with bleomycin, etoposide and *cis*-platin (BEP). Br J Cancer 47:613, 1983

11. Garnick MB, Canellos GP, Richie JP, Stark JJ: Sequential combination chemotherapy and surgery for disseminated testicular cancer: *Cis*-dichlorodiammine platinum (II), vinblastine, and bleomycin remission-induction therapy followed by cyclophosphamide and adriamycin. Cancer Treat Rept 63:1681, 1979

12. Ray B, Hajdu SI, Whitmore WF, Jr: Distribution of retroperitoneal lymph node metastasis in testicular germinal tumors. Cancer 33:340, 1974

13. Whitmore WF, Jr: Surgical treatment of adult germinal testis tumors, Sem Oncol 6:55, 1979

14. Raghavan D, Peckham MJ, Heyderman E, Tobias JS, Austin DE: Prognostic factors in clinical Stage I non-seminomatous germ cell tumours of the testis. Br J Cancer 45:167, 1982a

15. Raghavan D, Vogelzang NJ, Bosl GJ, et al: Tumor classification and size in germ-cell testicular cancer: Influence on the occurrence of metastases. Cancer 50:1591, 1982b

16. Pizzocarro G: The case for radical surgery and combined therapy in testicular non-seminoma. p. 315. In Anderson CK, Jones WG, Ward AM (eds): Germ Cell Tumours. Taylor & Francis, London, 1982

17. Mostofi FK, Price EB, Jr: Tumors of the Male Genital System. p. 76. A.F.I.P. Atlas of Tumor Pathology, Fascicile 8, second series, A.F.I.P., Washington, DC, 1973

18. Pugh RCB: Relative malignancy of tumours. p. 441. In Pugh RCB (ed): Pathology of the Testis. Blackwell Scientific Publications, Oxford, 1976

19. Pugh RCB, Cameron KM, Teratoma. p. 199. In Pugh RCB (ed): Pathology of the Testis. Blackwell Scientific Publications, Oxford, 1976

20. Sandeman TF, Matthews JP: The staging of testicular tumors. Cancer 43:2514, 1979

21. Raghavan D, Neville AM: The biology of testicular tumours. p. 785. In Chisholm GD, Innes Williams D (eds): Scientific Foundations of Urology. William Heinemann Medical Books, London, 1982

22. Caldwell WL: Why retroperitoneal lymphadenectomy for testicular tumors? J Urol 119:754, 1978

23. Glatstein E: Optimal management of clinical Stage I non-seminomatous testicular carcinoma: One oncologist's view. Cancer Treat Rept 66:11, 1982

24. Peckham MJ, Barrett A: Radiotherapy in testicular teratoma. p. 174. In Peckham MJ (ed): The Management of Testicular Tumours. Edward Arnold, London, 1981

25. Van der Werf Messing B, Hop WCJ: Radiation therapy of testicular non-seminomas. Int J Rad Oncol Biol Phys 8:175, 1982

26. Donohue JP, Einhorn LH, Perez JM: Improved management of non-seminomatous testis tumors. Cancer 42:2903, 1978

27. Fraley EE, Lange PH, Kennedy BJ: Germ-cell testicular cancer in adults. N Engl J Med 301:1370, 1420, 1979

28. Skinner DG, Scardino PT: Relevance of biochemical tumor markers and lymphadenectomy in management of non-seminomatous testis tumors: Current perspective. J Urol 123:378, 1980
29. Walsh PC, Kaufman JJ, Coulson WF, Goodwin WE: Retroperitoneal lymphadenectomy for testicular tumors. JAMA 217:309, 1976
30. Ekman EP, Edsmyr F: Chemotherapy in non-seminomatous testicular tumours Stage I. Br J Urol 53:184, 1981
31. Barrett A, Stedronska J, Hendry WF, Peckham MJ: Fertility of patients with testicular tumours and the effects of treatment—a preliminary report. p. 395. In Anderson CK, Jones WG, Milford Ward A (eds): Germ Cell Tumours. Taylor and Francis, London, 1982
32. Cockburn A, Vugrin D, Macchia R, Warden S, Whitmore W, Jr: Concerning the emergence of new malignancies in patients treated for germ cell tumors of the testis. Proc Am Soc Clin Oncol 2:139, 1983
33. Rustin GJS: Follow-up, fertility and second tumours: p. 267. Clinics in Oncology. W.B. Saunders, Philadelphia, London, 1983
34. Babaian RJ, Johnson DE: Management of Stages I and II non-seminomatous germ cell tumors of the testis. Cancer 45:1775, 1980
35. Donohue JP, Rowland RG: Complications of retroperitoneal lymph node dissection. J Urol 125:338, 1981
36. Sago AL, Ball TP, Novicki DE: Complications of retroperitoneal lymphadenectomy. Urology 13:241, 1979
37. Drasga RE, Einhorn LH, Williams SD, Patel DN, Stevens EE: Fertility after chemotherapy for testicular cancer. J Clin Oncol 1:179, 1983
38. Narayan P, Lange PH, Fraley EE: Ejaculation and fertility after extended retroperitoneal lymph node dissection for testicular cancer. J Urol 127:685, 1982
39. Peckham MJ, Barrett A, Husband JE, Hendry WF: Orchidectomy alone in testicular Stage I non-seminomatous germ cell tumours. Lancet ii:678, 1982
40. Sogani PC, Whitmore WF, Jr, Herr HW, et al: Orchiectomy alone in treatment of clinical Stage I non-seminomatous germ cell tumor of testis (NSGCT). Proc Am Soc Clin Oncol 2:140, 1983
41. Sturgeon JFG, Herman JG, Jewett MAS, et al: A policy of surveillance alone after orchidectomy for clinical Stage I nonseminomatous testis tumors. Proc Am Soc Clin Oncol 2:142, 1983
42. Jewett MAS: Expectant versus surgical therapy for clinical Stage I non-seminomatous germ cell tumor: An equivocal view. World J Urol 2:57, 1984
43. Read G: Follow-up policy in Stage I teratoma of testis—First years experience. p. 289. In Anderson CK, Jones WG, Ward AM (eds): Germ Cell Tumours. Taylor and Francis, London, 1982
44. Raghavan D: Expectant versus surgical therapy for clinical Stage I non-seminomatous germ cell tumors of the testis: Qualified support for a policy of surveillance. World J Urol 2:59, 1984
45. Whitmore WF, Jr: Germinal tumors of the testis. p. 219. Sixth National Cancer Conference Proceedings. J.B. Lippincott, Philadelphia, 1970
46. Mead GM, Green JA, Macbeth FR, Williams CJ, Whitehouse JMA: Second malignancy after cisplatin, vinblastine, and bleomycin (PVB) chemotherapy: A case report. Cancer Treat Rep 67:410, 1983
47. Sandeman TF: Symptoms and early management of germinal tumours of the testis. Med J Aust 2:281, 1979

48. Bosl GJ, Vogelzang NJ, Goldman A, et al: Impact of delay in diagnosis on clinical stage of testicular cancer. Lancet, ii:970, 1981

49. Holland JC: Psychologic aspects of cancer. p. 1175. In Holland JF, Frei E III (eds): Cancer Medicine. Lea and Febiger, Philadelphia, 1982

50. Vugrin D, Cvitkovic E, Whitmore WF, Jr, Cheng E, Golbey RB: VAB-4 combination chemotherapy in the treatment of metastatic testis tumors. Cancer 47:833, 1981

51. Hope-Stone JF, Irradiation as adjuvant therapy in the management of testicular tumours. Rec Res Cancer Res 68:178, 1979

52. Maier JG, Mittemeyer B: Carcinoma of the testis. Cancer 39:981, 1977

53. Staubitz WJ, Early KS, Magoss IV, et al: Surgical management of testis tumors. J Urol 111:205, 1974

3 | Treatment of Seminoma

Stephen D. Williams
Lawrence H. Einhorn

The successes in the management of disseminated nonseminomatous germ cell tumors (NSGCT) are well established. In excess of 70 percent of such patients will be cured with appropriate therapy. The proper integration of chemotherapy and surgery for early-stage patients has likewise given survival rates of 98 to 99 percent. Less well defined is the role and outcome of treatment with chemotherapy of patients with advanced seminoma and the appropriate integration of chemotherapy and radiation in certain patients with stage II disease. This review will summarize available chemotherapy data from several series and discuss the implications of this information for earlier stage patients.

ADVANCED DISEASE

For many years, alkylating agents were the mainstay of therapy for disseminated seminoma. These agents unquestionably have activity, but earlier studies were flawed by poorly defined patient populations and response criteria. These studies were discussed in detail in a previous publication from our institution,[1] but suffice it to say that durable complete responses (CR) are extremely unusual, and traditional alkylating agents do not have a clearly defined role in patients with seminoma.

For several years, patients with advanced seminoma at our institution have been treated on exactly the same protocols as their counterparts with NSGCT. These regimens basically have been combinations of cisplatin, vinblastine, and bleomycin, with or without adriamycin (PVB ± A).[2-4] During this same time

37

Table 3-1. Response to Therapy

Institution	No.	CR (%)	Radiotherapy[a]
Indiana	31	21 (68)	0
Netherlands Cancer Inst. ⎫			
Leyden U. ⎬	29	20 (70)	4
Utrecht U. ⎭			
Madrid	13	10 (77)	2
Total	73	51 (70)	6

[a] Number receiving consolidation radiotherapy.

period, similar treatment regimens were employed by investigators at several institutions in the Netherlands (Amsterdam, Leiden, Utrecht) and Madrid. Data from these hospitals and Indiana University were recently compiled by van Oosterom et al.[5] Several Indiana patients have been previously reported.[1]

In this compiled series, 73 patients were treated with PVB ± A. Patients received three to four courses of induction chemotherapy, given, in most instances, every three weeks. Twenty-four patients also received maintenance therapy with vinblastine and cisplatin. Some patients also received consolidation radiotherapy to residual masses or areas of bulk disease at beginning of treatment. Minimum follow-up is one year.

Table 3-1 shows the results of therapy in these patients. Overall, 70 percent attained complete remission, with similar results in all participating institutions. Of the 21 complete responders from Indiana, 2 relapsed and 2 died in CR (one of toxicity, one of intercurrent illness).

Table 3-2 shows results of treatment related to previous therapy. Patients with no previous therapy have a substantially higher CR rate than previously irradiated patients. It is not known whether this represents an inherent biological difference between these groups or whether this is related to lower chemotherapy doses given previously irradiated patients. The former explanation would appear most likely, however.

These data are quite similar to our experience with NSGCT, and there appears to be no difference in chemotherapy responsiveness or curability of seminoma as compared to NSGCT. It is also likely that current patients will fare somewhat better than earlier patients. There appears to be a tendency for more careful follow-up evaluation after primary treatment, and recent patients tend to have had less extensive radiation and no previous chemotherapy.

Several other institutions have now reported their initial experience with cisplatin-based therapy for advanced seminoma. Many of these publications are prelimi-

Table 3-2. Response Related to Prior Therapy

Prior Therapy	Number	Complete Response (%)
None	33	27 (81)
RT[a]	32	21 (65)
RT + Chemotherapy	8	2 (25)

[a] RT, radiotherapy.

nary, or published only in abstract. Investigators at Memorial Hospital treated 31 patients with either cisplatin + cyclophosphamide (9 patients) or VAB-6 (22 patients).[6,7] With the first regimen, five patients were chemotherapy CR's and three others became disease-free with post-chemotherapy radiation. Six remained disease-free. Of note, the three patients who had not had previous radiation all became disease-free. 19/22 VAB-6 patients achieved CR with chemotherapy alone.

Ball et al., at the Royal Marsden Hospital,[8] treated eight patients with PVB and one patient with cisplatin + VP-16 + bleomycin (BEP). The BEP patient achieved CR with chemotherapy alone. There were four CR and four PR with PVB; five received subsequent radiation and all eight were disease-free at the time of the report. Overall, all nine patients were disease-free from 8+ to 34+ months.

Simon et al. treated 10 patients with VAB-6.[9] All 10 attained CR with chemotherapy alone; 3 later relapsed and again became disease-free with additional chemotherapy and radiation.

Oliver treated 12 patients with PVB.[10] Durable CRs were seen in 7/8 previously untreated patients and ¾ who recurred after prior radiotherapy.

Two groups have recently reported a very high level of activity of cisplatin as a single agent. Samuels et al., from M. D. Anderson Hospital, treated 32 patients with cisplatin 100 mg/m²/week[11]; of these, 30/32 are in continuous CR with 22 followed in excess of 2 years. These patients in general had advanced disease, although the exact extent of disease and prior therapy is not stated. Oliver treated 14 patients with cisplatin 50 mg/m² days 1 and 2 every 3 weeks[10]; of these, 9/10 previously untreated patients and 1/4 failing prior radiation were CR with a median follow-up of 15 months. Of patients failing cisplatin, 3/4 are disease-free after combination chemotherapy.

Table 3-3 summarizes the results from all of these series. As can be seen, a substantial number of patients treated with modern chemotherapy programs will

Table 3-3. Results of Cisplatin Chemotherapy

Institution	Regimen	Number	Complete Response (%)[a]	Presently NED[b] (%)	Reference
Indiana, Netherlands Group, Madrid	PVB ± A	73	51 (70)	NS[c]	5
Memorial Sloan-Kettering	Cisplatin + cyclophosphamide	9	8 (89)	6 (67)	6
Memorial	VAB-6	22	19 (86)	18 (82)	7
Royal Marsden	PVB	8	8 (100)	8 (100)	8
Royal Marsden	BEP	1	1	1	8
Sao Paulo	VAB-6	10	10 (100)	10 (100)[d]	9
Urology Inst.	PVB	12	10 (83)	10 (83)	10
M. D. Anderson	Cisplatin	32	30 (94)	30 (94)	11
Urology Inst.	Cisplatin	14	10 (71)	13 (93)[e]	10
Total		181	147 (81)		

[a] Some patients received "consolidation radiotherapy."
[b] NED, no evidence of disease.
[c] NS, not stated.
[d] Three patients required additional treatment.
[e] Three patients became NED with combination chemotherapy after cisplatin.

achieve durable complete remission. Previous radiation therapy for reasons not clear may adversely affect treatment outcome. The superior regimen or, for that matter, the superiority of combination chemotherapy (versus cisplatin alone) is unclear.

Several additional points deserve emphasis. Several of these investigators employed post-chemotherapy radiation if a radiographically visible mass remained. It appears that a number of partial responders have achieved CR with such treatment. The role of radiotherapy, however, is questioned by the results in similar patients following surgical resection. In our experience, the pathological findings have almost invariably been fibrosis/necrosis. In fact, the desmoplastic response may be so intense that the surgery is extremely difficult and only subtotal excision achieved. Similarly, surgery in 7/7 of Simon's patients[9] and 10/10 of Memorial patients[7] confirmed CR and revealed only fibrosis/necrosis. It appears that radiotherapy in the vast majority of patients may be unnecessary.

The extent of previous radiotherapy is related to subsequent chemotherapy toxicity. Patients who receive mediastinal radiation in addition to infradiaphragmatic treatment seem to have much more toxicity from subsequent chemotherapy, should it be required.[12] Potential problems include worsened myelosuppression and an increased likelihood of bleomycin-induced pulmonary disease. The implications of these findings will be discussed further in a subsequent section.

One other group has employed non-cisplatin chemotherapy plus planned post-chemotherapy radiation.[13] Nine patients with stage B_3 (retroperitoneal mass $\geq$ 10 cm) and six stage C patients received two to three courses of vincristine + actinomycin-D + cyclophosphamide. Only one had been irradiated previously. After chemotherapy, all patients were irradiated (14 abdomen, 14 mediastinum, 1 bone). All 15 have been disease-free from 14 months to 9 years. These results are excellent, and the authors emphasize the low chemotherapy toxicity. However, the short- and long-term effects on these extensively treated patients can be substantial, and it seems that equally good results could have been obtained in many of them with only one treatment modality. Also, although not absolutely proven, it is likely that this chemotherapy regimen would be inferior to those regimens containing cisplatin.

USE OF RADIOTHERAPY

There is a vast amount of published data regarding the radiotherapeutic management of seminoma. Most patients present with clinical stage I or limited stage II (radiographically positive retroperitoneal nodes) disease and have an extremely high cure rate. Most of the published data, however, is from an earlier time period and uniform staging procedures and systems were not employed. Few patients had radioimmunoassay marker determinations. Table 3-4 shows the compiled results of five large series of seminoma patients treated with radiation therapy.[14-18] It should be noted that technique in these studies varied: three groups employed prophylactic mediastinal treatment (PMI), whereas two did not. Similarly, the definition of stage II_B disease varied from a retroperitoneal mass greater than 5 cm to a palpable mass.

Table 3-4. Radiotherapy of Seminoma[a]

Stage[b]	Number	Died of Seminoma (%)
I	768	24 (3)
II$_A$	151	15 (10)
II$_B$	107	33 (31)
III and IV	67	41 (61)

[a] Pooled data from references 14 to 18.
[b] Stage I, clinically negative retroperitoneal nodes; II$_A$, positive nodes variously defined ranging from <5 cm to non-palpable; II$_B$, variously defined greater than II$_A$; III, positive supradiaphragmatic nodes; IV, visceral metastases.

As can be seen, the cure rate of stage I disease with infradiaphragmatic radiation therapy is excellent, with little room for improvement. Similarly, patients with less than bulky stage II disease (various definitions) do quite well. The impact of prophylactic mediastinal treatment (PMI) will be discussed below.

The situation, however, is more difficult for patients who have supradiaphragmatic nodal seminoma with or without abdominal involvement at diagnosis. In the previously mentioned radiotherapy series, plus one additional group,[19] there were 32 such patients clearly defined. Of these, 19 (59 percent) were cured with radiation. These results would seem to be substantially inferior to those achievable with modern chemotherapy. In addition, if radiotherapy is used initially, a substantial number of patients ultimately will require chemotherapy, with the resultant significant morbidity in this heavily irradiated patient population.

Turning our attention to the management of stage II disease, we must first consider the appropriate extent of radiation. It has been the dogma of radiation oncologists that PMI must be applied in such patients. However, the evidence for the usefulness of such is weak. For patients with less than bulky stage II disease (variously defined), isolated mediastinal recurrences in patients irradiated below the diaphragm only are 0/40,[14] 0/6,[15] 2/47,[17] 0/8,[14] and 0/6.[20] In a recent review of Canadian experience from 18 institutions, 197 II$_A$ patients were treated (some of these were included in the previous figures) with only 8 mediastinal recurrences; only 2/197 patients died of seminoma.[21] In the modern chemotherapy era, such patients clearly can be treated with conservative radiotherapy without PMI, followed closely with marker determinations and chest radiographs, and should relapse occur, they can be treated with appropriate chemotherapy with an expected cure rate that approaches 100 percent with acceptable treatment morbidity. There is no justification for PMI.

For bulky stage II disease, the situation is somewhat more difficult. Isolated mediastinal failure in patients treated below the diaphragm are reported in 10/46,[14] 0/5,[15] 7/19,[17] and 0/2.[18] Once again, the validity of PMI seems to be in question, particularly since, in the first-mentioned group, 7 of the 10 failures were salvaged with further irradiation. Doornbos et al.[15] from M. D. Anderson Hospital recommend PMI for all stage II patients. Yet, their experience is based on 11 patients without such treatment, of whom 2 failed in the mediastinum. Both, however, also had extranodal relapses and both were salvaged with subsequent radiation.

Of note, two other extensively irradiated patients in this series developed acute leukemia. Dosoretz et al.[18] also recommend such treatment. Yet, 0/12 patients in their series not having PMI failed in the mediastinum. Thus, the concept of PMI is unfounded, even in patients with bulky stage II disease.

Confirmatory information is again obtained from the Canadian series,[21] in which 20/109 patients failed in the mediastinum, but 17 were controlled with further treatment. Overall, 9/109 died of seminoma. Even in II$_B$ patients, PMI may improve relapse-free survival, but, even prior to the modern chemotherapy era, it had a negligible impact on overall survival.

A significant number of patients with bulky stage II seminoma, however, will not be cured with radiation. Overall, around 40 percent will develop recurrent disease. The same comments for this group of patients regarding the relative merits of chemotherapy versus irradiation as initial treatment can be made as for the previously mentioned patients with stage III disease. However, the situation is not totally analogous, since these patients will be less extensively irradiated, assuming PMI is not given. It is likely that the cure rate would be very high with initial radiation and close follow-up with prompt chemotherapy at the first sign of relapse. The situation is similar to that of stage II nonseminomatous testicular cancer treated with lymphadenectomy and observation, with chemotherapy given at relapse.[22] A reasonable alternate approach is initial chemotherapy, which also will give excellent results.

Some guidance in this situation has recently been provided by the Royal Marsden Group.[8] They arbitrarily divided stage II into three substages: II$_A$, involved nodes $\leq$ 2 cm; II$_B$, nodes 2 to 5 cm; and II$_C$, nodes > 5 cm. Sixty-six patients were treated with infradiaphragmatic radiation $\pm$ PMI; two also received initial single agent chemotherapy. Of 32 II$_A$ patients, there were three recurrences (9.4 percent); 2/11 II$_B$ patients relapsed (18.2 percent). Among 23 II$_C$ patients, there were nine recurrences (39.1 percent; II$_C$ versus II$_A$ + II$_B$, p = 0.023). The authors conclude that abdominal radiation (without PMI) is indicated for II$_A$ and II$_B$, whereas II$_C$ patients should be treated initially with cisplatin-based combination chemotherapy.

A word should be said about the influence of marker status and histology on treatment decisions. It is generally agreed that elevation of alphafetoprotein represents the presence of nonseminomatous elements.[23] The best evidence, however, is that neither anaplastic histology[24] nor human chorionic gonadotropin elevation[25] adversely alters treatment results.

One novel approach has recently been proposed by Thomas and Herman[26] and Oliver[10] for clinical stage I seminoma. These investigators have suggested omitting radiotherapy entirely in such patients. The incidence of occult retroperitoneal metastases in clinical stage I patients is unknown, but thought to be 10 to 20 percent. As seen, prophylactic radiation therapy gives excellent results. Treatment is very well tolerated, but is associated with transient oligospermia in many patients and prolonged oligospermia in some.[27] There is little data in patients treated with orchiectomy alone. In the only available series,[10] 5/6 are disease-free after orchiectomy and the other is in complete response after cisplatin chemotherapy. Obviously, such an approach should be pursued only in a carefully controlled clinical setting.

SUMMARY AND CONCLUSIONS

There is evidence that modern chemotherapy will induce a large number of durable complete responses in patients with advanced and recurrent seminoma. The optimum treatment regimen or the indications for post-chemotherapy radiation are uncertain; however, cisplatin appears to be a very important component.

Radiation therapy is the mainstay of treatment for stage I and stage II disease. Modern radiographic techniques have allowed precise delineation of various degrees of retroperitoneal involvement. Patients with minimal or moderate retroperitoneal lymphadenopathy appear to be best treated with radiation with close observation and chemotherapy at relapse. There no longer is any justification for prophylactic mediastinal treatment. The management of advanced retroperitoneal disease (variously defined) is less clear, but initial chemotherapy ($\pm$ "consolidation" radiation) seems most appropriate.

ACKNOWLEDGMENTS

This work was supported in part by the Southeastern Cancer Study Group (CA 19657) and PHS MO1 RR00 750–06.

REFERENCES

1. Einhorn LH, Williams SD: Chemotherapy of disseminated seminoma. Cancer Clin Trials 3:307, 1980
2. Einhorn LH, Donohue JP: *Cis*-diamminedichloroplatinum, vinblastine, and bleomycin combination chemotherapy in disseminated testicular cancer. Ann Int Med 87:293, 1977
3. Einhorn LH, Williams SD: Chemotherapy of disseminated testicular cancer: A random prospective study. Cancer 46:1339, 1980
4. Einhorn LH, Williams SD, Troner M, Greco FA, Birch R: The role of maintenance therapy in disseminated testicular cancer. New Engl J Med 305:727, 1981
5. van Oosterom AT, Williams SD, Cortes-Funes H, ten Bokkel Huinnink WW, Vendrik CPJ: Treatment of seminomas with chemotherapy. Kurth KA (ed): Progress and Controversies in Oncological Urology, Alan R. Liss, Inc. Publishers, New York, 1984
6. Vugrin D, Whitmore WF, Batata M: Chemotherapy of disseminated seminoma with combination of *cis*-diamminedichloroplatinum (II) and cyclophosphamide. Cancer Clin Trials 4:423, 1981
7. Morse M, Herr H, Sogani P, Bosl G, Whitmore W: Surgical exploration of metastatic seminoma following VAB VI chemotherapy. Proc Am Soc Clin Oncol 2:143, 1983 (Abstract).
8. Ball D, Barrett A, Peckham MJ: The management of metastatic seminoma testes. Cancer 50:2289, 1982
9. Simon SD, Srougi M, Goes GM: Treatment of advanced seminoma with vinblastine, actinomycin-D, cyclophosphamide, bleomycin and *cis*-platinum. Proc Am Soc Clin Oncol 2:132, 1983 (Abstract).
10. Oliver RTD: Surveillance for stage I seminoma and single agent *cis*-platinum for metastatic seminoma. Proc Am Soc Clin Oncol 1984 (Abstract).

11. Samuels ML, Logothetis CJ: Follow-up study of sequential weekly pulse-dose cisplatinum for far advanced seminoma. Proc Am Soc Clin Oncol 2:137, 1983 (Abstract).
12. Peckham MJ, McElwain TJ, Barrett A, Hendry WF: Combined management of malignant teratoma of the testis. Lancet ii:267, 1979
13. Crawford ED, Smith RB, DeKernion JB: Treatment of advanced seminoma with pre-radiation chemotherapy. J Urol 129:752, 1983
14. Thomas GM, Rider WD, Dembo AJ, et al: Seminoma of the testis: Results of treatment and patterns of failure after radiation therapy. Int J Rad Oncol Biol Phys 8:165, 1982
15. Doornbos JF, Hussey DH, Johnson DE: Radiotherapy for pure seminoma of the testis. Radiology 116:401, 1975
16. Calman FMB, Peckham MJ, Hendry WF: The pattern of spread and treatment of metastases in testicular seminoma. Brit J Urol 51:154, 1979
17. Jackson SM, Olivotto I, McLaughlin MG, Coy P: Radiation therapy for seminoma of the testis: Results in British Columbia. Can Med Assoc J 123:507, 1980
18. Dosoretz DE, Shipley WV, Blitzer PH, et al: Megavoltage irradiation for pure testicular seminoma. Cancer 48:2184, 1981
19. Read G: The treatment of supradiaphragmatic metastatic seminoma. Clin Rad 31:349, 1980
20. Sause WT: Testicular seminoma analysis of radiation therapy for stage II disease. J Urol 130:702, 1983
21. Herman J, Sturgeon J, Thomas GM: Mediastinal prophylactic irradiation in seminoma. Proc Am Soc Clin Oncol 2:133, 1983 (Abstract).
22. Williams SD, Einhorn LH: Clinical stage I testis tumors: The medical oncologist's view. Cancer Treat Rept 66:15, 1982
23. Raghavan D, Sullivan AL, Peckham NJ, Neville AM: Elevated serum alphafetoprotein and seminoma. Cancer 50:982, 1982
24. Cockbarn A, Vugrin D, Hajdu S, et al: The prognostic significance of undifferentiated histology in seminoma. Proc Am Soc Clin Oncol 1:114, 1982 (Abstract).
25. Mauch P, Werchselbaum R, Batnick L: The significance of positive chorionic gonadotropins in apparently pure seminoma of the testis. Int J Rad Oncol Biol Phys 5:887, 1979
26. Thomas GM, Herman JG: The role of radiation in the management of seminoma. Kurth KA (ed): Progress and Controversies in Oncological Urology. Alan R. Liss, Inc. Publishers, New York, 1984
27. Hahn EW, Feingold SM, Simson L, Batata M: Recovery from aspermia induced by low-dose radiation in seminoma patients. Cancer 50:337, 1982

4 Treatment of Germ Cell Tumors at Memorial Sloan-Kettering Cancer Center: 1960 to Present

George J. Bosl

Germ cell tumors (GCT) have become the most curable solid tumor in the past decade. Combination chemotherapy regimens including cisplatin now cure 70 to 80 percent of all patients with metastatic disease. This success story has evolved over three decades with the discovery of new drugs, the application of the principles of combination chemotherapy, and the contributions of many investigators at several institutions. This report summarizes the steps leading to and the results of the VAB regimens developed at Memorial Sloan-Kettering Cancer Center (MSKCC).

1960–1970

An interest in the treatment of GCT has existed since the 1950s at MSKCC, and its physicians continue to see large numbers of patients with this disease each year. In 1960, Li et al. reported on 36 patients treated with different combinations of an alkylating agent, an antimetabolite, and actinomycin-D. Twenty-three patients were treated with chlorambucil, methotrexate, and actinomycin-D ("triple therapy"). Three patients achieved a durable complete remission (CR).[1] This was quite a remarkable result in an era when few patients with malignancy responded to therapy. The simultaneous use of three drugs was also novel at the time, and Li drew upon the experience of combination antibiotic therapy for pulmonary tuberculosis, synergistic activity of multiple drugs against animal tumors, and the emerging use of drug combinations in human acute leukemia.

In 1966, MacKenzie summarized the experience of MSKCC in 154 patients with GCT, including Li's patients. Although the original CR rate reported by Li for triple therapy was confirmed in a large number of patients, CR were also seen using actinomycin-D alone. Chlorambucil as a single agent was active only in patients with pure seminoma, and MacKenzie concluded that actinomycin-D "by itself may be the most effective means of treating metastatic testis cancer other than seminoma."[2]

1970–1975

Although regression of disease was regularly observed in patients treated with actinomycin-D or mithramycin,[3] clinical trials at this time with vinblastine and bleomycin led to the next series of combination chemotherapy trials, not only at MSKCC, but also at other institutions.

Samuels reported using vinblastine alone or with melphalan in 32 patients. Vinblastine was administered to 21 patients at doses of 0.4 to 0.8 mg/kg. These large doses produced four CR two of which were still ongoing at 13+ and 45+ months. Perhaps equally as important, two of four patients with pure seminoma achieved partial remissions (PR). Toxicity consisted of myalgias and myelosuppression, with 12/21 patients having white blood cell counts less than 1,000 leukocytes/mm³.[4]

Bleomycin entered clinical trials in the late 1960s. The European Organization for Research on the Treatment of Cancer (EORTC) reported four responses in six patients with GCT,[5] and Yagoda reported three responders in eight patients.[6] It was clear that bleomycin was an active agent in addition to vinblastine and actinomycin-D.

In 1972, investigators at MSKCC combined vinblastine, actinomycin-D, and bleomycin (VAB-1). Wittes et al. reported a CR + PR rate of 34 percent, with seven CR (15 percent) (Table 4-1). Of these seven, five were free of disease without relapse. Toxicity was tolerable.[7] Whether this result was better than actinomycin-D alone or actinomycin-D with methotrexate and chlorambucil was unknown. However, only 4/72 patients treated with "triple therapy" had a durable CR in MacKenzie's report,[2] as opposed to 5/47 in VAB-1, and five patients previously treated with actinomycin-D again responded to VAB-1.[7] Thus, there was a reasonable hope that this combination was superior to single-agent therapy.

Several avenues of investigation led to VAB-2. Higby et al. reported the activity of cisplatin against GCT[8] and continuous infusion was found to be superior to intermittent administration of bleomycin.[9] In June 1974, VAB-2 was opened and subsequently reported by Cheng et al. for 50 patients. Cisplatin was administered

Table 4-1. Summary of Treatment Trials in Testicular Cancer from 1972–1979 (VAB-1 through VAB-5)

Trial	Patients (%)		Complete Response (%)			NED[a] (%)	Reference
	Previous Chemotherapy	No Previous Chemotherapy	Previous Chemotherapy	No Previous Chemotherapy	Overall		
VAB-1	30 (64)	17 (36)	3 (10)	4 (24)	7 (15)	5 (11)	7
VAB-2	25 (50)	25 (50)	15 (60)	10 (40)	25 (50)	74 (28)	10
VAB-3	42 (57)	32 (43)	22 (52)	23 (72)	45 (61)	33 (44)	18
VAB-4	—	41 (100)	—	33 (80)	33 (80)	28 (68)	19
VAB-5	50 (50)	15 (50)	13 (87)	5 (33)	18 (60)	15 (50)	20

[a] NED, no evidence of disease

at a dose of 1.2 mg/kg. Overall, a 50 percent CR (84 percent CR + PR) rate was noted[10] (Table 4-1). Second-look procedures were undertaken in 15 patients, adding a new dimension to the treatment of patients with GCT. Obviously, the treatment result was gratifying and far better than VAB-1. However, about 50 percent of patients achieving CR relapsed, indicating that better therapy was needed. Concurrent with VAB-2, Samuels reported the improved activity of infusion over intermittent administration of bleomycin when combined with vinblastine.[11]

1975–1981

Cisplatin rapidly emerged as the single most important drug against GCT. Initially, cisplatin was limited in its usefulness by nephrotoxicity and ototoxicity;[12] however, Higby et al. had shown that five daily doses of 20 mg/m² could be administered without undue toxicity, with adequate intravenous hydration. Supported by preclinical trials in dogs,[13] Hayes et al. at MSKCC reported that doses of cisplatin of 120 mg/m² could be safely administered with concomitant hydration and mannitol-induced diuresis.[14] Even more importantly, five of nine previously treated patients with GCT achieved PR status.

The VAB-3 regimen, opened in 1975, was an outgrowth of these phase I studies with cisplatin. Cyclophosphamide was added during the induction based on the data of Buckner et al.,[15] and doxorubicin was added to the maintenance periods based on data reported by Monfardini et al.[16] The schedule for this regimen required two major inductions five to six months apart, separated by consolidation therapy every three weeks. This approach was used in an attempt to minimize cisplatin-induced toxicity.[17] Maintenance chemotherapy lasted for two years. Most patients achieved a CR or PR with this regimen; five patients were rendered free of disease by surgical procedures.[18] A relapse rate of 26 percent was noted,[18] with many of these relapses occurring between the two major inductions.[17] In an attempt to minimize this relapse rate, VAB-4 was initiated in September 1976. The only change from VAB-3 was the addition of a third induction cycle at 16 weeks after the start of therapy, with the third at 32 weeks. The CR rate was similar to that of VAB-3, but the relapse rate was only 12 percent[19] (Table 4-1).

During these few years, it became apparent that CR was the only acceptable outcome to therapy for patients with advanced GCT, since nearly all patients failing to achieve CR eventually died of disease.[18] Several possible prognostic variables were present, including pretreatment values of serum tumor markers, histopathology, prior treatment, and bulk of disease. In July 1977, a trial of more intensive therapy (VAB-5) was opened for patients with poor prognostic features, including bulky metastases over 5 cm in diameter, palpable retroperitoneal metastases, liver metastases, brain metastases, involvement of two parenchymal organs or more, pure choriocarcinoma, serum alphafetoprotein (AFP) or human chorionic gonadotropin (hCG) values greater than 1,000 ng/ml, serum values of lactate dehydrogenase (LDH) over 400 units/liter, and failure of prior chemotherapy. The overall CR rate was 47 percent, with an expected lower CR rate in previously treated

Table 4-2. Summary of VAB-6 Trials

	Patients	CR (%)	Relapse (%)	NED[a] (%)	Reference
Maintenance	25	23 (92)	2 (9)	21 (88)	22
No maintenance	34	31 (91)	3 (10)	28 (82)	23
Randomized	75	59 (79)	Too early		

[a] NED, no evidence of disease

patients (Table 4-1). Toxicity was substantial, including severe myelosuppression, mucositis, and moderate nephrotoxicity.[20] Whether this regimen was any improvement over prior regimens was debatable, and the heightened toxicity, lack of CR in patients with extragonadal primary tumors, and a complicated schedule led to a search for better therapy.

It was evident from the VAB-3, VAB-4, and VAB-5 regimens that the initial induction was the most effective part of therapy. In addition, a randomized trial of vinblastine, bleomycin, and cisplatin (VBP), with or without doxorubicin, showed that doxorubicin was unnecessary.[21] Chlorambucil, which had been part of the consolidation and maintenance schedule in VAB-3 through VAB-5, was also eliminated because of its marginal activity. These steps led to the VAB-6 trial, with three consecutive inductions at monthly intervals. The doses and schedule of cyclophosphamide, vinblastine, actinomycin-D, and cisplatin were unchanged. The duration of the bleomycin infusion was reduced from seven to three days. This last change was made because of the frequent mucositis that followed prolonged bleomycin infusions. Surgical intervention (discussed below) after three months of therapy, if necessary, was followed by two additional months of therapy if residual malignant elements were found in the operative specimen.

The VAB-6 trials, which ran from January 1979 through November 1982, had three phases. During the first phase, there was one year of maintenance chemotherapy with vinblastine and actinomycin-D; in the second, there was no maintenance therapy. During the last phase, patients achieving CR were randomly assigned either to receive or not to receive maintenance chemotherapy.

Results from the first two phases have been published.[22,23] A complete review of the MSKCC experience during those 45 months is currently underway. Of note, the randomized trial was closed because patients refused to be randomized. However, it is highly unlikely that maintenance chemotherapy prevents relapse or prolongs survival (Table 4-2). Einhorn has published the results of a randomized trial in a cooperative group setting of maintenance versus no maintenance chemotherapy after VBP and reported no difference in survival or relapse rate.[24] Other nonrandomized studies support these observations, which is not surprising given the absence of cisplatin from the maintenance regimens and the small increment of survival advantage that would need to be detected.

It was evident from these trials that the VAB-6 regimen was very active and had a low relapse rate. It had become the standard therapy at MSKCC, against which future treatment regimens would be compared.

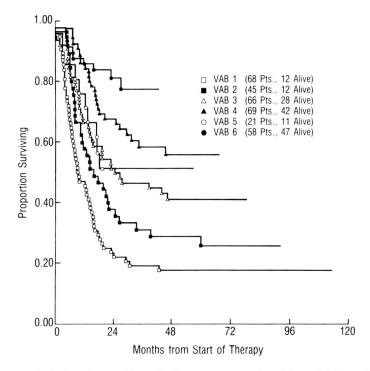

Fig. 4-1. Survival of patients with testicular cancer treated at Memorial Sloan-Kettering Cancer Center from 1972–1982.

SURGICAL INTERVENTION

Surgical intervention has become an integral part of the management of patients with advanced GCT. During early chemotherapy trials against GCT at MSKCC, several patients had apparent disease resected; pathologically, it was benign teratoma.[25] Unlike other malignancies, disease could remain after chemotherapy, but be benign. Whether this observation was a result of differentiation induced by the therapy or of the destruction of malignant elements, with the benign elements left behind, is unimportant clinically.

Three possibilities exist for apparent residual disease: (1) necrotic debris and/ or fibrosis; (2) benign teratoma; (3) either or both of the above, with residual malignant disease. Exploratory surgical procedures, usually a retroperitoneal node dissection or thoracotomy, was of both therapeutic and diagnostic value. If benign, there was no further therapy, if malignant, and all disease was resected, then two additional cycles of therapy were administered.

For patients with incomplete regressions, but considered candidates for cytoreductive surgery, most can have all disease resected. This represents a selected patient population, chosen on the basis of decreasing or absent markers and usually some reduction of disease. Patients showing progression and/or no decrease in markers are not considered surgical candidates. Brenner et al. reviewed the experience of several institutions and reported that in patients so chosen, 38 percent were found to have only necrotic debris or fibrosis, 30 percent had benign teratoma, and 32 percent were found to have residual malignant elements. Only 8/112 (7 percent) patients with necrotic debris, fibrosis, or benign teratoma had relapsed as opposed to 61 percent of patients with residual malignant elements. However, only 2/11 patients with malignant residual elements treated at MSKCC had relapsed.[26]

A review of the survival and relapse rate of patients achieving CR at MSKCC was recently reported by Scher et al.[27] For the purpose of that review, a CR to chemotherapy plus surgery was defined as a CR achieved after chemotherapy and complete resection of residual tumor shown to have malignant elements. If only necrotic debris, fibrosis, scar, and benign teratoma were found in the surgical specimen, then the patient was said to have achieved a CR to chemotherapy alone. Some patients required more than one surgical procedure for multiple disease sites. Patients with residual, but totally resected malignant tumor were treated with additional chemotherapy postoperatively; in the VAB-6 regimen, two additional cycles were administered. The relapse rate and survival of patients achieving CR to chemotherapy plus surgery was similar to that of patients achieving CR to chemotherapy alone.[27] Careful staging of all sites of disease after induction chemotherapy, complete resection of apparent residual tumor, and two additional months of chemotherapy if surgery revealed residual malignant elements afforded these patients a likelihood of survival that was essentially the same as a CR to chemotherapy alone.

An additional observation from Scher's review of patients achieving CR was the appearance of four patients with a late relapse (more than two years after starting chemotherapy). This observation has also been made at the Walter Reed Army Medical Center[28] and at the University of Minnesota (personal communication, Dr. B.J. Kennedy). Although this is a small percentage of all patients achieving CR, the occurrence of late relapses implies that patients will need to be followed carefully for long periods of time with serial assays of tumor markers, interval chest X-rays, physical examination, and other tests as indicated.

ADJUVANT CHEMOTHERAPY

Since a CR could be achieved even in the presence of widespread metastatic disease, a logical extension was to treat patients with pathological stage II nonseminomatous disease after retroperitoneal node dissection (RPLND). Table 4-3 summarizes nine years of trials with various adjuvant programs at MSKCC.[29,30,31] The first trial defined the important risk factors in predicting relapse after RPLND. The patients at highest risk had six or more positive lymph nodes, extranodal extension of tumor, or one or more nodes more than 2 cm in diameter. After 1975, only patients with these poor prognostic features received adjuvant chemotherapy. Only one recent patient has relapsed after adjuvant chemotherapy. This

Table 4-3. Adjuvant Chemotherapy of Patients with Pathological
Stage II Nonseminomatous Testicular Cancer

Trial	Patients	Relapses (%)	Reference
"Mini-VAB"	62	10 (18)	29
Good risk	33	0	
Poor risk	29	10 (35)	
VAB-3	29	0	30
VAB-6	24	0	31

patient had a malignant teratoma[32] (embryonal rhabdomyosarcoma in conjunction with a tumor consisting of other germinal elements) and pulmonary nodules that appeared three months after adjuvant chemotherapy and were found to be embryonal rhabdomyosarcoma.

Given the high cure rate of patients with metastatic disease, and the high probability of CR in patients with minimal disease, Williams et al. reported a "watch and wait" approach in patients with pathological stage II disease; essentially all patients entered CR when treated at the time of relapse.[33] Thus, the need for adjuvant chemotherapy was questioned and a national adjuvant study was started. This study is currently accruing patients. It is hoped that, at its conclusion, firm recommendations about which patients require adjuvant chemotherapy after RPLND (if indeed, it is necessary at all) can be made. In the meantime, patients at MSKCC with pathological stage II disease are offered the possibility of participating in the randomized national adjuvant study.

SEMINOMA

Patients with seminoma sufficiently extensive to require systemic chemotherapy are rare. Only 10 percent of patients with seminomas present with stage III disease. Two regimens have been used during the past seven years at MSKCC (Table 4-4). The CR rate was greater than 80 percent in patients treated with VAB-6.[36] Patients with extragonadal seminoma were also treated with VAB-6, and the results of treatment were similar.[37] Thus, similar CR rates were observed for patients with either nonseminomatous or seminomatous tumors.

Currently, our recommendations for the systemic treatment of patients with seminoma are (1) all patients with stage III disease; (2) all patients with extragonodal primary tumors; (3) all patients with retroperitoneal disease more than 10 cm in

Table 4-4. Treatment Results in Patients with Pure Seminoma[a]

	Patients	CR (%)	Relapses (%)	Reference
VBP	19	12 (63)	0	34
CYC + P	9	8 (89)	1 (13)	35
VAB-6	26	21 (8)	2 (10)	36

[a] Abbreviations: CR, complete response; VBP, see text; D, doxorubicin; CYC, cyclophosphamide; VAB-6, see Ref. 22.

diameter. Since this last group has a 40 percent chance of relapsing after radiation therapy,[38] we feel that they should receive chemotherapy first. Debate over the use of chemotherapy as first therapy for patients with bulky but apparently localized seminoma continues. However, the augmented myelosuppression that can be expected following radiation therapy may cause drug dose attenuation at relapse.

SALVAGE CHEMOTHERAPY

In 1980, Williams et al. reported the efficacy of treatment programs based on VP-16 and cisplatin, with or without doxorubicin and bleomycin.[39] A high CR rate was obtained in patients not responding to prior chemotherapy, including some patients previously treated with cisplatin. In February 1981, a program of VP-16 plus cisplatin was initiated at MSKCC. Doxorubicin and bleomycin were not used because of the substantial toxicity reported with the use of four drugs in combination,[39,40] the almost invariable previous exposure to bleomycin, the absence of benefit of doxorubicin in a randomized study,[21] and the absence of benefit of doxorubicin plus cisplatin as salvage therapy.[41]

The preliminary results of this study confirmed the activity of VP-16 plus cisplatin, but the CR rate was not nearly as high.[42] In addition, no patient who did not achieve a CR to prior high-dose cisplatin-based regimens achieved a CR to this salvage regimen.[43] Results similar to these, with a low CR rate, have been reported by others.[44,45] Significant factors prognostic of a CR to salvage therapy were the lack of prior exposure to cisplatin and relapse after a prior CR. One factor possibly prognostic of CR to salvage therapy was a first CR lasting longer than two months.[46] As with the data reported for salvage therapy in patients with resistant Hodgkin's disease,[47] reported response rates for VP-16 plus cisplatin will vary depending upon the patient selection. Nonetheless, therapy based on VP-16 plus cisplatin is active, but probably not really non-cross–resistant.

EXTRAGONODAL GERM CELL TUMORS

In the past decade, the treatment for mediastinal and retroperitoneal GCT and testicular GCT has been the same at MSKCC. Unlike Hainsworth et al.,[48] the MSKCC experience with extragonadal nonseminomatous GCT is not equivalent to that of testicular GCT. Our results[20,49] are more like those of Garnick et al.,[50] in which patients with primary extragonadal germ cell tumors did poorly. It is likely that these differences are a result of dissimilar patient populations. At least two patient populations exist: (1) patients with seminoma and (2) patients with nonseminomatous disease. Within this second group, patients with primary extragonadal yolk sac tumors (endodermal sinus tumor) appeared to do particularly poorly.[51] Our favorable results with primary extragonadal seminomas have already been mentioned.[37] Further data are required if dissimilarity between reports on the survival of patients with extragonadal germ cell tumors is to be understood.

1982 TO PRESENT

A plateau has been reached in the ability of current regimens to improve survival. Alterations in therapy could lead to new toxicities for the majority of patients who are likely to be cured. Nonetheless, some patients still die of this disease. These considerations led to studies of prognostic variables and new agents and a renewed interest in the biology of human germ cell tumors.

Many clinical variables exist in the patient with advanced GCT. During the past three years, these have been reviewed at MSKCC, in a univariate as well as in a multivariate fashion. Considering embryonal carcinoma, teratocarcinoma, and choriocarcinoma, histopathological cell type did not appear to be an important prognostic variable.[52] However, malignant teratoma, defined as a teratoma in which one or more mature elements are malignant, has a poor prognosis if it is metastatic.[32] Serum tumor marker values did not initially appear to be important.[53] Several points led to a multivariate analysis of this large data set. First, the variables were often interdependent. Second, arbitrary cutoffs for marker values (such as "normal" versus "abnormal") ignored the continuity of these values. Third, other investigators had reported that histopathology, as well as other variables, was prognostically important.

A logistic regression analysis of several prognostic variables was performed. The variables considered included serum tumor marker values, histopathology, prior treatment, and extent of disease. Several models were developed, using different definitions of serum tumor marker values, extent of disease, and prior treatment history. In the best model, three variables contributed in a statistically significant fashion: (1) log (LDH + 1), (2) log (hCG + 1), and (3) number of sites of metastases.[54] The logarithmic transformation was required because of the markedly skewed distribution of marker values[53] and the value (+1) was added to eliminate the possibility of logarithm (0), for which no value exists, and logarithms of values between 0 and 1, which are negative numbers. This model was tested against two independent data sets,[55] including 49 patients treated with VBP at the University of Minnesota and 54 patients treated at MSKCC.

The model appears to clarify several issues. It confirmed that embryonal carcinoma, elements of choriocarcinoma, and teratocarcinoma do not have prognostic value. Serum tumor markers are important, with hCG being more important than AFP. Progressively higher values of both hCG and LDH imply an increasingly worse prognosis. More subtle is the recognition that a palpable abdominal mass without elevations of LDH or hCG or both is not a poor prognostic feature. This is in contrast to the Samuels staging system,[11] in which patients with a palpable abdominal mass are classified as "advanced abdominal," regardless of marker status. Equally important, patients with multiple metastatic sites without marker elevations generally achieve CR. This partly relates to large tumor masses consisting of benign teratoma in some of these patients. Thus, this model can distinguish between good- and poor-risk patient populations.

Ongoing studies at MSKCC do differentiate between good- and poor-risk patients. A review of the predicted and actual CR rates showed that patients with a probability of CR less than 0.5 had a low CR rate when viewed as a group. In

Table 4-5. Phase II Trials Conducted at Memorial Sloan-Kettering Cancer Center

Drug[a]	Patients (N)	CR/PR	Reference
Vindesine	19	0/3	56
DACCP	9	0/0	—
13 Cis-retinoic acid	15	0/0	57
Methyl GAG	7	0/0	Ongoing

[a] DACCP, 1,2-diaminocyclohexane (4-carboxyphthalato) platinum II; Methyl GAG, methylglyoxal bis(guanylhydrazone).

the data set that generated the model, only 7/28 patients with probabilities less than 0.5 eventually achieved a CR.[54] Thus, patients with testicular cancer entering current prospective studies at MSKCC are determined to be either a good or a poor risk on the basis of the probability of CR predicted by the model, and separate trials exist for these two patient populations. This stratification assures reasonable patient uniformity in each trial, and minimizes the risk of toxicity in the good-risk group. For patients most likely to achieve a CR, a randomized trial compares VP-16 plus cisplatin and VAB-6; for patients not likely to achieve a CR, alternating cycles of VP-16 plus cisplatin and VAB-6 for six months are recommended. Timely surgical intervention remains an integral part of combined modality treatment of patients with advanced GCT.

Phase II trials will be extremely important in planning future treatment, particularly for poor-risk patients. Phase II trials in GCT conducted at MSKCC are summarized in Table 4-5. Although none of these drugs appears to be active against GCT, the search for new active agents must continue if improvement in the treatment of this disease is to occur.

Studies of tumor biology will become important. Screening for surface antigens with monoclonal antibodies led to the identification of neuroectodermal antigens on the cell surface of some cultured human GCT.[58] Monoclonal antibodies developed against antigens specific to GCT may have diagnostic and therapeutic value. Differentiation induced by 13-cis-retinoic acid in cultured lines of murine embryonal carcinoma cells,[59,60] and an increased life-span of mice inoculated with F9 embryonal carcinoma cells and treated with 13-cis-retinoic acid[61] led to a Phase II trial of 13-cis-retinoic acid in patients with GCT. Unfortunately, this drug was inactive in heavily pretreated GCT patients.[57] This is not surprising, since most of the work done on differentiation has been done in murine lines.

CONCLUSION

The success of the 1970s in the treatment of patients with GCT will be surpassed in the 1980s if disease can be detected earlier and treatment can be made less toxic for the majority and more successful for the minority. Issues of delayed toxicity, such as the report of Raynaud's phenomenon by Vogelzang,[62] will become more important. Laboratory studies of differentiation in GCT may provide important data not only to oncologists, but also to developmental biologists. We will continue to work toward these ends.

DEDICATION

This report would not be complete without acknowledging the many investigators who participated in these trials over the years. Even more important has been the steady presence of Dr. Robert B. Golbey and Dr. Willet F. Whitmore, Jr. Their contributions to the management of this disease are universally recognized and their continued presence at MSKCC provides a perspective not available at any other institution. To them, this report is dedicated.

ACKNOWLEDGMENT

This work was supported in part by grant CA 05826 and contract No-1-CM07337 from the National Cancer Institute.

REFERENCES

1. Li MC, Whitmore WF, Golbey RB, Grabstald H: Effects of combination drug therapy on metastatic cancer of the testis. JAMA 174:145, 1960
2. MacKenzie AR: Chemotherapy of metastatic testis cancer. Results in 154 patients. Cancer 19:1369, 1966
3. Kennedy BJ: Mithramycin therapy in testicular cancer. J Urol 107:429, 1972
4. Samuels ML, Howe CD: Vinblastine in the management of testicular cancer. Cancer 25:1009, 1970
5. Clinical Screening Co-operative Group of the European Organization for Research on the Treatment of Cancer: Study of clinical efficiency of bleomycin. Br Med J 2:643, 1970
6. Yagoda A, Mukherji B, Young C, Etcubanas E, LaMonte C, Smith JR, Tan CTC, Krakoff IH: Bleomycin, an antitumor antibiotic. Ann Int Med 77:861, 1972
7. Wittes RE, Yagoda A, Silvay O, Magill GB, Whitmore WF, Krakoff IH, Golbey RB: Chemotherapy of germ cell tumors of the testis. I. Induction of remission with vinblastine, actinomycin-D, and bleomycin. Cancer 37:637, 1976
8. Higby DJ, Wallace J, Holland JF. *Cis*-diamminedichloroplatinum (NSC-119875). Cancer Chemother Rept Part 1. 57:459, 1973
9. Cvitkovic E, Currie V, Ochoa M, Pride G, Krakoff IH: Continuous intravenous infusion of bleomycin in squamous cancer. Proc Am Assoc Cancer Res Am Soc Clin Oncol 15:179, 1974
10. Cheng E, Cvitkovic E, Wittes RE, Golbey RB: Germ cell tumors (II). VAB II in metastatic testicular cancer. Cancer 42:2162, 1978
11. Samuels ML, Lanzoti VJ, Holoye PY, Boyle LE, Smith TL, Johnson DE: Combination chemotherapy in germinal cell tumors. Cancer Treat Rev 3:185, 1976
12. Rossof AH, Slayton RE, Perlia CP: Preliminary clinical experience with *Cis*-diamminedichloroplatinum (II) (NSC-119875, CACP). Cancer 30:1451, 1972
13. Cvitkovic E, Spaulding J, Bethune V, Martin J, Whitmore WF: Improvement of *cis*-dichlorodiammineplatinum (NSC-119875) therapeutic index in an animal model. Cancer 39:1357, 1977
14. Hayes DM, Cvitkovic E, Golbey RB, Scheiner E, Helson L, Krakoff IH: High dose

cis-platinum diammine dichloride. Amelioration of renal toxicity by mannitol diuresis. Cancer 39:1372, 1977

15. Buckner CD, Clift RA, Fefer A, et al: High-dose cyclophosphamide (NSC-26271) for the treatment of metastatic testicular neoplasms. Cancer Chemother Rept 58:709, 1974

16. Monfardini S, Basetta E, Musumeli R, et al: Clinical use of adriamycin in advanced testicular cancer. J Urol 108:293, 1972

17. Golbey RB, Reynolds TF, Vugrin D. Chemotherapy of metastatic germ cell tumors. Semin Oncol 6:82, 1979

18. Reynolds TF, Vugrin D, Cvitkovic E, Cheng E, Braun DW, O'Hehir MA, Dukeman ME, Whitmore WF, Golbey RB: VAB-3 combination chemotherapy of metastatic testicular cancer. Cancer 48:888, 1981

19. Vugrin D, Cvitkovic E, Whitmore WF, Cheng E, Golbey RB: VAB-4 combination chemotherapy for testicular cancer. Ann Int Med 95:288, 1981

20. Vugrin D, Whitmore WF, Golbey RB: VAB-5 combination chemotherapy in prognostically poor risk patients with germ cell tumors. Cancer 51:1072, 1983

21. Einhorn LH: Testicular cancer as a model for a curable neoplasm. The Richard and Hinda Rosenthal Foundation Award Lecture. Cancer Res 41:3275, 1981

22. Vugrin D, Herr HW, Whitmore WF, et al: VAB-6 combination chemotherapy in disseminated cancer of the testis. Ann Int Med 95:59, 1981

23. Vugrin D, Whitmore WF, Golbey RB: VAB-6 combination chemotherapy without maintenance in treatment of disseminated cancer of the testis. Cancer 51:211, 1983

24. Einhorn LH, Williams SD, Troner M, Birch R, Greco FA: The role of maintenance chemotherapy in disseminated testicular cancer. N Engl J Med 305:727, 1981

25. Hong WK, Wittes RE, Hajdu ST, Cvitkovic E, Whitmore WF, Golbey RB: The evolution of mature teratoma from malignant testicular tumors. Cancer 40:2987, 1977

26. Brenner J, Vugrin D, Whitmore WF: Cytoreductive surgery for advanced nonseminomatous germ cell tumors of the testis. Urology 19:571, 1982

27. Scher H, Bosl GJ, Geller N, Cirrincione C, Whitmore WF, Golbey RB: Long-term follow-up of patients with testicular germ cell tumors achieving complete remission after chemotherapy (CT) alone or CT plus surgery. Proc Am Assoc Cancer Res 24:157 (Abstract 621), 1983

28. Terebelo HR, Geyer L, Brown A, Martin N, Stutz FH, Taylor HG, Blom J: Late relapses of testicular cancer. J Clin Oncol 1:566, 1983

29. Vugrin D, Cvitkovic E, Whitmore WF, Golbey RB: Adjuvant chemotherapy in resected nonseminomatous germ cell tumors of testis: Stages I and II. Semin Oncol 6:94, 1979

30. Vugrin D, Whitmore W, Cvitkovic E, Grabstald H, Sogani D, Golbey RB: Adjuvant chemotherapy with VAB-3 of Stage IIB testicular cancer. Cancer 48:233, 1981

31. Vugrin D, Whitmore WF, Herr HW, Sogani P, Golbey RB: VAB-6 combination chemotherapy in resected Stage IIB testis cancer. Cancer 51:5, 1983

32. Ahmed TA, Bosl GJ, Hajdu S: The importance of recognizing malignant teratoma. (submitted for publication).

33. Williams SD, Einhorn LH, Donohue JP: High cure rate of state I or II testicular cancer with or without adjuvant therapy. Proc Am Assoc Cancer Res Am Soc Clin Oncol 21 (Abstract C-407), 1980

34. Einhorn LH, Williams SD: Chemotherapy of disseminated seminoma. Cancer Clin Trials 3:307–313, 1981

35. Vugrin D, Whitmore WF, Batata M: Chemotherapy of disseminated seminoma with combination of *cis*-diamminedichloroplatinum (II) and cyclophosphamide. Cancer Clin Trials 4:423, 1981

36. Stanton GF, Bosl GJ, Vugrin D, Whitmore WF, Myers WPLM, Golbey RB: Treatment

of patients with advanced seminoma with cyclophosphamide, bleomycin, actinomycin D, vinblastine and cisplatin (VAB-6). Proc Am Soc Clin Oncol 2:141 (Abstract C-551), 1983

37. Jain KK, Bosl GJ, Bains MS, Whitmore WF, Golbey RB: The treatment of extragonadal seminoma. J Clin Onc 2:820, 1984

38. Batata MA, Chu FC, Hilaris BS, Papantoniou PA, Whitmore WF, Golbey RB: Therapy and prognosis of testicular carcinomas in relation to TNM classification. Int J Radiat Oncol Biol Phys 8:1287, 1982

39. Williams SD, Einhorn LH, Greco FA, Oldham R, Fletcher R: VP-16-213 salvage chemotherapy for refractory germinal neoplasms. Cancer 46:2154, 1980

40. Vogelzang NJ, Kennedy BJ: Salvage chemotherapy for refractory germ cell tumors. Proc Am Assoc Cancer Res AM Soc Clin Oncol 22:471 (Abstract C-540), 1981

41. Einhorn LH, Williams SD: Combination chemotherapy with cisdichlorodiammineplatinum (II) and adriamycin for testicular cancer refractory to vinblastine plus bleomycin. Cancer Treat Rept 62:1351, 1978

42. Bosl GJ, Yagoda A, Whitmore WF, Sogani P, Herr H, Vugrin D, Dukeman M, Golbey RB: VP-16-213 and cisplatin in the treatment of patients with refractory germ cell tumors. Am J Clin Oncol (in press).

43. Bosl GJ, Yagoda A, Vogelzang NJ, Whitmore W, Golbey RB: VP-16 plus cisplatin "salvage" chemotherapy for patients (pts) with germ cell tumors (GCT) who fail to achieve a complete remission (CR). Proc Am Assoc Cancer Res 24:150 (Abstract 594), 1983

44. Mortimer J, Bukowski RM, Montie J, Hewlett JS, Livingston RB: VP-16-213, cisplatinum, and adriamycin salvage therapy of refractory and/or recurrent nonseminomatous germ cell neoplasms. Cancer Chemother Pharmacol 61:99, 1982

45. Lederman GS, Garnick MB, Richie JP, Canellos GP: VP-16-213 and *cis*-platinum as secondary therapy in patients with refratory testicular and extragonadal germ cell cancer. Proc Am Assoc Cancer Res 24:146 (Abstract 576), 1983

46. Williams SD, Turner S, Loehrer PJ, Einhorn LH: Testicular cancer: Results of reinduction therapy. Proc Am Soc Clin Oncol 2:137 (Abstract C-536), 1983

47. Bonadona G, Santoro A: ABVD chemotherapy in the treatment of Hodgkin's disease. Cancer Treat Rev 9:21, 1982

48. Hainsworth JD, Einhorn LH, Williams SD, Stewart M, Greco FA: Advanced extragonadal germ-cell tumors. Successful treatment with combination chemotherapy. Ann Intern Med 97:7, 1982

49. Vugrin D, Martini N, Whitmore WF, Golbey RB: VAB-3 combination chemotherapy in primary mediastinal germ cell tumors. Cancer Treat Rept 66:1405, 1982

50. Garnick MB, Canellos GP, Richie JP: Treatment and surgical staging of testicular and primary extragonadal germ cell cancer. JAMA 250:1733, 1983

51. Kuzur ME, Cobleigh MA, Greco FA, Einhorn LH, Oldham RK: Endodermal sinus tumor of the mediastinum. Cancer 50:766, 1982

52. Bosl GJ, Geller N, Cirrincio C, Hadju S, Whitmore W, Nisselbaum J, Vugrin D, Golbey RB: Interrelationships of histopathology and other clinical variables in patients with germ cell tumors of the testis. Cancer 51:2121, 1983

53. Bosl GJ, Geller NL, Cirrincione C, Nisselbaum J, Vugrin D, Whitmore WF, Golbey RB: Serum tumor markers in patients with metastatic germ cell tumors of the testis. Am J Med 75:29, 1983

54. Bosl GJ, Geller NL, Cirrincion C, Vogelzang NJ, Kennedy BJ, Whitmore WF, Vugrin D, Scher H, Nisselbaum J, Golbey RB: Multivariate analysis of prognostic variables in patients with metastatic testicular cancer. Cancer Res 43:3403, 1983

55. Bosl GJ, Geller N, Cirrincione C, Scher H, Whitmore WF, Golbey RB. A multivariate analysis of prognostic variables in patients (pts) with metastatic germ cell tumors of the testis (GCT). Proc Am Soc Clin Oncol 2:141 (Abstract C-552), 1983

57. Gold E, Bosl GJ, Whitmore WF, Myers WPL, Golbey RB: Phase II trial of 13 *cis*-retinoic acid in the treatment of patients (PTS) with advanced germ cell tumors. Proc Am Assoc Cancer Res, 24:150 (Abstract 595), 1983

58. Fradet Y, Houghton AN, Bosl GJ, Bronson D, Whitmore WF: Cell surface antigens of human teratocarcinoma cell lines identified with monoclonal antibodies. Cold Spring Harbor Symposium on Cell Proliferation. Volume X. Teratocarcinoma. (In press).

59. Strickland S, Madhavi V: The induction of differentiation in teratocarcinoma stem cells by retinoic acid. Cell 15:393, 1978

60. Jones-Villeneuve E, McBurney MW, Rogers KA, Kalnins VI: Retinoic acid induces embryonal carcinoma cells to differentiate into neurons and glial cells. J Cell Biol 94:253, 1982

61. Strickland S, Sawey MJ. Studies on the effect of retinoids on the differentiation of teratocarcinoma stem cells in vitro and in vivo. Dev Biol 78:76, 1980

62. Vogelzang NJ, Bosl GJ, Johnson K, Kennedy BJ: Raynaud's phenomenon. A common toxicity after combination chemotherapy for testicular cancer. Ann Intern Med 95:288, 1981

5 Diagnosis and Management of Extragonadal Germ Cell Tumors

Mehmet F. Fer
John D. Hainsworth
F. Anthony Greco

The development of curative therapy for metastatic germ cell tumors during the past decade has rendered imperative the accurate recognition and appropriate management of these diseases.[1,2] Although controversy exists regarding the cure rates of extragonadal germ cell tumors (EGCT), in comparison to highly curable testicular germ cell cancers, all would agree that a substantial number of these patients can enjoy durable remissions. In contrast to testicular germ cell neoplasms, which are easily recognized, EGCT can present in a variety of unusual locations and may be more difficult to diagnose, particularly if they have poorly differentiated histology or negative serum tumor markers. In fact, some patients with "poorly differentiated carcinoma" or "carcinoma of unknown origin" possess clinical characteristics similar to germinal neoplasms and experience dramatic responses to chemotherapy.[3-6] Although the nature of these tumors is unclear, their clinical and biological behavior has led to the speculation that they are unrecognized EGCT. This chapter will first review the clinical approaches to histologically well-defined EGCT, followed by a discussion of atypical or suspected cases.

CLINICAL CHARACTERISTICS

Extragonadal germ cell tumors have been postulated to arise from primordial germs cells from either the endoderm (yolk sac) or the urogenital ridge (extending in the embryo from the sixth cervical to the second sacral vertebra), which have failed to migrate into the scrotum.[7-10] The similar spectrum of histological types seen in EGCT and testicular germinal tumors supports this hypothesis (Table 5-1).[10]

Major histological types include seminomas, embryonal carcinomas, teratomas, choriocarcinomas, and yolk sac tumors, which occur either as the sole histological type or in combination. Classically, seminomas comprise approximately 40 percent of testicular malignancies and approximately 50 percent of mediastinal germ cell tumors. Histopathological considerations are described in detail elsewhere,[10,11] and will not be discussed further here.

Extragonadal germ cell neoplasms occur predominantly in young adults, with seminomas being most common in the fourth decade of life and nonseminomatous germ cell tumors in the third. As in gonadal germinal tumors, these neoplasms are more common in men than in women. In three recent series totaling 44 patients, no female patients were reported.[12-14] In a combined series from Vanderbilt and Indiana Universities, only 2 of the 32 patients were women.[15]

Most EGCT occur in either the mediastinum or the retroperitoneum, although other sites are occasionally reported (Table 5-2). Initial signs and symptoms are usually related to mass effect at the primary site; mediastinal and retroperitoneal tumors, however, are usually quite large before symptoms occur. Metastases are common at diagnosis, and preferentially involve the lung, lymph nodes, and the liver.

In spite of their frequent occurrence in the mediastinum, EGCT account for

Table 5-1. Relative Frequency of Histopathological Types of Extragonadal Germ Cell Tumors

Authors	Location	Seminoma	Embryonal Carcinoma	Endodermal Sinus Tumor	Chorio-carcinoma	Terato-carcinoma	Mixed Tumors
Utz and	Mediastinum	6	1		1		4
Buscemi[9]	Retroperitoneum	1	2		1		1
	Pineal gland	1					
Recondo and	Mediastinum	5	1		1	4	6
Libshitz[38]							
Johnson	Mediastinum	5			1	2	1
et al.[39]	Retroperitoneum	3			2	2	1
	Pineal gland	1				1	
	Presacral area		1				
Beattie[24]	Mediastinum	10	4				16
Hainsworth		6	9		7	7	
et al.[15]							
Garnick		1	6	1			7
et al.[14]							
Feun et al.[13]	Mediastinum	2	4		1	3	1
	Retroperitoneum	2	2		1	1	
	Other				1		1

Table 5-2. Frequent Locations of Extragonadal Germ Cell Tumors

Authors	Medias-tinum	Retro-peritoneum	Pituitary Gland	Pineal Gland	Lung	Presacral Area	Lymph Node	Other
Utz and Buscemi[9]	12	5		1				
Johnson et al.[39]	7	8		2		1		
Hainsworth et al.[15]	17	13					1	1
Garnick et al.[14]	8	6*	1					
Feun et al.[13]	12	6			1			

a Abdominal mass

only a small percentage of mediastinal tumors. In a retrospective review of 186 patients with mediastinal tumors, Rubush et al. found six malignant teratomas.[16] In a review of the literature, the same authors found that 39 of the reported 1,037 mediastinal tumors (3.8 percent) were malignant teratomas. In another review, 19 of 1687 mediastinal mass lesions (1.1 percent) were germinal tumors.[17] It is probable that some mediastinal germinal tumors have been unrecognized in the past, but they nevertheless must be considered to be relatively rare.

The production of the serum tumor markers beta-human chorionic gonadotro-pin (beta-hCG) and alphafetoprotein (AFP) by EGCT is frequent, as it is by gonadal germinal tumors. The frequency of tumor marker production according to histologi-cal subtype of EGCT based on the combined Vanderbilt–Indiana experience is summarized in Table 5–3.[15] In this series, only 8 of 32 patients had negative markers, and the remaining 24 had one or both markers elevated in their serum. Since serum levels of these markers are not universally elevated in patients with EGCT, their use as diagnostic tests in patients presenting with mass lesions remains limited. Nevertheless, an elevated serum AFP or beta-hCG should alert one to the possibility of an EGCT.

EVALUATION OF THE PATIENT

After an initial diagnosis of EGCT has been made, a thorough pathological review of multiple sections is important. This is especially critical with the diagnosis of pure seminoma since examination of other areas can reveal that a mixed tumor is present and radically alter treatment plans (vida infra).

Table 5-3. Correlation of Histological Patterns with Serum Marker Status[15][a]

	No. of Patients	Elevated AFP	Elevated hCGβ	Both Markers
Embryonal carcinoma	9	4	6	2
Choriocarcinoma	7	1	7	0
Teratocarcinoma	7	6	3	1
"Seminoma"	6	0	3	3

a Endodermal sinus tumors, usually associated with alphafetoprotein production, were not included in this series.

Modified from Hainsworth JD, Einhorn LH, Williams SD, Stewart M, Greco FA: Advanced extragonadal germ cell tumors. Successful treatment with combination chemotherapy. Ann Int Med 97:7, 1982

Staging procedures should include routine laboratory tests (chemistry profile, complete blood count), chest X-ray, computerized tomography (CT) of the chest and abdomen, and measurement of serum beta-hCG and AFP. Marked hCG elevation (>100 mg/ml) or *any* elevation of AFP indicates the presence of nonseminomatous elements, even if the histological sections show "pure seminoma." Although metastases to the central nervous system (CNS) imply a poor prognosis, they are unusual in patients with EGCT, and routine CT scanning of the brain and/or lumbar puncture is not recommended. When involvement of the CNS is suspected, tumor marker studies in the cerebrospinal fluid (CSF) can be useful.[18] In trophoblastic choriocarcinoma, a CSF beta-hCG exceeding 2 percent of the serum level correlates well with the presence of CNS metastasis, and this may apply to germinal neoplasms as well.[19] Beta-hCG seems to be a more useful marker in the CSF compared to alpha-fetoprotein or CEA, possibly because its smaller molecular weight might allow its easier passage into the CSF.

A question that is often raised during the evaluation of patients with EGCT without a palpable testicular mass is whether there might be an occult testicular primary lesion.[9] In the past, the concern for locating a primary lesion has led to orchiectomies in these patients, with occasional discovery of occult testicular primaries.[20,21] In other cases, scar tissue, thought to represent regressed tumor foci, was found.[20] The concept that germinal tumors can arise in extragonadal locations is now widely accepted, based on both clinical observations in large numbers of these patients, and autopsy data in which examination of the testicles failed to reveal tumor.[17] Orchiectomy or blind testicular biopsies in patients with clinically normal testicles and normal testicular ultrasound should, therefore, not be performed. The removal of a clinically undetectable primary lesion of the testicle in the presence of metastatic disease has no value, since the survival of these patients depend on their response to systemic chemotherapy. Although the testicles may provide a "sanctuary site" for malignant cells in childhood leukemia, there is no indication for a similar phenomenon in germinal neoplasms.

THERAPY OF EXTRAGONADAL SEMINOMAS

The great majority of patients with mediastinal seminomas can be cured by extended field radiotherapy. Since seminomas are highly sensitive to radiotherapy, and doses in the range of 2,500 to 3,500 rads over three to four weeks produce high cure rates in patients with localized extragonodal seminomas.[22] There is no evidence to suggest that extragonadal seminomas differ from testicular seminomas with respect to their radiosensitivity.

However, when bulky disease is present, such as retroperitoneal tumors over 5 cm in diameter, close to 40 percent of patients relapse after radiotherapy.[22,23] Thus, patients with bulky disease should be considered for chemotherapy, in addition to radiotherapy. Other patients with elevated beta-hCG or AFP, which suggests the presence of nonseminomatous components, and patients with widely metastatic seminoma require chemotherapy. Einhorn et al. have reported that treatment of advanced testicular seminomas with vinblastine, bleomycin, and *cis*-platinum gives a complete remission rate exceeding 75 percent.[1] These results are comparable to those observed in the treatment of advanced nonseminomatous germ cell tumors. In the series reported by Hainsworth et al., four of the six patients with advanced extragonadal seminomas achieved complete responses (CR) with combination chemotherapy (described below).

THERAPY OF NONSEMINOMATOUS EXTRAGONADAL GERM CELL TUMORS

In a retrospective surgical series reported prior to the development of modern chemotherapy, Beattie reported that 19 of the 20 patients in his review had metastases early in their course and that all these patients died within 16 months of their diagnosis.[24] Thus, surgery as the only mode of therapy cannot be recommended for EGCT, although the role of surgery as a debulking procedure needs to be clarified. It is generally recommended that if tumors are easily and safely resectable, this should be done. After this procedure, patients with seminomas can be approached as described above, although patients with nonseminomatous tumors should receive combination chemotherapy. Like surgery, irradiation of the primary lesion in nonseminomatous tumors would be of limited benefit due to the high incidence of systemic metastases.

The chemotherapy of germinal neoplasms has evolved substantially over the past decade. Cure rates have steeply increased in patients with testicular germ cell cancers after the introduction of *cis*-platinum combination chemotherapy regimens.[1,2] However, the success of comparable regimens against EGCT has remained controversial, and several groups have reported survival rates far less than those observed in testicular cancers.[12,13,14] One of the reasons for this might be that EGCT often present with more bulky and advanced disease, whereas testicular lesions may be recognized earlier because of their superficial location. Nevertheless, a certain subset of patients with EGCT are curable with effective combination chemotherapy. In a recently published combined series from Vanderbilt and Indiana, the durable remission rate for patients with EGCT were comparable to those with testicular primaries of similar advanced stages, with the exception of mediastinal endodermal sinus tumors and possibly choriocarcinomas.[15,25]

Results of combination chemotherapy from recently reported series are summarized in Table 5–4. The largest series reported by Hainsworth et al., combining the patients treated at Vanderbilt and Indiana Universities, utilized a combination of vinblastine, bleomycin, and *cis*-platinum with or without doxorubicin, as outlined in Table 5–5. The mean age of the patients was 30 years, with a range of 16 to 52 years. Thirty patients were men and two were women. Eight patients had previously received other forms of therapy, six with radiotherapy and two with radiotherapy and chemotherapy. All patients initially received full doses of the agents described in Table 5–5 and dose reductions were made in subsequent courses for severe myelosuppression (leukocytes less than 1,000/mm² three weeks after chemotherapy) or documented bacterial sepsis. After completing four cycles of

Table 5-4. Results of Combination Chemotherapy in Extragonadal Germ Cell Tumors

Authors	No. of Patients	Complete Response	Partial Response	Stable Disease	Progression	Mean Duration of Response	Toxic Death	Long-Term Remissions
Feun et al.[13]	19	3	6	2	8	2	1	0
Vugrin et al.[12a]	10	2			8			2
Hainsworth et al.[15b]	31	21	10				1	18
Garnick et al.[14c]	15	10			5[d]		1[e]	4
Funes[38]	14	6						5

[a] No histological classification/breakdown provided in this paper.
[b] Mediastinal endodermal sinus (yolk sac) tumors were not included in this series.
[c] Nine of ten patients achieved CR after resection of residual tumor.
[d] ⅗ initially showed a brief PR.
[e] Death 2° to postoperative complication

chemotherapy, patients were evaluated for response with tumor markers and a repeat of all previously abnormal studies. Patients achieving complete remission either received no further therapy or maintenance vinblastine, 0.3 mg/kg body weight every four weeks for two years. Of the 31 evaluable patients in this series, 21 achieved a complete remission and the remaining 10 had a partial response (PR). Of the 21 complete responders, 18 have remained continuously disease-free, and all have now been followed for over 24 months after completion of therapy.

When response rates were analyzed according to histological subtype, the CR rate for choriocarcinoma was lower than the other types. Complete response rates were 29 percent for choriocarcinoma, 67 percent for metastatic seminoma, 78 percent for embryonal carcinoma, and 83 percent for teratocarcinoma. Toxicity was significant, with severe myelosuppression occurring in most patients and documented bacteremia in two. Restrictive lung disease, presumably due to bleomycin,

Table 5-5. Chemotherapy Regimens for Extragonadal Germ Cell Tumors[15]

Cis-platinum-bleomycin-vinblastine
Cis-platinum (20 mg/m²) IV, days 1 through 5
Bleomycin (30 U) IV, on day 2 and weekly
Vinblastine 0.15 mg/kg IV, days 1 and 2
    Cycle length, 3 weeks

Cis-platinum-bleomycin-vinblastine-doxorubicin
Cis-platinum (20 mg/m²) IV, days 1 through 5
Bleomycin (30 U) IV, on day 2 and weekly
Vinblastine (0.2 mg/kg) IV, on day 1
Doxorubicin (50 mg/m²) IV, on day 2
    Cycle length, 3 weeks

Modified from Hainsworth JD, Einhorn LH, Williams SD, Stewart M, Greco FA: Advanced extragonadal germ cell tumors. Successful treatment with combination chemotherapy. Ann Int Med 97:7, 1982 occurred in four patients, and was mild to moderate in three patients, but fatal in the fourth. Platinum-induced renal failure was not a major problem, probably because of vigorous hydration prior to and during *cis*-platinum therapy.

Of note is that patients with mediastinal endodermal sinus (yolk sac) tumors were not included in this report. A series of patients with this histology treated at Vanderbilt and Indiana Universities with comparable chemotherapy, but without success, has been previously reported.[25] In this series reported by Kuzur et al., 9 of the 10 patients with mediastinal endodermal sinus tumors relapsed after transient initial responses, and there was only 1 long-term survivor. Interestingly, ovarian endodermal sinus tumors respond well to similar chemotherapy. Julian et al. have reported complete remissions documented by second-look laparotomies in all three of their patients treated with vinblastine, bleomycin, and *cis*-platinum.[26] Primary mediastinal choriocarcinoma has been previously reported to carry a poor prognosis prior to the development of current effective regimens, and it is discouraging that this trend continued to some extent in this series.[27]

Other recent series utilizing comparable chemotherapy regimens have not produced equally encouraging results. A study by the Southwest Oncology Group reported by Feun et al.[13] included 19 patients with metastatic EGCT treated with a combination of vinblastine (12 mg/m²) on day 1, Bleomycin (15 mg/m²), IV or IM twice weekly, and *cis*-platinum (15 mg/m²) on days 1 through 5 in 28-day cycles. After four cycles, all responders were placed on a maintenance regimen of vinblastine alternating with actinomycin-D and chlorambucil. Of the 19 patients included in this study, there were three CR and six PR. The mean duration of response was only two months (range one to eight months); there were no long-term survivors. One of the three complete responders died of drug toxicity while in remission and a second one was lost to follow-up. The histological types included in this study were four seminomas, three choriocarcinomas, six embryonal carcinomas, four teratocarcinomas and one mixed tumor. All patients were men, with a median age of 32 (range 19 to 52). There were no patients with mediastinal endodermal sinus tumors in this group. Although the chemotherapy regimen used in this study is similar to those used at Vanderbilt and Indiana, there are some major differences in the two studies. First of all, 8 of the 19 patients had received prior radiotherapy and 3 patients had prior chemotherapy. This may have been a factor that limited tolerance to chemotherapy or possibly resulted in drug resistance. Second, the chemotherapy used in these patients was considerably less intensive. The *cis*-platinum dose was 15 mg/m² daily for five days, as opposed to 20 mg/m² used at Vanderbilt and Indiana, and the chemotherapy cycles were given every four rather than every three weeks. These factors may have jeopardized the outcome of therapy in these kinetically active tumors.[28] The median performance status in this series was 40 percent, and 80 percent of the patients had bulky tumors; both factors imply a poor prognosis.

Another series of patients from Memorial Sloan-Kettering Cancer Center was reported by Vugrin et al.[12] In this series, 10 patients were treated with the VAB-3 regimen, consisting of alternating chemotherapy including cyclophosphamide, vinblastine, actinomycin-D, bleomycin, and *cis*-platinum sequentially used with vinblastine, doxorubicin, and chlorambucil. Histological types were not specified. All nine patients with measurable lesions showed tumor regression in this series, but seven subsequently relapsed. The remaining two patients were free of recurrent tumor at 40 months following chemotherapy. In this regimen, *cis*-platinum, probably the most active drug against these tumors, was given only every six weeks, with less effective agents used in alternating cycles.

Garnick et al. recently reported the results of therapy in 15 patients with EGCT and compared it with the outcome of 39 other patients with metastatic testicular carcinoma.[14] The median age in this group was 26 (range 14 to 55), and only two had received radiation or chemotherapy. The predominant histology was seminoma in one, embryonal carcinoma in six, and endodermal sinus tumor in one. Other patients had mixed histology. Remission-induction chemotherapy included vinblastine (0.15 to 0.2 mg/kg) IV on days 1 and 2; bleomycin (30 units) IV on days 1, 8, and 15; and *cis*-platinum (20 mg/m^2) IV on days 1 through 5, with saline hydration. Cycles were repeated every 21 days. Although 10 of these patients achieved CR, only 4 remained in continuous complete remission. Of note is that of the 10 complete responders, only 1 achieved complete remission by chemotherapy alone; the other 9 had PR after which remaining lesions were resected. Of the patients rendered disease-free at surgery, four had fibrosis alone, one had residual teratoma and the remaining patients had embryonal carcinoma. Of the four CR patients who remained in remission, two had fibrosis at the time of exploration, one had teratoma, and the other embryonal carcinoma. In this study, patients with residual malignancy found at surgery after chemotherapy received consolidation therapy with cyclophosphamide and doxorubicin every three weeks for a total of five cycles. Patients who had fibrosis or teratoma received no further therapy. In this series, there were four patients with endodermal sinus tumor elements, none of whom remained in remission in spite of initial responses. The poor prognosis associated with this disease may account for some of the differences in overall survival rates in this series compared with the series from Vanderbilt and Indiana. All four patients in this series who had mixed tumors with choriocarcinoma components died with progressive disease.

It appears from this review that patients with extragonadal mediastinal endodermal sinus tumors or choriocarcinomas have a poor prognosis, whereas patients with other histologies (embryonal carcinoma, teratocarcinoma, and metastatic seminomas) may have a prognosis comparable to patients with testicular primaries. Although triple drug therapy with vinblastine, bleomycin, and *cis*-platinum may be sufficient for good-prognosis patients, poor-prognosis patients (i.e., those with bulky tumor or unfavorable histologies) may require more intensive investigational approaches. An agent suitable for incorporation into such intensive regimens could be VP-16.[29-32] Williams et al. observed that 29 of 33 patients with testicular germ cell tumors refractory to platinum-based therapy had responses to VP-16 with 14 complete remissions.[29] However, Lederman et al. have recently pointed out that the value of this agent may be greater in the treatment of testicular germ cell cancers compared to EGCT.[32] In their series of 18 patients with advanced germ cell cancers refractory to vinblastine, *cis*-platinum, and bleomycin, 5 of 12 patients with primary testicular carcinoma achieved a complete response and were free of disease following VP-16–based chemotherapy. In contrast, none of the six patients with EGCT had achieved a complete remission and only two had a PR. In this study, VP-16 was given at a dose of 100 mg/m^2 daily on days 1 through

5, in combination with bleomycin (30 mg) IV on days 1, 8 and 16 and doxorubicin (40 mg/m^2) on day 1, with cycles repeated every 21 days. Although discouraging, these results do not demonstrate that combinations incorporating VP-16 in the initial chemotherapy regimen will necessarily fail.

A novel approach to the administration of this agent might be to use higher doses (up to 2,400 mg/m^2) with autologous bone marrow transplantation.[30] In a phase I study of high-dose VP-16 with autologous bone marrow rescue, Wolff et al. used escalating doses ranging from 1,500 to 2,700 mg/m^2. Six patients with germ cell carcinomas were treated, resulting in five responses, one of which was a CR.[30] Dose-limiting toxicity was mucositis, which was severe above 2,400 mg/m^2. Interestingly, of four patients with germ cell malignancy who had failed with standard doses of VP-16, three responded to these escalated doses, suggesting that there may be a dose–response relationship. Based on this experience, a phase II study of high-dose VP-16 for refractory germinal malignancies was conducted.[31] In this study, of six patients previously resistant to standard doses of VP-16, two responded to high-dose therapy (one CR and one PR, lasting five and three months, respectively).[31] Thus, it is conceivable that higher doses of VP-16 might prove more effective against EGCT. The incorporation of high-dose VP-16 into combination regimens for poor prognostic categories of EGCT could be evaluated in specialized centers where toxicities of such therapy can be effectively treated.

In patients who achieve CR, maintenance therapy is of questionable value. Einhorn et al. have prospectively randomized 113 patients with testicular carcinoma in complete remission to receive maintenance doses of vinblastine or no further therapy.[33] The relapse rates were 9 percent during maintenance therapy and 7 percent without it. This information may or may not apply to EGCT. However, many patients have a limited ability to tolerate additional chemotherapy after the intensive induction regimens, and continued low-dose therapy would be unlikely to make a substantial impact. An exception may be in patients achieving a PR who are rendered disease-free at surgery. These patients would be at high risk for relapse and may, at that point, have the best chance for eradicating residual micrometastases. These patients should continue to receive either the same regimen that placed them in remission, or switch to a non-cross–resistant combination. The optimal duration of continued therapy for these patients is undetermined, but is generally limited by patient tolerance.

The approach to advanced EGCT often requires intensive combination chemotherapy, administered by experienced specialists in centers equipped to treat the complications of therapy. Myelosuppression with sepsis and thrombocytopenia, pulmonary toxicity, or potential renal complications all require skilled supportive care.

THE EXTRAGONADAL GERM CELL CANCER SYNDROME

Within the heterogeneous group of patients diagnosed as having "poorly differentiated carcinoma" or "poorly differentiated adenocarcinoma of unknown origin," a certain subset of patients have tumors compatible with germinal malignancy, based on both their natural history and response to therapy. It has been recently proposed by our group and others that these patients may have germinal neoplasms with undifferentiated or atypical histology.[3-6] Although the clinical features in this group are heterogeneous, most patients have been young men with tumors in midline locations (mediastinum, retroperitoneum, lymph nodes). In addition, some patients have had elevated serum levels of beta-hCG or AFP. Some patients with these characteristics have had CR and long-term survival following treatment with chemotherapy regimens effective against germinal neoplasms. These patients may not receive effective therapy, since many physicians will have a negative outlook when dealing with the diagnosis of "metastatic poorly differentiated carcinoma" or "metastatic poorly differentiated adenocarcinoma of unknown origin." When such patients are approached conventionally, they often receive therapies that are relatively nontoxic, but also ineffective against germinal neoplasms. Although the cure rate for EGCT may or may not be as high as those observed for testicular carcinomas, we feel that patients with suspected germinal neoplasms should receive therapeutic trials with regimens oriented toward germinal cancers. This is particularly important since many of these patients are young and may enjoy a normal life-span if therapy proves effective.

As recently described by Greco et al., diagnosis of a germ cell neoplasm has been considered in young adults with poorly differentiated neoplasms seen at Vanderbilt University since 1976.[6] This interest was stimulated by the initial observation that a young man with a poorly differentiated carcinoma of the mediastinum metastatic to the supraclavicular nodes was free of disease two years following combination chemotherapy in 1974 with cyclophosphamide, adriamycin, bleomycin, and vincristine. Shortly after this, several similar patients achieved CR following treatment with chemotherapy regimens effective against germinal tumors. These patients have recently been described in detail by Richardson et al. and Greco et al.[5,6] Independently, Fox et al. made similar observations and reported another series from Australia.[4]

An update of the Vanderbilt series, which has been expanded to 81 patients, was recently reported,[34] and some of the patient characteristics and treatment results will be summarized here. Patients with poorly differentiated carcinoma or poorly differentiated adenocarcinoma were included in this series if they had at least one of the following features: (1) age less than 50, (2) tumor in such midline locations as the mediastinum or retroperitoneum or metastatic tumor in lymph nodes or lungs, (3) elevated serum beta-hCG or AFP. Most patients were given therapeutic trials either with vinblastine, bleomycin, and *cis*-platinum (51 cases) or with these three drugs plus doxorubicin (9 cases). Seven patients had received therapy with other regimens before systematic treatment was initiated. Response was evaluable in 67 patients, with a response rate of 64 percent and CR in 34 percent. Of the 20 patients who achieved CR, 13 remained disease-free 9 to 60 months following chemotherapy (median, 37 months). The prognosis was better and response rates higher in patients who had the multiple features listed above, compared to those with only one of the features. Forty-two patients with an initial histological diagnosis of "poorly differentiated carcinoma" had more responsive tumors (response 81 percent overall, 44 percent CR, and 29 percent long-term survivors) than did 25 patients with the diagnosis "poorly differentiated adenocarcinoma" (36 percent overall response rate, 8 percent CR, and 4 percent long-term survivors). Response rates were higher when tumor involved lymph nodes, mediastinum, or retroperitoneum (79 percent responses, 54 percent complete remissions) than when visceral sites were involved (65 percent total response, 16 percent CR). Age, sex, or marker status were not predictors of response.

The question has often been raised of whether these patients actually have atypical or histologically undifferentiated germinal neoplasms or undifferentiated tumors that simply respond to the chemotherapy regimens used or an altogether different type of previously unrecognized neoplasm. Although this speculation is interesting, from a practical point of view the questions are primarily of a semantic nature. Irrespective of what one may call these tumors, a subset of these patients have responsive tumors to germ cell tumor-oriented chemotherapy. Until accurate predictors of response become available, these patients should be given therapeutic trials with such regimens. Obviously, only responding patients should be continued on therapy after an initial trial. At this point we are not aware of any specific predictors of response, although as stated above, patients with extensive visceral involvement appear to do poorly. Interestingly, a certain subset of patients who have had no markers detected in the serum have had beta-hCG and/or AFP demonstrated in immunocytochemical stains of tumor tissues.[5,6] These stains are not recommended as a diagnostic tool, since their ability to predict prognosis or response is not yet clear. Additionally, their specificity is limited, since a number of non-germinal tumors can produce these markers.[35,36]

We currently view these patients as having a clinical syndrome characterized by a constellation of findings, for which there is no specific diagnostic test. It is possible that through such improved diagnostic procedures as the definition of antigenic markers, genetic analysis, or electron microscopy, certain subsets responsive to therapy can be identified without resorting to therapeutic trials. With the accumulating clinical experience, multivariate analysis of presenting features may also provide accurate predictors of the prognosis. In vitro testing of tumor cells for sensitivity to drugs by the clonogenic assay may provide more accurate predictions of outcome, although this laboratory procedure is still far from practical.[37]

CONCLUSION

The therapy of germinal neoplasms have undergone a rapid evolution over the past decade. Although the majority of patients with testicular germ cell tumors are cured by platinum-based combination chemotherapy, controversy exists regarding the efficacy of similar regimens against EGCT. Although the overall cure rates are lower for patients with EGCT than with testicular germinal neoplasms, this difference is probably related to tumor stage at diagnosis rather than to intrinsic biological differences. Most evidence indicates that EGCTs are as responsive as testicular germinal neoplasm of comparable stage. Certain poor prognostic categories of EGCT, such as patients with extremely bulky disease, endodermal sinus tumor histology, and possibly, choriocarcinomas, may be responsible, in part, for the poor results in some series, whereas patients with other histological types respond well to therapy, at least in our experience. Consequently, we feel that all these patients should be treated aggressively with regimens offering the best chance of a durable remission. This also applies to patients with the "extragonadal germ cell cancer syndrome," in which germinal neoplasms with atypical features and histology may exist.

ACKNOWLEDGMENTS

The expert secretarial assistance of Ms. Pam Kaufman and Ms. Carol Ferguson is greatly appreciated.

REFERENCES

1. Einhorn LH, Donohue J: *Cis*-diamminedichloroplatinum, vinblastine and bleomycin combination chemotherapy in disseminated testicular cancer. Ann Int Med 87:293, 1977
2. Anderson T, Waldmann TA, Javadpour N, Glatstein E: Testicular germ cell neoplasms: Recent advances in diagnosis and therapy. Ann Int Med 90:373, 1979
3. Richardson RL, Greco FA, Wolff S, Hande KR, Oldham RK: Extragonadal germ cell malignancy: Value of tumor markers in metastatic carcinoma in young males. Proc Am Soc Clin Oncol 20:825 (Abstract), 1979
4. Fox RM, Woods RL, Tattersall MHN, McGovern VJ: Undifferentiated carcinoma in young men: The atypical teratoma syndrome. Lancet i:1316, 1979
5. Richardson RL, Schoumacher RA, Fer MF, et al: The unrecognized extragonadal germ cell cancer syndrome. Ann Int Med 94:181, 1981
6. Greco FA, Oldham RK, Fer MF: The extragonadal germ cell cancer syndrome. Semin Oncol 9:448, 1982
7. Schlumberger HG: Teratoma of the anterior mediastinum in the group of military age. Arch Pathol 41:398, 1946
8. Witschi E: Migration of the germ cells of human embryos from the yolk sac to the primitive gonadal folds. p. 67. Contributions to embryology, No. 209, Carnegie Institution of Washington. Vol. 32. Publication 575. Carnegie Institution, Washington, D.C., 1948
9. Utz DC, Buscemi MF: Extragonadal testicular tumors. J Urol 105:271, 1971
10. Hajdu SI: Pathology of germ cell tumors of the testis. Semin Oncol 6:14, 1979
11. Mostofi FK, Price EB: Tumors of the male genital system. Armed Forces Institute of Pathology, Washington, D.C., 1973
12. Vugrin D, Martini N, Whitmore W, Golberg RB: VAB-3 combination chemotherapy in primary mediastinal germ cell tumors. Cancer Treat Rept 66:1405, 1982
13. Feun LG, Samson MK, Stephens RL: Vinblastine (VLB), bleomycin (BLEO), *cis*-diamminedichloroplatinum (DDP) in disseminated extragonadal germ cell tumors. A Southwest Oncology Group Study. Cancer 45:2543, 1980
14. Garnick MB, Canellos GP, Richie JP: Treatment and surgical staging of testicular and primary extragonadal germ cell cancer. JAMA 250:1733, 1983
15. Hainsworth JD, Einhorn LH, Williams SD, Stewart M, Greco FA: Advanced extragona-

dal germ cell tumors. Successful treatment with combination chemotherapy. Ann Int Med 97:7, 1982

16. Rubush JL, Gardner IR, Boyd WC, Ehrenhaft JL: Mediastinal Tumors: Review of 186 cases. J Thorac Cardiovasc Surg 65:216, 1973

17. Luna MA, Valenzuela-Tamariz J: Germ-cell tumors of the mediastinum: Post-mortem findings. Am J Clin Pathol 65:450, 1976

18. Schold SC, Vugrin D, Golbey RB, Posner JB: Central nervous system metastases from germ cell carcinoma of testis. Semin Oncol 6:102, 1979

19. Bagshawe KD, Harlane S: Immunodiagnosis and monitoring of gonadotropin-producing metastases in the central nervous system. Cancer 38:112, 1976

20. Wacksman J, Case G, Glenn JR: Extragenital gonadal neoplasia and metastatic testicular tumor. Urology 5:221, 1975

21. Asif S, Uehling DT: Microscopic tumor foci in testes. J Urol 99:776, 1968

22. Maier JC, Sulak MH: Radiation therapy in seminoma. Cancer 32:1212, 1973

23. Paulson DF, Einhorn LH, Peckham MJ, Williams SD: Cancer of the testis. p. 794. In DeVita VT, Hellman S, Rosenberg SA (eds): Principals and Practice of Oncology. J.B. Lippincott, Philadelphia, 1982

24. Beattie EJ, Jr: Mediastinal germ cell tumors (Surgery). Semin Oncol 6:109, 1979

25. Kuzur MD, Cobleigh MA, Greco FA, Einhorn LH, Oldham RK: Endodermal sinus tumor of the mediastinum. Cancer 50:766, 1982

26. Julian CG, Barrett JM, Richardson RL, Greco FA: Bleomycin, vinblastine and *cis*-platinum in the treatment of advanced endodermal sinus tumor. Obstet Gynecol 56:396, 1980

27. Sickles EA, Belliveau RE, Wiernik PH: Primary mediastinal choriocarcinoma in the male. Cancer 33:1196, 1974

28. Shackney SE, McCormack GW, Cuchural GJ, Jr: Growth rate patterns of solid tumors and their relation to responsiveness to therapy. Ann Int Med 89:107, 1978

29. Williams SD, Einhorn LH, Greco FA, Oldham RK, Fletcher R: VP-16-213 salvage therapy for refractory germinal neoplasms. Cancer 46:2154, 1983

30. Wolff SN, Fer MF, McKay CM, et al: High-dose VP-16-213 and antologous bone marrow transplantation for refractory malignancies: A phase I study. J Clin Oncol 1:701, 1983

31. Wolff SN, Johnson DH, Hainsworth JD, Greco FA: High-dose VP-16-213 monotherapy for refractory germinal malignancies. A phase II study. J Clin Oncol (In press)

32. Lederman GS, Garnick MB, Canellos GP, Richie JP: Chemotherapy of refractory germ cell cancer with etoposide. J Clin Oncol 1:706, 1983

33. Einhorn LH, Williams SD, Troner M, Birch R, Greco FA: The role of maintenance therapy in disseminated testicular cancer. N Engl J Med 305:727, 1981

34. Hainsworth JD, Fer MF, Oldham RK, Greco FA: Advanced poorly differentiated carcinoma (PDC) and adenocarcinoma (PDA): Further documentation of a treatable syndrome. Proc Am Soc Clin Oncol C-542 (Abstract), 1983

35. Rosen S, Weintraub S, Vaitukaitis J, et al: Placental proteins and their subunits as tumor markers. Ann Intern Med 82:71, 1975

36. Skrabanek P, Kirrane J, Powell D: A unifying concept of chorionic gonadotropin production in malignancy. Invest Cell Pathol 2:75, 1979

37. Selby P, Buick RN, Tannock I: A critical appraisal of the "Human Tumor Stem Cell Assay." N Engl J Med 308:129, 1983

38. Funes HC, Mendez M, Alonso E, et al: Mediastinal germ cell tumors treated with cis-platinum, bleomycin, vinblastine (PVB). Proc Am Assoc Cancer Res 22:474, 1981 (abstract)

6 | Origin of Seminomatous Germ Cell Tumors

Perinchery Narayan
Clarke F. Millette
William DeWolf

Seminomas arise from germ cells. Evidence of this has been established by several studies based on morphological criteria as defined by light and electron microscopy. We have utilized two-dimensional electrophoresis to study the protein composition of seminoma cells, and germ cells at different stages of development. Our results provide further evidence that seminomas arise from germ cells, probably from the premeiotic pachytene stage of spermatogenesis, and represent the first molecular evidence for germ cell origin of seminomatous tumors at a specific stage during spermatogenesis. This chapter will discuss the existing morphological data for the germ cell origin of seminomas, the molecular evidence linking seminomas to pachytene germ cells, and the significance of these findings.

BACKGROUND

Early History of the Origin of Seminomatous Germ Cell Tumors. Seminomas were first recognized as a distinct entity from nonseminomatous tumors by Coats in 1895.[1] Chevassu, in 1906, was the first to describe the germ cell origin of seminomas.[2] He gave the tumor the name "seminome" (Latin semen, seed). Since then, several investigators have noted that seminomas first begin as intratubular malignances of germ cells in the seminiferous epithelium. At least four lines of evidence indicate that seminomas arise from germ cells in the seminiferous tubules.

Dixon and Moore, in 1950, performed some of the classical studies on histogenesis of germ cell tumors, which included seminomas.[3] They examined 1,000 testicular tumors at the Armed Forces Institute of Pathology and noted a 23 percent incidence of intratubular occurrence of seminomatous tumors. They also noted the resemblance of seminoma cells to spermatogonia. Based on these findings, it was concluded that seminomas arise from intratubular germ cells.

This concept was reinforced by the description of intratubular malignant cells in testicular biopsies of infertile patients and their subsequent development of invasive testes cancer. For example, Skakkebek found carcinoma in situ in two biopsies of 500 infertile men who both went on to develop invasive carcinoma within five years.[4,5]

Additionally, carcinoma in situ, which later becomes invasive, has been found in the contralateral testes of men with ipsilateral testicular seminomas. For example, Berthelson et al.[6] noted carcinoma in situ in biopsies of the contralateral testes in 3 of 21 men with seminomas; 1 of these patients, who had follow-up for more than a year, developed invasive testicular cancer.

This is perhaps related to the finding that malignant cells may occur within normal-appearing tubules located at the periphery of solid tumors.[7] For example, in the periphery of some seminomatous tumors in the basal layer of "normal" seminiferous tubules, dark-staining cells interspersed with normal-appearing spermatogonia have been noted. These dark-staining cells have some ultrastructural features of germ cells, but mostly resemble tumor cells. It is postulated that these cells are the precursors of the solid tumor cells and eventually break through the basement membrane of the seminiferous tubules to form classical seminomas.[8] Thus, at present, several lines of morphological evidence suggest that seminomatous tumors arise by virtue of malignant conversion of intratubular seminiferous epithelial germ cells.

Cell Types of Seminomas.   Seminomas are composed of several cell types that differentiate along spermatogenic lineage. Histologically, three variants of seminoma are recognized: (1) classical, (2) anaplastic, and (3) spermatocytic.[9,10] The classical variant comprises over 90 percent of all seminomas. Grossly, these tumors are homogeneous on cut section, with few areas of necrosis or hemorrhage. Microscopically, these tumors consist of large cells arranged in sheets separated by septa. The cells have abundant clear or finely granular cytoplasm and rounded nuclei with large nucleoli. The cells are relatively uniform and give a monotonous appearance to the tumor. The stroma between the cell lobules shows lymphocyte infiltration in 80 percent of these tumors.

The anaplastic variety of seminomas comprises less than 5 percent of all seminomas. They are distinct histologically from the classical seminomas. Microscopically, the cells are variable in size and contain less cytoplasm, and under light microscopy, the nuclear chromatin is pleomorphic, with numerous mitotic figures.

Upon ultrastructural examination, however, the nuclei of these cells resemble the nuclei of classical seminomas and the distinction seen under light microscopy is no longer evident.[11] Nuclei of both types of seminomas show about the same degree of irregularity of the nuclear membrane, chromatin of the same granular nature, and nucleoli of similiar configuration. Mitosis are noted in about the same frequency as noted by light microscopy. These tumors are diagnosed by the histological finding of more than three mitoses per high power field.[10] Initially, these tumors were thought to indicate a poorer prognosis than classical seminomas, but more recent reports on the survival of patients with anaplastic seminomas reveal that this may not be the case.[12,13] At present, most pathologists and clinicians regard anaplastic seminomas as more of a histological variant than a clinically important finding.

The third type of seminoma variant is the spermatocytic seminoma that accounts for approximately 3 percent of testicular seminomas.[14,15] First described by Masson in 1946,[16] the tumor is composed of polygonal cells of unequal size, the smaller cells resembling spermatogonia and the larger cells resembling primary spermatocytes; the cytoplasm is densely eosinophilic and free of glycogen. The nuclei are rounded and contain uniform-appearing chromatin, in contrast to other variants of seminoma in which the chromatin is more irregular. The stroma shows no lymphocytic infiltration, and multinucleated cells are frequent. The striking feature of these tumors is the variability in size of the cells and nuclei. The cells in classical seminomas are relatively similar and close to 20μ in diameter, whereas in spermatocytic seminomas, the cells vary between 10 and 20μ in diameter. These tumors are also biologically different from the other two types of seminoma variants. Whereas the classical seminomas reach their peak age of incidence in the fourth decade and are infrequent after the age of 50, the average age of patients with spermatocytic seminomas is 50 and 50 percent of the tumors occur in men over 50. Also, unlike the other seminoma variants, spermatocytic seminomas occur only in testes and never in the retroperitoneum or other sites where extragonadal germ cell tumors have been noted. They also do not occur as mixed tumors along with nonseminomatous tumor elements. Spermatocytic seminoma tumors have a better prognosis than classical seminomas and have not been associated with tumor invasion or metastasis. Five-year survival after orchiectomy approaches 100 percent.[14,15] Masson[16] and Scully[17] maintain that these tumors are distinct pathologically and clinically from other seminoma variants. More than the other types, spermatocytic seminomas appear to represent a malignancy of the more mature type of germ cell elements. However, more data are necessary before this question can be resolved.

Cell Variants Among Classical Seminomas. Although the literature describes the classical seminoma as a homogeneous tumor composed of a single type of cells, several investigators have found that these tumors have more than one cell type. Holstein and Korner,[7] for example, in a study of six classical seminomas, found that three types of cells were present. In the center of the tumor were the typical clear cells characteristic of classical seminomas. However, at the periphery and also scattered in the interstitium and in the basal layer of otherwise normal-appearing seminiferous tubules were cells with clear cytoplasm with distinct characteristics. Electron microscopy of these cells revealed that whereas typical seminoma cells had few figured elements in the cytoplasm, few mitochondria, and scarce glycogen, the intratubular and interstitial type of seminoma tumor cells had larger nuclei, flocculent granular chromatin, abundant free ribosomes, and glycogen granules. Both types of tumor cells had microfilaments and cell expansions.

Also, unlike normal seminiferous epithelium, seminomatous tumor cells had no desmosome structures between cells. A third type of cell, intermediate between the two described above, was also found in the periphery and interstitium of classical seminomatous tumors.

The presence of more than one cell type in classical seminomatous tumors was also noted by Pierce in a study of 13 classical seminomas.[18] He noted that, under light microscopy, seminomas had at least three types of cells: those with clear cytoplasm, those with partial dark-staining cytoplasm, and a minority of cells that had uniformly dark-staining cytoplasm. Upon ultrastructural examination, these cells were noted to have a variety of cell organelles. No single tumor cell had all the organelles. These findings for seminoma tumor cells suggest that these cells are in a spermatogenic line of differentiation and express incomplete formed elements of various germ cell stages, including spermatozoa.

Stem Cell Origin of Seminomatous Tumors. Based on the morphological data detailed here, there is substantial evidence that seminomas arise from germ cells. First, seminomas arise in the intratubular seminiferous epithelium. Second, they possess some of the characteristics of germ cells under the light microscope. Ultrastructural studies have revealed a number of cell organelles in seminomatous tumor cells that relate to all stages of spermatogenesis. The presence of microtubules and cell evaginations suggest a similarity to migrating gonocytes and primordial germ cells, whereas the presence of glycogen, mitochondria, and ribosomes relate to spermatogonia and spermatocytes. Abortive acrosomal elements have also been noted, suggesting that differentiative changes towards spermatids and spermatozoa formation occur among these tumor cells. Apart from electron-microscopic morphological studies, no other technique has been utilized to study the stem cell origin of seminoma. Because of recent advances in cell separation and molecular analysis of normal germ cells, we examined this issue further.

Advances in Germ Cell Separation and Molecular Analysis. Recent advances in cell separation techniques have allowed the isolation and purification of germ cells of a number of laboratory animal models. The purity of these isolated germ cells have allowed biochemical analysis and characterization of different stages of spermatogenesis. Adapting procedures already established in germ cell separations in these animal models, we have been able to isolate and purify human germ cells at two major stages of spermatogenesis.

Human testes tissue for study was obtained from patients with cancer of the prostate undergoing therapeutic orchiectomy. Cut sections of tissue were examined and confirmed to be normal. Testes were decapsulated, minced, and by a process of enzymatic digestion and mechanical agitation, a single cell suspension of mixed germ cells was obtained. Cells were loaded onto a medium STA-PUT chamber and separated by sedimentation at unit gravity according to procedures developed for murine spermatogenic cell separations.[19,20] Cell populations were pooled using morphological criteria previously established by examining individual fractions by Nomarski differential interference microscopy.[21,22] Following unit gravity sedimentation, pooled populations of human round spermatids and particularly pachytene spermatocytes remained contaminated by significant numbers of Leydig cells.

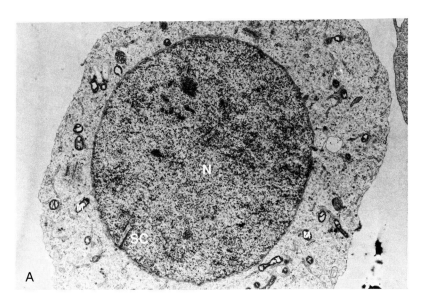

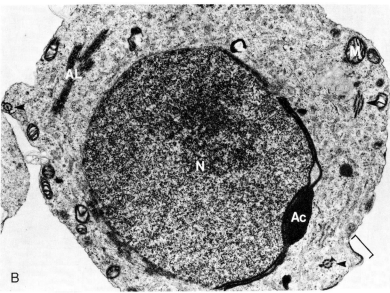

Fig. 6-1. Ultrastructural examination of isolated human spermatogenic cells indicated that these cells retain their normal in situ morphology. (A) Isolated primary pachytene spermatocyte containing vacuolated mitochondria (M) typical of meiotic cells in the testis. A prominent section of a synaptonemal complex (SC) is visible in the nucleus (N). Other images of synaptonemal complexes are also visible upon close inspection. ×40,200. (B) Isolated developing spermatid showing the acrosome (Ac) spreading over the anterior third of the nucleus (N) which has not yet started condensation. Annulate lamellae (AL) and vacuolated mitochondria (M) are visible in the spermatid cytoplasm. Note sections of the elongating spermatid flagellum (arrowheads). The thickened region of the plasma membrane, which is bracketed, represents the remnant of the cytoplasmic bridge that connected adjacent spermatids in vivo. ×132,300.

Contaminating Leydig cells were removed from isolated germ cells, using a modification of a Percoll centrifugation procedure first described by Schumacher et al.[23] This procedure essentially consists of density centrifugation of germ cells in discontinuous Percoll gradients. Following Percoll centrifugation, highly homogeneous populations of human germ cells in purities ranging from 89 to 96 percent for round spermatids and 90 to 95 percent for pachytene spermatocytes are obtained (Fig. 6-1).

EXPERIMENTAL FINDINGS

Two-dimensional electrophoresis separates proteins on the basis of charge and molecular size.[24] Each spot on a gel analyzed by this technique presumably represents a separate polypeptide, since both the first and second dimensions are performed under separate reducing and denaturing conditions. Using this technique, the total polypeptide composition of separated human germ cells was analyzed to compare human and other mammalian germ cells (species-specificity); samples of human spermatocytes were compared from different individuals (allospecificity), and pachytene spermatocytes and round spermatids from the same patient (stage-specificity) were analyzed.

Species, Stage, and Allospecific Protein Expression in Germ Cells. Comparison of mouse and human pachytene spermatocytes revealed extensive differences in the number and patterns of proteins between the two species. Certain proteins appear to be markers of human pachytene spermatocytes. These proteins, including a group at P45/5.1 (Fig. 6-2) and P67/5.2 (P45 represents protein of molecular weight 45,000 daltons and 5.1 the isoelectric point of migration in an electrophoretic gel), are usually present in human samples and have never been seen in isolated mouse pachytene cells. Comparison of two-dimensional gels of germ cells from several other species, including the monkey, calf, and rat, indicate that the P45/5.1 protein is not present in the germ cells of these species.

Comparison of polyacrylamide gel patterns between human pachytene cells and round spermatids reveals that about 80 percent of total cellular proteins are common between the two cell types. However, the group of proteins at P45/5.1 that were markers of pachytene spermatocytes was absent in human round spermatids.

The two-dimensional gel pattern of mature sperm was very distinct from that of germ cells. There was only about a 60 percent homology of proteins of spermatocytes and spermatids. Again, the P45/5.1 group of proteins were absent. The polyacrylamide gel patterns of human pachytene cells from different individuals was also compared, and about 90 percent of the spots were found to be electrophoretically identical. The P45/5.1 group of proteins, however, appear to be variable in some individuals. These differences were probably not related to technique, since the gels were run under identical conditions; it is more likely that the differences are due to genetic or pathological differences.

The results suggested that although great overall similarity is seen in the protein compliment of human spermatocytes and round spermatids, reproducible

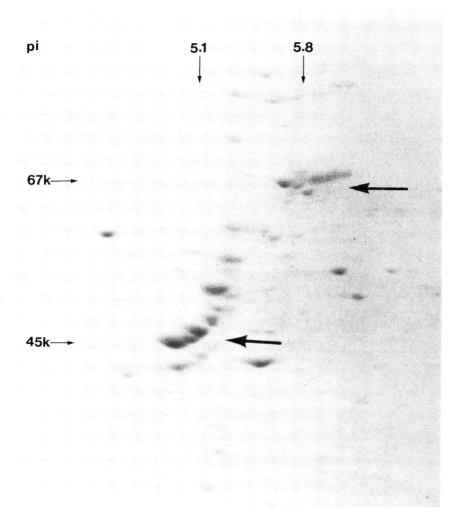

Fig. 6-2. A complete two-dimensional electrophoretic pattern of total cellular homogenate of purified (>95 percent) human pachytene spermatocyte (premeiotic) germ cells obtained from a surgical orchiectomy specimen. The lower arrow indicates the P45/5.1 group of marker proteins of seminoma present, along with additional proteins in the same molecular weight range and isoelectric point in early germ cells. The upper arrow indicates a second group of proteins at P67/5.8, which are markers of early (premeiotic), but not late (post-meiotic) germ cells. Separation in the horizontal dimension is by isoelectric point. In this and all subsequent figures, the acid side of the gel is to the left. Separation in the vertical dimension is by molecular weight. All gels are stained with Coomasie Brilliant Blue R.

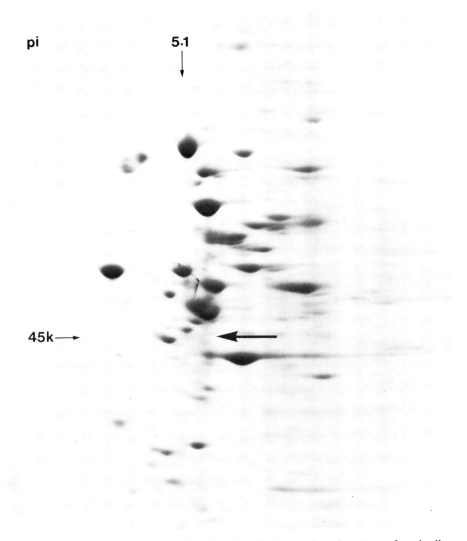

Fig. 6-3. A complete two-dimensional polyacrylamide electrophoretic pattern of total cellular homogenate obtained from isolated seminoma cell suspensions. The arrow indicates the group of proteins at P45/5.1, which are marker proteins of seminoma.

differences do exist and represent stage-specific marker proteins for these cell types. Having obtained this information, we proceeded to examine the molecular composition of a number of seminomatous tumors to try to relate the protein composition of a particular germ cell type to seminoma.

Comparisons of Protein Expression Between Seminomatous Tumors and Germ Cells. Morphological comparisons between isolated germ cells and isolated seminoma cells were initially conducted on three classical seminomatous tumors. The majority of cells revealed a close similarity, both in size and appearance, by

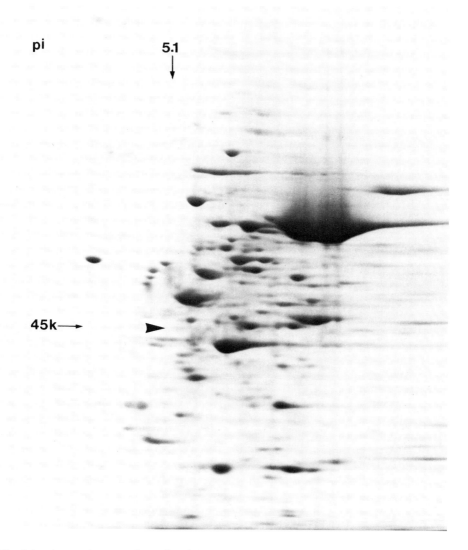

Fig. 6-4. A complete two-dimensional electrophoretic pattern of total cellular homogenate of primary embryonal carcinoma, with yolk sac and teratoma elements obtained from a surgical specimen. The arrowhead indicates where the P45/5.1 group of proteins would be expected to be seen. These proteins are absent in nonseminomatous tumors.

light microscopy, to pachytene germ cells. There were, however, several large cells seen among seminomatous tumors that were unlike pachytene cells or any other type of germ cells.

Two-dimensional electrophoresis of 11 seminomatous tumors was performed. Protein expression was found to be homologous between the various seminomatous tumors. Especially prominent among all seminomas were four proteins in the molecular weight range of 45,000 to 50,000, with an isoelectric point of 5.1 (Fig. 6-3).

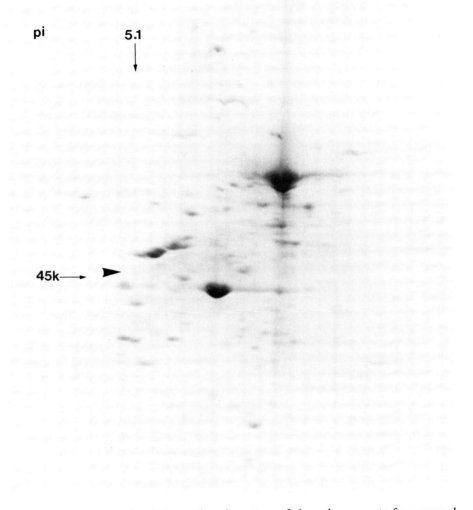

Fig. 6-5. A two-dimensional electrophoretic pattern of tissue homogenate from normal lung. The arrowhead indicates where the P45/5.1 group of proteins would be expected to be present. These proteins are absent in all normal and tumor tissues examined, except germ cells and seminomatous tumors.

These proteins were similar in molecular weight and isoelectric point to the marker proteins of human pachytene spermatocytes (Fig. 6-2). Comparison of seminoma polypeptides and germ cell polypeptides revealed a greater homology between pachytene (early germ cells) and seminoma than round spermatids (late germ cells). There was also less homology with mature sperm.

Comparison of Protein Expression with Nonseminomatous Germ Cell Tumors. Two-dimensional electrophoretic analysis of five human teratocarcinoma cell lines maintained in our laboratory was also carried out. These were lines

HT-A (1156Q), HT-C (12550), HT-D (1218E), HT-E (833K), and HT-H (2061H). These lines are established and characterized.[25-27] Two-dimensional electrophoresis revealed approximately 40 percent protein homology between seminomas and nonseminomatous tumors. However, the P45/5.1 group of proteins was absent in all nonseminomatous tumors (Fig. 6-4). Comparison to two fresh nonseminomatous tumor specimens also revealed a similar absence of the P45/5.1 proteins.

Comparison with Other Human Tumors and Normal Tissues. Two-dimensional electrophoretic analysis of seven human tumors, including breast, colon, adrenal cortical, melanoma, bladder, and prostate, failed to reveal the presence of the P45/5.1 marker proteins (Fig. 6-5). In addition, eight human organs (lung, liver, spleen, stomach, kidney, prostate, bladder, and lymphoid tissue) were examined and these marker proteins were not found.

IMPLICATIONS

Evidence from this report suggests that the p45/5.1-associated proteins detected on two-dimensional gels of seminomatous germ cell tumors are marker proteins that are specific for tissues of early germ line origin. The evidence is based on their absence on numerous tissues tested, including germ cells from four other species, seven human tumors, and tissue from eight normal human organs. Although experiments are currently in progress to extend this tissue analysis, evidence thus far points to the p45/5.1-associated proteins as species- (human) and germ line-specific. We have, therefore, tentatively called them "seminoma marker proteins" (SMP).

The results of these experiments present an entirely new basis and approach to study problems of germ cell pathology. The first and most important is whether the stem cell of origin of seminomas and nonseminomatous tumors are one and the same. There is strong evidence that both tumors originate from germ cells. Intratubular malignancy of seminiferous epithelium has been noted among nonseminomatous germ cell tumors and in seminomas. The presence of carcinoma in situ in seminiferous tubular biopsies and the subsequent development of invasive carcinoma in testes with nonseminomatous tumors also suggest that nonseminomas arise from germ cells. Ultrastructural studies, however, that show seminomas that originate from germ cells have not been substantiated in nonseminomatous tumors, because nonseminomatous tumors differentiate along trophoblastic and embryonic lines. The cells observed in these tumors bear no morphological resemblance to germ cells. This has led the British pathologists to maintain that teratomas and other nonseminomatous tumors are tumors of "uncertain origin."[28]

Comparison of protein expression among germ cells and nonseminomatous germ cell tumors, however, reveals sufficient homology to suggest that nonseminomatous tumors originate from germ cells. There is more homology of nonseminomas to germ cells than to several other normal human tissues examined. The absence of the marker proteins of pachytene germ cells in nonseminomatous tumors suggests that nonseminomatous tumors probably do not differentiate along spermatogenic lines. Alternatively, the malignant transformation of germ cells to nonseminomas may in some way suppress the protein expression of these cells. Further study is needed to elucidate these observations.

All pathologists agree, however, that seminomas originate from germ cells. As detailed here, there is extensive morphological data on the origin of seminomatous germ cell tumors from early germ cells; there is also evidence that seminoma tumor cells differentiate along spermatogenic lines. The experiments described here provide the molecular data to substantiate the origin of seminoma from premeiotic human germ cells, and furthermore, the presence of shared marker proteins in seminoma and pachytene germ cells may further localize the stage during spermatogenesis when germ cells undergo malignant transformation to seminomatous tumors.

Although germ cell origin of seminomas is accepted, the exact stage at which malignant transformation occurs has not been resolved by morphological data. This is because various seminomas undergo incomplete differentiation along spermatogenic lines, and several cell types at various stages of differentiation may be present in one tumor. The study of protein expression of germ cells may elucidate these observations and help stratify the origin of seminoma at certain stages of germ cell development. The fact that the p45 proteins are localized in the pachytene spermatocytes may provide some preliminary evidence as to stage. However, other cells, such as spermatogonia, have not been analyzed in detail. The fact that seminomas are rare in children may be a clue that these tumors do not arise in spermatogonia, since testes in boys below 10 years of age are mostly composed of immature germ cells and spermatogonia.

Chromosomal studies of seminomatous tumors also provide some evidence suggesting seminomas arise from premeiotic germ cells, at the pachytene stage of spermatogenesis. For example, several studies have noted that seminomas contain both X and Y chromosomes.[29,30] This implies that the tumor cells arose from germ cells prior to reduction division. Martineau[30] has also noted that the total number of chromosomes in a seminoma cell is usually hypotriploid or tetraploid. During normal spermatogenesis, spermatogonia contain a diploid number of chromosomes; spermatocytes contain diploid or tetraploid number of chromosomes depending on the stage of development. Spermatids contain a haploid number of chromosomes. No cells other than spermatocytes, however, contain a tetraploid number of chromosomes at any stage during development. The presence of double Y bodies in seminoma cells,[31] but not in nonseminomatous tumors, also strengthens the conclusion that seminomas probably arise from the later spermatocyte stage of germ cell development at or just prior to reduction division. The origin of extragonadal tumors is also an issue that may be addressed more meaningfully in light of these SMP. Extragonadal tumors in at least three locations have been described as resembling seminomas. These include pineal tumors,[32] thymic tumors,[33] and retroperitoneal tumors. It has been theorized that these tumors arise from germ cells that were left behind or did not migrate into the sex cords of the developing embryo during the second month of intrauterine life.[9] Because ultrastructural studies of these tumors have shown their resemblance to classical seminomatous tumors, this is an acceptable hypothesis. It would be informative to analyze these tumors for the presence of the germ line marker proteins to determine their cell of origin.

Another potential use of these proteins, and perhaps the most important clinically, is their application as clinical tumor markers. Because these proteins are not found on somatic tissues or spermatozoa there is a strong possibility that they are never exposed to the general circulation under normal conditions and therefore fulfill one of the basic criteria for a tumor marker. This is offset by the fact that these SMP are not membrane-associated proteins and, therefore, probably not amenable to in vivo immunolocalization studies. Preliminary evidence, however, suggests that SMP are immunogenic because these proteins can be detected by rabbit polyvalent antisera to germ cell preparations. Experiments are currently underway in our laboratory to make SMP-specific antibodies.

We have noted that the p45/5.1 group consists of at least seven germ cell proteins. Seminomas, however, seem to express, reproducibly, only four of these proteins. Preliminary results from experiments presented here demonstrate differences in the protein expression at the P45/5.1 area by these seminomatous tumor subtypes. Results suggesting a heterogeneity among seminomas has also been obtained in other studies as shown by reactive patterns with monoclonal antibodies. For example, placental alkaline phosphatase monoclonal antibodies react with nonuniform patterns among different seminomas.[34] This may account for the clinical dissimilarity of seminomas, especially with respect to their biological behavior. Further investigations of the SMP and other proteins are currently underway and may resolve some of these problems.

The data presented here also indicate that SMP are species-specific. The fact that SMP are not evolutionary conserved molecules parallels the general phenomenon that humans are uniquely different from other species in their response to immune challenge by reproductive tissues. For example, autoimmune orchitis exists in animals, but not in humans.[35] Again, it has been found that atherosclerosis is accelerated in primates following vasectomy.[36] At least three major epidemiological studies have found no change in the incidence of atherosclerosis or cardiovascular disease in men following vasectomy.[37,38] Numerous other examples of differences between human and other species in germ cell physiology and pathology may be cited. For example, gossypol, an antifertility agent that affects spermatogenic cell function in man,[39,40] has no similar antifertility effect on mice, the model most commonly used for studying mammalian spermatogenesis. Studies in our laboratory and others have also found that gene expression in human sperm is different from that of murine sperm.[41] Our laboratory is currently studying the cellular immune properties of human germ cells to determine if they have suppressive capability in immune response experiments, as has been suggested in animal models.[42] Similar experiments have not yet been conducted using human germ cells. At present, there is no evidence that this phenomenon occurs in humans. Thus, there are significant evolutionary differences in spermatogenic development and function between man and other species. The p45/5.1-associated group of proteins may be part of the molecular evidence for such differences. Further investigations of these proteins may provide better tools for the bedside.

REFERENCES

1. Coats J: A manual of Pathology. p. 1047 3rd ed. Longmans Green and Co, London, 1895
2. Chevassu M: Tumeurs du Testicule. Steinhill G, Paris, 1906
3. Dixon FJ, Moore RA: Tumors of the Male Sex Organs A.F.I.P. Atlas of Tumor Pathology VIII 31b and 32, Washington D.C., 1952
4. Skakkebek NE: Abnormal morphology of germ cells in two infertile men. Acta Pathol Microbiol Scand A80:374, 1972a
5. Skakkebek NE: Possible carcinoma in situ of the testis. Lancet 2:515, 1972
6. Berthelson JG, Skakkebek NE, Mogenson P, Sorensen BL: Incidence of carcinoma in situ of germ cells in contralateral testes of men with testicular tumors. Br Med J 2:363, 1979
7. Holstein AF, Korner F: Light and electron microscopical analysis of cell types in human seminoma. Virchows Arch Pathol Anat Histol 363:97, 1974
8. Schulze, C, Holstein AF: On the histology of human seminoma. Cancer 39:1090, 1977
9. Mostofi FK: Testicular tumors. Epidemiologic, etiologic, and pathologic features. Cancer 32:1186, 1973
10. Mostofi FK, Price EB: Tumors of the male genital system. In Atlas of Tumor Pathology, 2nd series. Fasc. 8. AFIP, Washington D.C., 1973
11. Janssen M, Johnston WH: Anaplastic seminoma of the testis. Cancer 41:538, 1978
12. Javadpour N· The National Cancer Institute experience with testicular cancer. J Urol 120:651, 1978
13. Kademian M, Bosch A, Caldwell WL, Jaeschke W: Anaplastic seminoma. Cancer 40:3082, 1977
14. Maier JG, Sulak MH, Mittmeyer BT: Seminoma of the testis: Analysis of treatment success and failure. Am J Roentgenol 102:596, 1968
15. Thackray AC, Crane WAJ: Seminoma. p. 164. In Pugh RCB (ed): Pathology of the Testis. Blackwell Scientific Publications Oxford, 1976
16. Masson P: Etude sur le seminome. Rev Canad Biol 5:361, 1946
17. Scully RE: Spermatocytic seminoma of the testis. Cancer 14:788, 1961
18. Pierce GB, Jr: Ultrastructure of human testicular tumors. Cancer 19:1963, 1966
19. Romrell LJ, Bellve AR, Fawcett DW: Separation of mouse spermatogenic cells by sedimentation velocity. A morphologic characterization. Develop Biol 49:119, 1976
20. Bellve AR, Cavicchia JC, Millette CF, O'Brien BA, Bhatnagar YM, Dym M: Spermatogenic cells of the prepuberal mouse. Isolation and morphologic characterization. J Cell Biol 74:68, 1977
21. Narayan P, Scott BK, Millette CF, DeWolf WC: Human spermatogenic cell marker proteins detected by 2-dimensional electrophoresis. Gamete Res 7:227, 1983
22. Shepard RW, Millette CF, DeWolf WC: Enrichment of primary pachytene spermatocytes from the human testes. Gamete Res 4:487, 1981
23. Schumacher M, Schaffer G, Holstein AF, Hil ZH: Rapid isolation of mouse Leydig cells by centrifugation in Percoll density gradients with complete retention of morphological and biochemical integrity. FEBS Lett 91:333, 1978
24. O'Farrell PH: High resolution 2-dimensional electrophoresis of proteins. J Biol Chem 215:4007, 1975
25. Andrews PW, Bronson BL, Benham F, Strickland S, Knowles BB: A comparative study of 8 cell lines derived from human testicular teratocarcinoma. Int J Cancer 26:269, 1980

26. Wang N, Trend B, Bronson BL, Fraley EE: Nonrandom abnormalities in chromosome I in human testicular cancers. Cancer Res 40:796, 1980

27. Ducibella T, Anderson D, Aalberg J, DeWolf WC: Cell surface polarization, tight junctions and eccentric inner cells characterize human teratocarcinoma embryoid bodies. Develop Biol 94:197, 1982

28. Collins DH, Pugh RCB: The pathology of testicular tumors. Br J Urol suppl. p. 364, 1964

29. Theiss EA, Ashley D, Mostofi FK: Nuclear sex of testicular tumors and some related ovarian and extragonadal neoplasms. Cancer 13:323, 1960

30. Martineau M: Chromosomes in human testicular tumors. J Pathol 99:271, 1969

31. Atkin NB: High chromosome numbers of seminomata and malignant teratomata of the testis: A review of data on 103 tumors. Br J Cancer 28:275, 1973

32. Cravioto H, Dart D: The ultrastructure of pinealoma. J Neuropathol Exp Neurol 32:552, 1973

33. Levin GD: Primary thymic seminoma—a neoplasm ultrastructurally similar to testicular seminoma and distinct from epithelial thymoma. Cancer 31:729, 1973

34. Paiva J, Damjanov I, Lange PH, Harris H: Immunohistochemical localization of placental-like alkaline phosphatase in testes and germ cell tumors using monoclonal antibodies. Am J Pathol 111:156, 1983

35. Bigazzi PE: Immunopathological findings in vasectomized rabbits. P. 339. In Lepow IH, Crozie R (eds): Immunologic and pathophysiologic effects in animals and man. Academic Press, New York, 1979

36. Alexander NJ, Clarkson TB: Vasectomy increases the severity of diet-induced atherosclerosis in *Macaca fascicularis.* Science 201:538, 1978

37. Walker AM, Jick H, Hunter JR, et al: Vasectomy and nonfatal myocardial infarction. Lancet 1:13, 1981

38. Goldacre MJ, Holford TR, Vessey MP: Cardiovascular disease and vasectomy. N Engl J Med 308:805, 1983

39. Dai RX, Pang SN, Lin S, et al: The study of antifertility effects of cotton seed. Document of First National Conference on Male Antifertility Agents. Acta Biol Sin 11:1, 1978

40. Dai RX, Pang SN, Liuz L: Studies on the antifertility of Gossypol II. Morphologic analysis of the antifertility effects of Gossypol. Document of the 4th Int. Conf. on Male Antifertility Agents, Suzlou Acta Biol Exp Sin 11:27, 1978

41. Anderson DJ, Bach BL, Yunis EJ, DeWolf WC: Major histocompatibility antigens are not expressed on human epididymal sperm. J Immunol 129:452, 1982

42. Hurtenbach U, Shearer GM: Germ cell induced immune suppression in mice. J Exp Med 155:1719, 1982

7 Lymph Node Sampling in the Management of Prostate Cancer

Jerome P. Richie

Adenocarcinoma of the prostate is the second most common carcinoma in males in the United States and the third leading cause of male death from neoplastic disease. In the United States in 1983, 55,000 cases were diagnosed in whites (45/100,000 population) and 9,200 (80/100,000) in blacks. This incidence in blacks represents the highest incidence in the world. Nearly 20,000 men die yearly of carcinoma of the prostate in the United States alone. The cause of the disease is unknown, but the incidence of carcinoma of the prostate increases significantly with age. The incidence of patients harboring prostatic carcinoma increases approximately twofold when serial pathological sections of the excised gland are examined, reaching an incidence of 70 percent in males aged 80 to 89. Obviously, however, carcinoma of the prostate does not necessarily compete as a cause of death in all these patients. It is the physician's task to select those patients in whom carcinoma of the prostate is likely to interfere with survival and, hence, those patients who require further clinical delineation of the extent of tumor and appropriate therapy. It is the purpose of this chapter to reflect on the various modalities of clinical staging versus surgical staging techniques and their impact upon selection of therapeutic modalities for the treatment of carcinoma of the prostate.

DIAGNOSIS

Rectal examination frequently provides the clue to the diagnosis of carcinoma of the prostate. Prostate cancer produces an area of firmness within the prostate that is different than that of the surrounding tissue. Approximately 10 percent of the patients with newly diagnosed carcinoma of the prostate have a normal feeling prostate by rectal examination and are discovered only at the time of surgical removal of the prostate for the clinical symptoms of benign prostatic hyperplasia.

In patients with a clinically suspicious lesion in the prostate, the clinical diagnosis should be confirmed by histological review of tissue from the area under suspicion. A closed needle biopsy, either via the perineal or the transrectal route, provides tissue for histological diagnosis. Transrectal needle biopsy has the advantage of allowing the surgeon to position the needle accurately into a small suspicious area. Broad-spectrum antibiotic coverage, along with antibiotic enemas, has reduced the hazard of postbiopsy sepsis to a low level. In patients in whom surgical extirpation of the prostate has been performed for clinical benign obstruction, the extent of involvement, as well as histological differentiation, is extremely important in the determination of need for further therapy.

HISTOLOGY

Prostatic neoplasms are nearly always adenocarcinoma. Histologically, adenocarcinoma of the prostate is generally characterized by minimal cellular atypia. In well-differentiated tumors, the acinar pattern is preserved, but invasion into the stroma is observed. As the tumor becomes progressively less well differentiated, the glandular pattern may be lost entirely. Significant prognostic factors include invasion into vascular channels, penetration through the capsule of the prostate, and involvement of the seminal vesicles. However, appearance of tumor in perineural lymphatics is of little prognostic significance.

Although there is no universally accepted grading scheme, most centers have divided carcinoma of the prostate into three grades of adenocarcinoma: well differentiated, moderately differentiated, and poorly differentiated. The most extensive grading system is that of Gleason, which describes five distinct patterns based upon description of tumor margins, glandular pattern, size, and distribution, as well as invasion into the stroma.[1] Gleason et al. assigned a numerical score of 1 to 5 to both the primary and secondary cellular characteristics of the tumors, based upon histological review of 2,911 patients with carcinoma of the prostate. Because the majority of tumors show at least two different grades, a primary and secondary designation and score are given. Each tumor was recorded as two digits and the total score, ranging from 2 to 10, was obtained by adding the two values. The histological patterns from Gleason's original work are demonstrated in Figure 7-1. Gleason's score seems to correlate reasonably well with the clinical behavior of the tumor and the presence of metastatic disease. Tumors with lower Gleason scores tend to be relatively indolent, whereas those with higher scores tend to progress more rapidly. Although the Gleason grading system is increasingly being used, many pathologists still continue to grade prostatic malignancies into well, moderately, or poorly differentiated tumors.

A new technique to predict metastic potential of human prostatic cancer has recently been described by Diamond et al.[2] These investigators focused on the

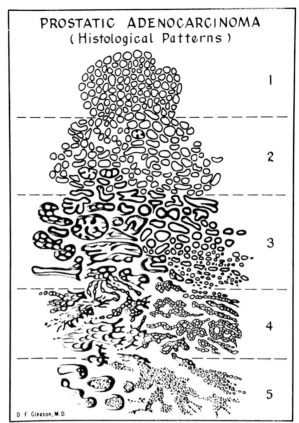

Fig. 7-1. Histological patterns of glandular differentiation for Gleason score. (Gleason, DF: Veterans Administration Cooperative Urological Research Group: Histologic grading and clinical staging of prostatic carcinoma. In Tannenbaum M (ed): Urologic Pathology: The Prostate. Lea & Febiger, Philadelphia, 1977.)

prostatic cancer cell nucleus and developed a computerized method to assess its shape. They described a nuclear roundness factor that could segregate, with a high statistical significance, those patients with cancer clinically limited to the prostate who subsequently had tumor recurrence versus those who did not. This promising work may provide another avenue of histological investigation that can predict biological activity of the cancer.

CLINICAL STAGING OF PROSTATE CANCER

Accurate staging to determine the extent of disease is essential in planning the proper therapeutic approach. Two staging classifications are in common usage, one from the American Urological Association and VA studies and the other a TNM system. These two systems are similar in that disease is classified as being confined to the prostate, having local spread, or distant spread. These two classifications are compared in Table 7-1.

Table 7-1. Comparison of Staging Systems

AUA Staging System (VA Studies)		TNM Staging System	
A1	Microscopic focus of well-differentiated adenocarcinoma in up to three foci of transurethral specimen or enucleation; clinically not apparent on rectal examination	T_0	No tumor palpable
A2	Tumor not well differentiated or present in more than three areas		
B1	Asymptomatic palpable nodule <1.5 cm; normal surrounding prostate; no capsular extension; normal acid phosphatase	T_1	Tumor intracapsular (normal gland surrounds tumor)
B2	Diffuse involvement of gland; no capsular extension; normal acid phosphatase	T_2	Tumor confined to gland; smooth nodule deforming contour
C	Extensive local tumor with penetration through the capsule, contiguous spread; may involve seminal vesicles, bladder neck, lateral side wall of pelvis; acid phosphatase may be elevated; normal bone scan	T_3	Tumor beyond capsule
D1	Metastases to pelvic lymph nodes below aortic bifurcation; acid phosphatase may be elevated	N_{1-2}	Regional lymph node metastases
D2	Bone or lymph node metastases above aortic bifurcation or other soft tissue metastases	M_1	Distant metastases

Stage A

Stage A prostate cancers refer to unsuspected latent or occult carcinomas prior to resection. Incidental carcinoma is probably the best designation for stage A disease because it is unapparent as well as unexpected. An important distinction exists between stage A cancers that are well differentiated and focal, designated stage A1, and those that are more diffuse yet undetected on rectal examination, designated stage A2. Stage A1 is reserved for those cases when a very small volume of the total tissue removed is cancerous. Stage A1 is defined as up to three foci of well-differentiated adenocarcinoma of the prostate. Any differentiation less than well differentiated is cause to classify the tumor as Stage A2. Stage A1 lesions are commonly found in men over the age of 45. These latent foci are usually 80 times or more prevalent than the palpable or symptomatic clinical prostatic cancer.[3]

Stage B

Clinically, this stage represents a nodule that is histologically and anatomically confined to the prostate gland and detectable on rectal examination. It constitutes about 15 percent of all prostatic carcinomas at the time of presentation. Stage B prostate cancer is subdivided into stages B1 and B2. A stage B1 tumor is a small discrete nodule, less than 1.5 cm in diameter, confined to a single lobe of the prostate. Stage B2 disease consists of a larger area in one lobe of the prostate or multiple nodules of the tumor confined within the prostate.

Stage C

Prostatic cancer that has extended through the prostatic capsule, but has not metastasized, constitutes approximately 40 percent of all prostate cancers at the time of diagnosis. The majority of patients with stage C prostate cancer have extension into the adjacent seminal vesicle. Stage C tumors are subdivided into stages C1 and C2, with the stage C1 tumor being less than 5 cm in diameter and the stage C2 tumor being more than 5 cm in diameter. Patients with stage C disease may or may not have an elevated serum prostatic acid phosphatase.

Stage D

Stage D represents metastatic prostatic cancer detected on clinical or pathological examination. Metastases are usually manifest by spread to regional and distant lymph nodes, as well as by bony metastases. There may be pelvic node metastases sometimes associated with ureteral obstruction. Metastases to other organs, such as the liver, can occur. The serum prostatic acid phosphatase is usually elevated. It is useful to divide stage D into D1 and D2 disease. Stage D1 disease is initially diagnosed as lower stage disease, but found to metastasize to the pelvic lymph nodes. Stage D2 disease refers to clinically evident metastatic cancer, usually to the bone or soft tissue.

NONSURGICAL METHODS OF STAGING

With increasing clinical stage of prostatic carcinoma, there is an increased likelihood that pelvic or distant lymph nodes will be involved with the disease. Because of the importance of pelvic lumph node involvement on prognosis and survival, attempts have been made to determine the status of the lymph nodes by a variety of methods. Numerous diagnostic modalities, other than operative intervention, have been utilized, in an attempt to assess the status of pelvic lymph node involvement.

Computerized Tomography Scanning

Computerized tomography (CT) scanning may not detect positive pelvic lymph nodes in patients with carcinoma of the prostate. The CT scan cannot accurately distinguish intranodal pathology, and unless the nodes are substantially enlarged, they will appear normal. The pelvic lymph nodes are difficult to visualize by CT scanning. Furthermore, conditions other than prostatic cancer may cause enlargement of the pelvic lymph nodes; hence, enlargement of nodes does not necessarily correlate with metastatic involvement of those nodes. Golimbu et al. studied 46 patients with carcinoma of the prostate, and found that the CT scanner had an accuracy of only 70 percent in assessing lymph node status and 47 percent in determining overall tumor extent.[4] Overall sensitivity of the test was poor in determining the status of lymph nodes and the extent of tumor. Most studies suggest that the overall sensitivity of CT scans in detecting lymph node metastases is not significantly better than that of lymphangiography.[5-7] Computerized tomography scanning can also be combined with fine needle aspiration cytology.

Bipedal Lymphangiography

Perhaps the most extensively evaluated imaging technique for staging of pelvic lymph nodes is lymphangiography.[8] Lymph node metastases from prostate cancer may distort the internal architecture of the lymph nodes and appear as filling defects or cutouts within the involved lymph nodes. False positive lymphangiograms, however, are seen in approximately 15 percent of patients with prostate cancer. Filling defects less than 1 cm in diameter should not be considered diagnostic for nodal metastases. Similarly, subtle findings, such as delayed filling of lymphatic channels, displaced channels, or enlarged nodes, should not be considered pathognomonic for metastatic cancer, since many other disease entities may produce similar changes. Perhaps the most serious objection to the routine use of lymphangiography is the observation that bipedal lymphangiography does not routinely visualize the internal iliac and obturator nodes that are the primary draining sites from carcinoma of the prostate. The major limitation of lymphangiography is its poor sensitivity in detecting nodal metastases. Lymphangiograms can detect metastases in only approximately 60 percent of patients with proven metastases. Lymphangiography fails to detect metastases in hypogastric and presacral nodes, which are frequently involved and not visualized on the bipedal lymphangiogram. Furthermore, lymphangiography is an invasive procedure that does carry some risks of thrombophlebitis and/or oil emboli to the lungs. In a study by Hoekstera and Schroeder, lymphangiography had an accuracy rate of 75 percent in 36 patients with documented carcinoma of the prostate. There was a 21 percent false positive rate, a 79 percent specificity rate, and a 67 percent sensitivity rate.[9]

Serum Acid Phosphatase

It has been conclusively shown that serum acid phosphatase determination is not a good screening test for prostatic cancer. Nonetheless, in patients with documented carcinoma of the prostate, determination of the acid phosphatase level by either enzymatic or radioimmunoassay methods may prove of some value in terms of staging and follow-up. In a recent study by Whitesel et al., 343 patients with carcinoma of the prostate had acid phosphatase sampling prior to staging lymphadenectomy.[10] Of these patients, 318 had a negative serum acid phosphatase and 70 (22 percent) had positive lymph nodes at the time of surgery. Thus, even in the presence of stage D disease, acid phosphatase levels may be in the normal range.

Of more importance, however, were 25 patients in whom the serum acid phosphatase was known to be elevated prior to surgery. Of these 25 patients, 15 had positive lymph nodes at the time of staging lymphadenectomy and 10 had no evidence of regional lymph node involvement. In the ensuing two years, 10 of 12 (83 percent) of those with positive lymph nodes developed evidence of metastatic disease. Importantly, five of six (83 percent) patients with negative lymph nodes also had evidence of metastatic disease by two years. These results indicate that even in the presence of a negative lymph node dissection, an elevated serum acid phosphatase in a patient with documented prostatic cancer is an important prognostic sign. These authors reinforce the suggestion that an elevation of the acid phosphatase strongly indicates metastatic disease and contraindicates radical treatment directed toward cure. It should be noted that these results only apply to acid phosphatase levels determined enzymatically. Experience with radioimmunoassays has not been sufficient nor have patients been followed long enough to draw similar conclusions. Moreover, the incidence of false positive tests in acid phosphatase determinations by the radioimmunoassay method is high.

Bone Marrow Acid Phosphatase

The role of bone marrow acid phosphatase in the staging of carcinoma of the prostate is uncertain. Because of limitations of the assay, most urologists do not perform bone marrow acid phosphatase routinely. In a study by Belleville, et al., 87 patients with documented carcinoma of the prostate were followed for a minimum of three years.[11] Only 3 of 86 men with negative serum and bone marrow acid phosphatase values showed progression of the disease, whereas 4 of 11 (36 percent) of those with normal serum acid phosphatase and elevated bone marrow acid phosphatase showed progressive disease during follow-up.

In spite of the limitations of acid phosphatase as a screening test, the bone marrow acid phosphatase may have some prognostic significance, although this is not universally accepted. This test remains more a research tool than a valuable prognosticator.

The Relationship to Histological Grading

In an attempt to predict the likelihood of nodal involvement based upon the histological grade of tumor, the Gleason classification has been used to predict the percentage of patients with lymph node metastases. Kramer et al have used Gleason histopathological grading to evaluate what percentage of their surgically staged patients could be predicted to have lymph node metastases.[12] This study was prompted by the inaccuracy of clinical staging as a predictor of the biological potential of prostate cancer. In the review of 228 patients with carcinoma of the prostate seen over a four-year period, 144 had no detectable bony disease and, therefore, underwent pelvic lymphadenectomy for staging. The primary prostatic biopsies were classified by the Gleason grading system, as noted. Of patients with Gleason scores 8 to 10, 93 percent had regional lymph node metastases, regardless of the primary clinical stage. No patient with a low Gleason score (2 to 4) had documented lymph node metastases. In this same series, false positive and false negative lymphangiograms were 29 and 35 percent, respectively. These authors concluded that the Gleason system was reproducible and did afford a better method of prediction of lymph node metastases.

The predictability of the Gleason score with surgical staging, however, has not met with uniform acceptance. Gaeta tried to correlate the Gleason score with surgical staging of the disease and found that there were patients with low Gleason scores of 3 to 4 who did have lymph node metastases.[13] Other recent reports have seriously challenged the predictability of the Gleason system and found that even in patients with a low Gleason number of 2 to 4 a significant percentage of patients may have positive nodes.[14,15] Furthermore, in patients with high Gleason scores of 7 to 9, as many as 40 percent will be free of nodal disease. Thus, the Gleason grading system cannot be used as an absolute indicator of nodal involvement.

Bone Scanning

The technetium-99 bone scan remains an important part of the staging of patients with adenocarcinoma of the prostate.[16] Bone scans are much more sensitive than radiographic skeletal surveys in detecting bony metastases.[17] Approximately 25 percent of patients with bony metastases will have normal acid phosphatase levels and be without symptoms of bony pain. The Uro-Oncology Research Group recently reported their experience in identifying the impact of radioisotopic bone scan, as well as lymphangiography, in determining disease extent among patients with carcinoma of the prostate.[16] Five hundred and nine patients with newly diagnosed prostate carcinoma were assigned a preliminary clinical stage based upon routine bone survey, acid phosphatase, and physical examination. Patients then underwent radioisotopic bone scan, bipedal lymphangiography, and subsequently, a staging pelvic lymph node dissection. Technetium-99 medronate bone scanning demonstrated bony extension of malignancy in approximately 25 percent of all patients judged to be free of disease by routine bone survey. Thus, the importance of the bone scan is obvious in excluding metastatic disease prior to consideration of staging pelvic lymphadenectomy.

Urinary Hydroxyproline Determination

Hydroxyproline, one of the constituents of collagen, has been shown to correlate with turnover of bone matrix. Urinary hydroxyproline excretion has been shown to be elevated in patients with bony metastases from breast cancer,[18] as well as in patients with stage D2 adenocarcinoma of the prostate.[19] Urinary hydroxyproline seems to be more reliable than serum acid phosphatase in detecting bony metastases from prostatic carcinoma and is probably as sensitive as the bone scan; however, it has not been universally accepted.

INCIDENCE OF LYMPH NODE METASTASES

Clinical stage seems to bear a direct relationship to the size of the local tumor and, hence, its malignant potential. The incidence of pelvic lymph node metastases increases with increasing stage of tumor. Table 7-2 summarizes the incidence of pelvic lymph node metastases according to clinical stage in a variety of series. The incidence ranges from 0 percent for stage A1 to 56 percent for stage C.

Table 7-2. Incidence of Surgically Proven Pelvic Lymph Node Metastasis Compared to Clinical Stage

Authors (Year)	Clinical Stage				
	A1	A2	B1	B2	C
Nicholson and Richie[20] (1977)	—	—	2/26[a]	2/14	2/6
Freiha et al.[21] (1979)	0/0	0/2	2/13	10/44	24/41
Brendler et al.[22] (1980)	0/1	3/22	11/58	14/27	10/17
Grossman et al.[23] (1980)	0/3	25/47	3/18	4/14	5/9
Lieskovsky et al.[24] (1980)	0/2	1/8	3/16	12/39	11/17
Smith et al.[25] (1983)	0/41	8/33	18/156	43/154	36/68
Total (%)	0/47(0)	37/112(33)	39/287(14)	85/292(29)	88/158(56)

[a] Number of patients with positive nodes/total number of patients

Note that A2 disease, "occult" cancer that is diffuse throughout the gland, has an incidence of lymph node metastases roughly equivalent to stage B2 disease; it is certainly much higher than stage B1 disease.

All the above studies point out our inability to stage patients with positive but unsuspected nodal involvement clinically. The identification and confirmation of positive nodes in patients with prostatic adenocarcinoma are important factors in consideration of treatment.

SURGICAL STAGING

The lymphatic spread of adenocarcinoma of the prostate occurs via the vasculature, which exits from the posterior aspect of the prostate and subsequently extends to the hypogastric, obturator, external iliac, and presacral lymphatics in that order. Nodes of the external iliac, common iliac, and paraaortic lymphatics are readily opacified by bipedal lymphangiography and account for the relatively high incidence of false negative lymphangiograms.

The limits of dissection of pelvic lymphadenectomy for staging of prostatic adenocarcinoma vary. Some surgeons prefer to dissect all the way to the bifurcation of the aorta, others include the presacral nodes in the nodal dissection. The mass of data that has accrued on areas of primary and secondary involvement would indicate that extension of the dissection to include the presacral nodes, common iliac area, or paraaortic area may increase the amount of nodal material removed, but does not significantly identify more patients with node-positive disease.

Technique

The pelvis may be entered through either a midline or a transverse lower abdominal incision. The dissection is carried out as an extraperitoneal dissection, which limits adherence of the bowel contents to the area of the dissection. The bladder should be mobilized laterally and both the common and external iliac arteries identified. Dissection is begun at the bifurcation of the common iliac vessels, just below the level where the ureter crosses the iliac artery, and is carried medial to the external iliac vasculature to the pelvic floor, across the pelvic floor to the inferior border of the prostate, and superiorly along the hypogastric vessels back to the bifurcation. The tissue surrounding the obturator nerve should be incorporated in the specimen. The obturator artery and vein may be ligated with clips. The limits of this dissection comprise a limited nodal dissection, which seems to identify nodal spread as accurately as a more extensive dissection. The more extensive dissection, which encompasses all the lymphatic vessels around the external iliac arteries or which goes superior to the bifurcation of the common iliacs to the bifurcation of the aorta, has been associated with delayed lower extremity and genital edema. This complication of edema is especially prevalent in patients who receive full-dose pelvic external beam radiotherapy.

Complications

Staging pelvic lymphadenectomy may be performed as an independent procedure or in conjunction with radical extirpative surgery on the prostate. The morbidity reported in the literature often relates to lymphadenectomy combined with other prostatic surgery and the incidence of complications from lymphadenectomy alone may not be as obvious. Paul et al., in a review of 150 patients who underwent staging pelvic lymphadenectomy as an independent procedure, reported intraoperative complications in 8.6 percent of their patients.[26] Wound morbidity occurred in 26 patients, with complications including superficial hematomas, superficial wound infections, or postoperative urinary tract infections. There were no instances of wound dehiscence or subsequent incisional hernia. Non-wound–related postoperative complications included epididymo-orchitis in six patients, atrial fibrillation in one patient, and lymphocele in one patient. Minor complications, such as atelectasis or prolonged ileus, occurred in seven patients. Delayed postoperative complications were noted in four patients, three of whom suffered lower extremity edema, one to two years postoperatively, requiring the use of support stockings. The overall complication rate was 33 percent, and the mean hospital stay for all patients was 11 days, with a range of 4 to 39 days.

Lieskovsky et al. reported 6 thromboembolic complications in 82 patients who underwent pelvic lymphadenectomy, 65 of whom also underwent radical prostatectomy.[25] These complications occurred in 52 patients who had not received anticoagulation, compared to 0 in 30 patients prophylactically anticoagulated with Coumadin. Lymphedema occurred in 15 patients, 10 of whom had received postoperative radiation therapy.

THE ROLE OF STAGING LYMPHADENECTOMY

The recognized complications ensuing from staging lymphadenectomy, especially when associated with external beam radiation therapy, have led to a reconsideration of the role of lymphadenectomy in the evaluation of patients with carcinoma of the prostate. Important questions in discerning the role of staging lymphadenectomy include (1) What is the prognostic value of staging pelvic lymphadenectomy in patients with prostatic cancer? (2) What is the therapeutic value of staging pelvic lymph node dissection in terms of planning for radiation therapy or additional therapy? (3) What is the role of pelvic lymph node dissection as a curative procedure? (4) What is the relative value of pelvic lymphadenectomy?

Prognostic Value of Staging Lymphadenectomy

Numerous studies have addressed the prognostic value of positive lymph nodes in patients with adenocarcinoma of the prostate. Whitmore et al. found that 40 percent of patients with positive lymph nodes who underwent pelvic lymphadenectomy and treatment with ^{125}I implantation had failed within two years of therapy.[27] As a further indication of poor prognosis, more than 75 percent of these patients had evidence of distant metastases within five years of therapy. Kramer et al., in the late 1970s, evaluated the outcome of radical prostatectomy in patients with node-positive or node-negative disease at Duke University.[28] Using, for the first time, evidence of treatment failure as the end point, 50 percent of the patients who had node-positive disease demonstrated evidence of distant metastases in less than two years, with a median time to failure of 19.5 months. This was in marked distinction to those patients with negative nodes, who had not yet approached the median time to failure by 68 months. In Whitmore's series of ^{125}I implantations, survival in patients with node-positive disease is much lower than in patients with node-negative disease.[29] Fewer than 50 percent of the patients with B2 disease who had node-positive disease confirmed by pelvic lymphadenectomy were free of disease at five years; none of the patients with stage C disease and positive nodes were without evidence of disease at five years. This study supports the contention that metastases to regional nodes is an ominous prognostic sign. Patients with nodal involvement are at increased risk of failure from distant metastases, regardless of the number of nodes involved.

Value of Lymph Node Dissection in Planning Radiation Therapy

One reason for staging pelvic lymph node dissection is to aid the radiation therapist in planning treatment fields. The rationale behind this recommendation is that node-negative involvement would require radiation to be given only in a small field to the prostate, whereas node-positive disease would require extension to full or whole-pelvis irradiation. However, Freiha et al. have presented data that bring into doubt the ability of radiation therapy to destroy metastatic prostatic cancer in the regional lymph nodes. Kramer et al. charted length of time after treatment to failure rate in 20 patients with extended field radiation and 24 patients with radical prostatectomy.[28] Even with extended pelvic irradiation of 7,000 rads to the prostate and 5,000 rads to the paraaortic and pelvic nodes, survival apparently was not prolonged, indicating that in patients with stage D1 disease, neither surgery nor radiation therapy could destroy involved pelvic lymph nodes. Thus, there appears to be little rationale for staging pelvic lymphadnectomy as an adjunct to radiation therapy, since whole-pelvis or extended field radiation therapy does not benefit patients with node-positive disease.

Can Pelvic Lymph Node Dissection Be Curative?

A report by Barzell et al., from Memorial Sloan-Kettering Cancer Center, supported the concept of pelvic lymph node dissection as a possible therapeutic maneuver.[30] In their study, patients with lymph node involvement of a total volume of less than 3 cm³ appeared to benefit therapeutically from lymph node dissection, and behaved prognostically as if they had negative nodes. However, subsequent reports from the same institution have not confirmed these findings. Reports from other institutions, such as Kramer et al. from Duke University, have shown that positive pelvic lymph nodes—even a single positive node—doom the patients to a 50 percent failure rate within 18 months. In 33 stage D1 patients treated with radiation therapy or delayed hormonal therapy, time to 50 percent failure was 19 months, compared to 18 months for radical perineal prostatectomy plus pelvic node dissection.[28] These data seem to imply that pelvic lymphadenectomy has very little impact on subsequent treatment failure of patients with stage D1 disease. If a single positive node was involved, the mean time of failure was 21.5 months, compared to 13.7 months with multiple nodes; the difference is not significant.

Thus, it would appear that pelvic lymphadenectomy is not curative for patients with stage D1 carcinoma of the prostate.

Relative Value of Pelvic Lymphadenectomy

It would seem that in routine clinical practice it is not essential to obtain pelvic lymph node staging data on patients whose management would not be influenced by the results of staging. This would generally mean patients for whom no immediate therapy, palliative therapy, or external beam radiation therapy is planned. However, in patients in whom radical therapy, such as radical prostatectomy, is likely to be useful for cure, staging pelvic lymphadenectomy can give important information about the selection of patients for radical therapy. With a staging pelvic lymphadenectomy limited to include the obturator nerve area, as described above, the dissection is about 85 percent accurate in detecting nodal metastases, as compared with more extensive pelvic dissections.

A strong argument can be made for the routine use of staging pelvic lymphadenectomy prior to subjecting a patient to either radical prostatectomy or curative radiation therapy. Since neither of these modalities has a high success rate in curing patients with stage D1 disease, it would seem to be reasonable to withhold these therapeutic modalities in such patients.

Given the inaccuracies of nonsurgical methods of staging, it would seem that pelvic lymphadenectomy is essential to achieve a high degree of staging accuracy. One must recall that lymphadenectomy is prognostic, but not therapeutic. Therefore, the decision concerning lymphadenectomy as opposed to noninvasive staging to determine nodal status should take into consideration the potential for cure in the patient at risk. Lymphadenectomy is the standard by which the accuracy of all nonsurgical methods for determining presence or absence of regional nodal involvement should be assessed. By the use of a limited node dissection for prognostic value, i.e., confining the dissection to the area around the obturator nerve and hypogastric vessels, it is possible to obtain accurate staging information with minimal postsurgical morbidity. Limited node dissection will reduce the incidence of delayed edema that is often seen after a more extensive pelvic dissection and full pelvic external beam radiation therapy.

As better predictors of nodal involvement are encountered, the need for a surgical procedure to assess involvement of the pelvic lymph nodes will diminish accordingly. At present, a patient with a very well-differentiated (Gleason score 2 or 3) B1 nodule has such a low incidence of pelvic node involvement that staging pelvic lymphadenectomy may be overlooked in the absence of a clinical study that demands accurate staging.[20] Similarly, the patient with a bulky stage C that is poorly differentiated and a Gleason score of 8 to 10 has such a high likelihood of nodal metastases that a CT scan with needle aspiration can confirm this and obviate the need for a staging lymphadenectomy. In the broad middle group of patients with stage A2–C lesions and an intermediate Gleason score, however, staging pelvic lymphadenectomy remains an important procedure to identify poor-prognostic variables that would preclude radical therapy.

REFERENCES

1. Gleason DF, Veterans Administration Cooperative Urological Research Group: Histologic grading and clinical staging of prostatic carcinoma. In Tannenbaum M (ed): Urologic Pathology: The Prostate. Philadelphia, Lea & Febiger, 1977
2. Diamond DA, Berry SJ, Jewett HG, Eggleston JC, Coffey DS: A new method to assess metastatic potential of human prostate cancer: Relative nuclear roundness. J Urol 128:729, 1982
3. Mostofi FK, Price EB: Tumors of the male genital system. Fascicle 8. Armed Forces Institute of Pathology, Washington, D.C., 1973
4. Golimbu M, Morales P, Al-Askari S, Shulman Y: CT scanning and staging of prostatic cancer. Urology 23:305, 1981
5. Lee JK, Stanley RJ, Sagel SS, et al: Accuracy of CT in detecting intraabdominal and pelvic lymph node metastases from pelvic cancers. Am J Roentogenol 131:675, 1978
6. Benson KH, Watson RA, Spring DB, et al: The value of computerized tomography in evaluation of pelvic lymph nodes. J Urol 126:63, 1981
7. Levine MS, Arger H, Coleman BG, et al: Detecting lymphatic metastases from prostatic carcinoma: Superiority of CT. Am J Roentgenol 137:207, 1981
8. Liebner EJ, Stefani S: Uro-Oncology Research Group: An evaluation of lymphangiography with nodal biopsy in localized carcinoma of the prostate. Cancer 45:728, 1980
9. Hoekstra T, Schroeder FH: The role of lymphangiography in the staging of prostate cancer. Prostate 2:433, 1981
10. Whitesel JA, Donohue RE, Mani JH, Mohr S, et al: Acid phosphatase: Its influence on the management of carcinoma of the prostate. J Urol 131:70, 1984

11. Belville WD, Mahan DE, Sepulveda RA, Bruce AW, Miller CF: Bone marrow acid phosphatase by radioimmunoassay: Three years of experience. J Urol 125:809, 1981
12. Kramer AS, Spahr J, Brendler CB, et al: Experience with Gleason's histopathologic grading in prostate cancer. J Urol 124:223, 1980
13. Gaeta JF: Glandular profiles and cellular patterns in prostatic cancer grading. Urology 17:33, 1981
14. Catalona WJ, Stein A, Fair WR: Grading errors in prostatic needle biopsies: Relation to the accuracy of tumor grade in predicting pelvic lymph node metastases. J Urol 127:919, 1982
15. Olsson CA, Tannenbaum M, Babian R, O'Brien M, DeVere White R: Prediction of pelvic lymph node metastases in adenocarcinoma of the prostate. AUA Annual Meeting, 1982
16. Paulson DF, Uro-Oncology Research Group: The impact of current staging procedures in assessing disease extent of prostatic adenocarcinoma. J Urol 121:300, 1979
17. Schaffer DL, Pendegrass HP: Comparison of enzyme, clinical, radiographic and radioneuclide methods of detecting bone metastases from carcinoma of the prostate. Radiology 121:431, 1976
18. Powels TJ, Leese CL, Bondy PK: Hydroxyproline excretion in patients with breast cancer. Br Med J 2:164, 1975
19. Bishop MC, Fellows GJ: Urinary hydroxyproline excretion—a marker of bone metastases in prostatic carcinoma. Br J Urol 49:711, 1977
20. Nicholson TC, Richie JP: Pelvic lymphadenectomy in stage B1 adenocarcinoma of the prostate: Justified or not? J Urol 117:199, 1977
21. Freiha FS, et al: Pelvic lymphadenectomy for staging prostatic carcinoma: Is it always necessary? J Urol 122:176, 1979
22. Brendler CB, et al: Staging pelvic lymphadenectomy for carcinoma of the prostate: Risk versus benefit. J Urol 124:849, 1980
23. Grossman IC, et al: Staging pelvic lymphadenectomy for carcinoma of the prostate: Review of 91 cases. J Urol 124:632, 1980
24. Lieskovsky G, Skinner DG, Weisenberger T: Pelvic lymphadenectomy in the management of carcinoma of the prostate. J Urol 124:635, 1980
25. Smith JA, Jr, Seaman JP, Gleidman JB, Middleton RG: Pelvic lymph node metastasis from prostatic cancer: Influence of tumor grade and stage in 452 consecutive patients. J Urol 130:290, 1983
26. Paul DB, Loening SA, Narayana AS, Culp DA: Morbidity from pelvic lymphadenectomy in staging carcinoma of the prostate. J Urol 129:1141, 1983
27. Whitmore WF, Jr, Batata MA, Hilaris BS: Prostatic irradiation: Iodine-125 implantation. p. 195. In Johnson DE, Samuels ML (eds); Cancer of the Genitourinary Tract. Raven Press, New York, 1979
28. Kramer SA, Cline WA, Jr, Farnham R, Carson CC, Cox EB, Hinshaw W, Paulson DF: Prognosis of patients with Stage D1 prostatic adenocarcinoma. J Urol 125:817, 1981
29. Whitmore WF, Jr: Interstitial radiation therapy for carcinoma of the prostate. Prostate 1:157, 1980
30. Barzell W, Bean MA, Hilaris BS, Whitmore WF, Jr: Prostatic adenocarcinoma: Relationship with grade and local extent to pattern of metastases. J Urol 118:278, 1977

8 | Gonadotropin-Releasing Hormone Analogues and Other New Hormonal Treatments of Prostate Cancer

L. Michael Glode

This chapter will review the most recent advances in the hormonal manipulation of prostatic adenocarcinoma. Before undertaking this task, however, it is necessary to pay tribute to the vast amount of work that preceded these advances, as well as to review the fundamental underpinning of hormonal therapy itself.

In 1941, Huggins and Hodges reported the results of castration and estrogen therapy in men with advanced carcinoma of the prostate.[1-3] These results led to the widespread use of estrogen for all stages of the disease in doses ranging from 1 to 500 mg/day.[4] A retrospective review of this experience evaluated patients who had received dosages of 1 to 5 mg of diethylstilbesterol (DES) daily and compared them with historical controls.[5] Although definite improvement in quality of life was undeniable, the essential conclusion, namely that hormonally treated patients lived longer, was appropriately challenged, since many of the control patients had been treated in the preantibiotic era. This led to the formation of the Veterans Administration Cooperative Urological Research Group (VACURG), which was organized in 1960 and which initiated three landmark studies during the next decade.

The first study was designed to answer the question of whether DES therapy, either alone or in combination with orchiectomy, was truly superior to placebo treatment for patients with locally extensive or metastatic disease. As with other VACURG studies, investigators were allowed to change the therapy when disease progression occurred, thus making some of the conclusions regarding the impact of treatment on survival difficult to interpret. In contrast to Nesbit and Baum's review,[5] this study showed no survival advantage for any form of hormonal manipulation.[6,7] Moreover, the study revealed an excess of cardiovascular deaths in patients receiving 5.0 mg DES/day.

In the second study, the cardiovascular risk of DES therapy was more critically analyzed. Patients were randomized to receive placebo, 0.2, 1.0, or 5.0 mg DES/day. After a few years, this study confirmed the cardiovascular risks of 5.0 mg DES/day; also the 1.0 mg/day dose was found to be as effective as 5.0 mg/day in delaying disease progression.[8] By this time, however, other studies appeared that suggested that 1.0 mg DES taken three times a day was more effective than 1.0 mg in suppressing plasma testosterone throughout a 24-hour period.[9] The 3.0-mg dose became a standard for therapy in the United States, although there was no evidence that it was either superior in cancer treatment or that it avoided the cardiovascular complications associated with the 5.0 mg/day dose.[10]

The third VACURG study is the most pertinent to this review, since it was designed to answer criticisms that DES was not a natural estrogen, which might have accounted for its increased cardiovascular toxicity. It also studied the possible benefits of using a progestational agent, medroxyprogesterone, which has some antiandrogenic activity. Although the final results of this study have not been presented in detail, preliminary reports indicate no advantage in the use of Premarin (a preparation of conjugated equine estrogens) or medroxyprogesterone.

GONADOTROPIN-RELEASING HORMONE ANALOGUES

The seminal observation for this category of drugs came in 1971 when Shally et al.[11,12] purified and determined the amino acid sequence of LH-RH/FSH-RH. Before this, it had been known that hypothalamic extracts could stimulate FSH and LH release from the anterior pituitary; however, it was assumed that different releasing hormones would be found to mediate the release of each gonadotropin. Final proof that a single peptide can release both hormones was obtained by injecting the synthetic peptide Glu-His-Trp-Syr-Tyr-Gly-Leu-Arg-Pro-Gly-NH$_2$ into animals and man. The observed release of both FSH and LH established the term "gonadotropin-releasing hormone" (GnRH).[13]

Because of the ease with which such small molecules are synthesized, it has been possible to construct numerous (now more than 2,000)[14] analogues of native GnRH.

Before reviewing the use of these analogues in the therapy of prostate carcinoma, we shall examine what is currently known about the normal action of GnRH at the pituitary level. The stimuli for hypothalamic GnRH release are as yet poorly understood. Two modes of release have been extensively studied, the pulsatile release, seen in normal and castrate animals, and the preovulatory release, brought about mostly by estrogen.[15] The physiological stimuli of light/dark cycles and stress are known to effect gonadotropin levels, probably through the hypothalamus. However, the neurotransmitters involved are myriad and include norepinephrine, serotonin, opioid peptides, dopamine, histamine, and acetylcholine, in addition to the sex steroids and prostaglandins. It is possible that a separate, as yet unidentified FSH-specific releasing hormone exists in the hypothalamus.[16]

Whatever the stimuli for GnRH release, GnRH enters the pituitary portal circulation in a pulsatile fashion, which, in turn, results in pulsatile gonadotropin secretion (Fig. 8-1). Both the frequency and amplitude of the GnRH pulse affect the pituitary response, and indeed, the differential effect of such alterations on FSH and LH release may explain how the single releasing hormone can control both FSH and LH secretion.[17] A second observation resulting from studies on pulse amplitude and frequency is that *continuous* infusion of native GnRH (or increased pulse frequency) actually inhibits, rather than stimulates gonadotropin secretion. As we shall see, this may explain the seemingly paradoxical effect of GnRH agonist administration in suppressing the hypothalamic–pituitary–gonadal axis. The effectiveness of these compounds in treating prostatic carcinoma is due to this suppression.

At the pituitary level, GnRH encounters specific receptors on gonadotrophs that synthesize and secrete FSH and LH (Fig. 8-1B). Only binding and the formation of a divalent bridge between two receptors appears to be necessary for gonadotropin release. Capping and internalization of receptor hormone complexes occurs, but is unnecessary for LH release.[18] Following the formation of a microaggregate or bridge between two receptor molecules, a calcium channel is opened and redistribution of calmodulin occurs. Calcium enters the cell to effect the release of preformed LH and FSH from the cell.[19]

The other consequence of GnRH binding to its receptor is desensitization for further stimuli. This may involve internalization of the receptor–hormone complexes, with loss in the number of receptors from the plasma membrane. This latter process is not calcium dependent and cannot be elicited by GnRH antagonists.[20]

The agonist analogues of GnRH are from 2 to 144 times as potent as natural GnRH in effecting LH release.[21] This activity crudely corresponds to their binding activity to the GnRH receptor. It is generally observed that substitutions of D-amino acids at position six, as well as modification of the *N*-terminus, increases both binding and biological potency. Such modifications also inhibit breakdown of the analogues and may account for their seemingly paradoxical inhibitory activity. Just as continuous infusion of GnRH effects a fall in LH and testosterone, so chronic agonist administration produces a chemical castration.

The first use of GnRH analogues in treating prostatic carcinoma was reported by Redding and Shally in rats in 1981.[22] These investigators found that administration of D-Trp[6]-GnRH significantly inhibited tumor growth in two separate testosterone-dependent tumors, 11095, and Dunning R-3327. A short time later, a report of this approach in man showed similar positive results with the same analogue and with D-Ser(TBU)[6],des-Gly-NH$_2$ ethylamide (Buserelin).[23]

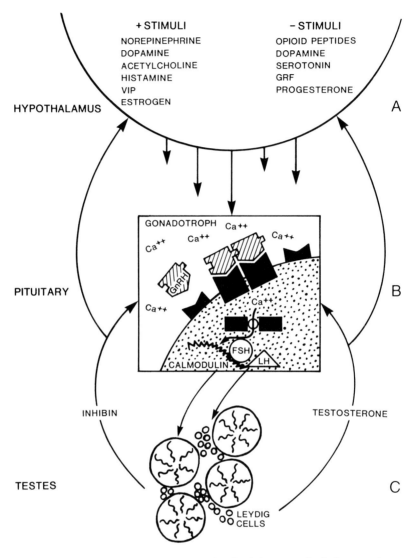

Fig. 8-1. The hypothalamic–pituitary–gonadal axis: (A) under the influence of numerous stimuli, GnRH is released in a pulsatile fashion; (B) GnRH molecules bind receptors on the surface of a gonadotroph in the anterior pituitary gland. Microaggregates consisting of as few as two hormone receptor complexes form and calcium channels are opened. Calcium influx and redistribution of calmodulin release preformed LH and FSH. (C) At the testicular level, LH binds to Leydig cells, with synthesis and release of testosterone that feedback negatively at the pituitary and hypothalamic levels. In rats, GnRH receptors on Leydig cells, when occupied, bring about down-regulation of LH receptors. The FSH binds to Sertoli cells to regulate spermatogenesis. Feedback inhibition of FSH is brought about by inhibin.

Table 8-1. GnRH (LHRH) Agonists

Chemical Name	Trade Name	Pharmaceutical Company
[D-Trp⁶] GnRH	Decapeptyl	Lederle/Cyanamid
[D-Ser(TBU)⁶, des-Gly¹⁰-NH₂] GnRH ethylamide	Buserelin	Hoechst AG
[D-Leu⁶, des des-Gly¹⁰-NH₂] GnRH-pro-ethylamide	Leuprolide	Takeda-Abbott Products
[D-Ser(TBU)⁶-azaglycinamide] GnRH	ICI 118630	ICI

At the time of writing this chapter, it became almost impossible to keep up with the large number of studies with GnRH analogues, which now appear almost monthly. To add to this problem, different investigators have used different response criteria and a number of different analogues at different doses. In spite of this confusion, the overall emerging picture is quite clear. Table 8-1 shows the chemical structures, trade names, and pharmaceutical companies for the GnRH agonist analogues that have been reported or which are in ongoing clinical trials at present. Table 8-2 is a partial listing of published clinical trials.[24-33] An attempt has been made to eliminate, when possible, separate publications which report on the same patients cited in the table; however, this may have inadvertently led to the omission of other patients who have received this form of therapy.

To date, it is not apparent that any of the compounds listed are superior to any of the others in terms of either response rates or side effects. Thus, the conclusions of our study, which reported the largest number of patients and used the response criteria of the NPCP probably apply in a general way to all studies and will be discussed in some detail to highlight the results of this form of treatment.[32]

Beginning in 1981, 118 patients with stage C or D prostatic carcinoma were entered in a study in which Leuprolide, one of the well-characterized GnRH analogues, was administered daily in doses of 1 or 10 mg by subcutaneous injection at 14 different U.S. institutions. As shown in Figure 8-2, subsequent evaluation of hormonal responses in these patients showed no difference for the two doses.[34] In all patients, there was an expected initial rise in FSH and LH in response to the agonistic activity of Leuprolide (Fig. 8-3). By the end of two weeks of treatment, however, the agonistic response was no longer evident, and the serum gonadotropin and testosterone levels had fallen dramatically.

The clinical response of 59 previously untreated patients was evaluated by blinded observers using the response criteria of the NPCP.[35] Table 8-3 shows that 40 of 58 evaluable patients benefited from therapy, with approximately equal numbers showing objective response and stabilization of disease. Thirteen patients did not respond and were taken off the study after objective evidence of progression was noted. The median response duration to this treatment is in excess of one year, but has not been adequately evaluated at present.

In Table 8-4, the maximum objective response of previously treated patients is shown. For patients treated previously with DES, therapy proved beneficial in 10 of 21 patients. There was a much higher rate of progression for patients who

Table 8-2. Trials Using GnRH Agonists for Prostatic Carcinoma

Author	Patient (No.)	Analogue	Response[a]			
			Previously Untreated		Previously Treated	
			Objective	Subjective	Objective	Subjective
Kautsilieris[26]	20	Buserelin	12/20	16/20	—	—
Borgmann[31]	9	Buserelin	—	—	—	—
Faure[30]	47	Buserelin	7/16	7/8	4/7	3/5
Borgmann[33 b]	21	Buserelin	17/21	—	—	—
Waxman[28]	12	Buserelin	1/12	8/12	—	—
Labrie[29 c]	88	Buserelin	29/30	31/35	14/30	34/39
Glode[32 d]	118	Leuprolide	40/53	27/30	16/47	21/58
Walker[25 e]	8	ICI 118630	5/8	7/8	—	—
Ahmed[24 f]	12	ICI 118630	7/12	7/8	—	—
Allen[27]	10	ICI 118630	8/10	5/5	—	—
Total	345		126/182(69%)	108/126(86%)	34/84(40%)	58/102(57%)

[a] "Response" includes each author's criteria of objectively stable, partial response, or complete response, but omits patients for whom inadequate data are presented, where possible.

[b] Locally advanced (stage C) patients. Response is by cytology only.

[c] Combined therapy with the nonsteroidal antiandrogen RU-23908. "Objective" responses indicate improvement in bone scan only. Three patients were previously treated.

[d] Data confirmed by external review; NPCP criteria was used.

[e] Response criteria unstated; 5/8 had a fall in prostatic acid phosphatase level to normal.

[f] Response criteria of British Prostate Group

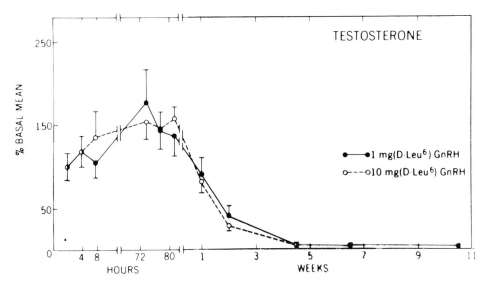

Fig. 8-2. Testosterone response to Leuprolide administration in patients receiving 1 or 10 mg of drug/day, SQ. Initial stimulation is followed by a fall in testosterone to castrate levels. No difference is seen between the two doses (Warner B, Worgul TJ, et al: Effect of very high dose D-leucine[6]-gonadotropin-releasing hormone proethylamide on the hypothalamic–pituitary–testicular axis in patients with prostatic cancer. J Clin Invest 71:1842, 1983. Reproduced from The Journal of Clinical Investigation, by copyright permission of The American Society for Clinical Investigation.)

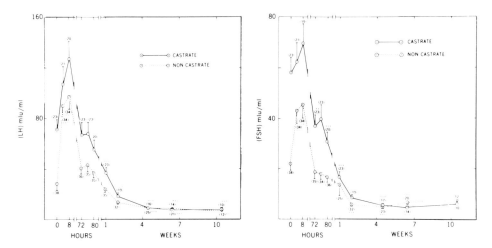

Fig. 8-3. The LH and FSH response to Leuprolide administration. The initial agonistic rise in gonadotropin secretion is followed by suppression with chronic administration of the GnRH analogue. (Warner B, Worgul TJ, et al: Effect of very high dose D-leucine[6]-gonadotropin-releasing hormone proethylamide on the hypothalamic–pituitary–testicular axis in patients with prostatic cancer. J Clin Invest 71:1842, 1983. Reproduced from The Journal of Clinical Investigation, by copyright permission of The American Society for Clinical Investigation.)

Table 8-3. Maximum Objective Response of Previously Untreated Patients to Leuprolide

No. Treated	No. Evaluable	Response (%)			
		Complete	Partial	Stable	Progressive
59	53	2 (4%)	17 (32%)	21 (40%)	18 (24%)

had undergone orchiectomy (20/26). Although the reason for this is not clear, it probably reflects the entrance criteria and the type of patients considered for study, rather than a true difference between the categories of patients. In the case of DES, many patients entered had not shown progression, but rather had suffered a thrombotic cardiovascular event. The bias of most investigators was that such side effects would be fewer with GnRH analogue therapy, and hence such patients were readily considered for entry into the study, regardless of their tumor status. On the other hand, most orchiectomy patients were probably considered for entry only after disease progression had been documented. In both categories, the reduced response rate, compared to previously untreated patients, is expected, since GnRH analogue therapy is merely another mechanism to reduce serum testosterone levels.

Subjective responses to GnRH analogue therapy have been high; however, they are not higher than might be expected with other forms of testosterone depletion (Table 8-2). Given the evidence from the VACURG studies cited above, which fail to show a survival benefit for hormonal manipulation, it may be that this is at least as important as the objective response data presented in Table 8-2. The ultimate role, therefore, of GnRH analogue therapy in prostatic carcinoma will depend on the maintenance of a comparable objective and subjective response rate with fewer side effects than conventional treatment. In this regard, the findings are not conclusive.

Figure 8-2 shows the LH and FSH response of some of the patients in our study.[34] There is an initial response to the agonistic effect of Leuprolide, which increases gonadotropin levels following injections during the first week of therapy. Figure 8-3 shows, in patients who had not had previous therapy, a rise in serum testosterone that was similar at doses of either 1 or 10 mg of analogue daily. During this time, there was a worsening of bone pain or a rise in acid phosphatase in 10 to 20 percent of the patients. During the subsequent period of depleted androgens, 40 percent of the patients experienced hot flashes, impotence, and decreased libido; 3 percent had skin irritation at the injection site; and 2 percent developed skin rashes. The two major side effects of DES therapy, gynecomastia and increased cardiovascular events, were not seen. Only a careful, prospective

Table 8-4. Maximum Objective Response of Previously Treated Patients to Leuprolide

Pretherapy	Evaluable	Complete	Partial	Stable	Progression	Unevaluable
DES ($N = 28$)	21	0	1 (15%)	9 (43%)	11 (52%)	7
Orchiectomy ($N = 31$)	26	0	0	6 (23%)	20 (77%)	5

randomized trial of DES and GnRH analogue therapy will show the relative incidence of thromboses, myocardial infarction, and stroke.

Four important practical questions remain regarding the use of GnRH analogues in prostatic carcinoma: dose, route of administration, cost, and benefit to patients who have failed other forms of hormonal administration. With regards to the dose, it would appear that treatment with 1.0 mg/day, at least during the initial period of therapy, lowers serum testosterone levels more than lower doses do.[31,34]

The route of administration, in turn, depends on the final dose desired. Although a number of the studies in Table 8-2 have explored intranasal administration, only 1 to 4 percent of the drug is absorbed, and cost considerations may make this method impractical.[35] Independent of this consideration, synthetic peptides may be inherently more expensive than DES to manufacture, especially if pharmaceutical companies expect to recoup some of the costs of research on this category of compounds to date.

Finally, the potential response of patients who have previously failed treatment is uncertain. In our study, which used the criteria of the NPCP,[36] a small percentage of patients in the orchiectomy group appeared to have their disease stabilized. This finding requires further study in a larger group of such patients. Recent studies by Heirowski et al. have documented the presence of GnRH-like membrane receptors in the Dunning rat tumor.[37] If similar receptors are present on human prostatic adenocarcinoma cells, the possibility exists for a direct extrapituitary effect on tumor growth.

Another group of GnRH analogues, the antagonists, will soon be available in sufficient quantity for clinical studies in prostatic carcinoma. These compounds, which contain modifications of positions 2,3,6, and in some cases 1 and 10, act at the same receptor site as the agonists, but do not cause the initial rise in gonadotropin secretion seen with the agonists. Schally et al. have recently demonstrated inhibition of rat prostatic carcinoma using an antagonist.[38] Interestingly, their study did not show the decrease in testicular weight that is commonly seen with agonist treatment. This finding may be related to the apparently unique presence of GnRH receptors in the rat testis and the resultant extrapituitary effects of the compounds in rats.

Although the final role of the GnRH analogues in therapy of prostatic carcinoma cannot now be determined, it is clear that they are efficacious and potentially less toxic than other currently available hormonal drugs. Jacobi has pointed out recent European data that confirm the risk of estrogen therapy in male patients in this age range.[39] In one study, 60 percent of patients receiving polyestradiol phosphate or estramustine phosphate (vide infra) experienced a cardiovascular complication.[40] Among patients with a previous history of cardiovascular disease, 15/86 (17 percent) actually died from a cardiovascular complication in this modern trial. The argument in favor of GnRH analogues versus orchiectomy is less clear. Potential advantages include the use of a reversible modality of therapy and the absence of psychological disturbances, although the latter has not been well studied and, in general, men accept orchiectomy when informed that the alternative modalities will produce the same degree of impotence and loss of libido.

ANTIANDROGENS

Three antiandrogens have received clinical trials in the therapy of prostatic carcinoma. The first Flutamide is an anilide (4-nitro-3-trifluoromethylisobutyranilide), which effectively competes for cytosolic androgen receptor sites. Clinically, it is administered to patients in doses of 750 to 1,500 mg/day. The response to such therapy, in some of the more recent trials, is shown in Table 8-5. In previously untreated patients, the 72 percent response seen in these trials is at least as good as that for DES or orchiectomy. Lower response rates are seen in patients who have had previous endocrine therapy. Side effects from Flutamide therapy include nausca, vomiting, and painful gynecomastia at rates that approach those seen in DES trials. Of interest, there is the apparent ability to maintain potency and libido among some patients without previous sexual dysfunction.[41-45]

A second antiandrogen, cyproterone acetate, has a more complex mode of action. This synthetic steroid posesses low estrogenic, androgenic, and corticoid activitiy but has pronounced progestational and antiadrogenic properties.[46] The mechanism for the effect appears to be inhibition of the desmolase activity in testicular Leydig cells, as well as cytoplasmic competition with dihydrotestosterone for androgen receptor protein.[47] Patients receiving cyproterone acetate experience a rapid fall in plasma testosterone similar to that observed with the GnRH analogues or long-acting estrogen compounds.[46] In his recent review of trials completed over the past 17 years with this compound, Jacobi tabulated a greater than 50 percent response rate among 101 previously untreated patients.[47] Among the 373 previously treated patients, objective response rates were lower. The difficulty in comparing response rates between trials was again noted. However, in his own direct prospective randomized study comparing the side effects of cyproterone and estradiol, Jacobi documented a much lower rate of gynecomastia and cardiovascular events with cyproterone. Similar results have been seen in a large study of 106 patients treated with orchiectomy and cyproterone by Giuliani et al.[48]

The third antiandrogen RU-23909 is a nonsteroidal drug similar to

Table 8-5. Selected Trials on Flutamide Therapy for Prostatic Carcinoma

Author	Patient (No.)	Response[a] Untreated Objective	Untreated Subjective	Previously Treated Objective	Previously Treated Subjective
Jacobi[41]	8	2/8	—	—	—
Stoliar[42]	18	1/1	1/1	6/16[b]	—
Sogani[43]	21	19/21	8/10	—	—
Prout[44]	13	7/13	5/6	—	—
Narayana[45]	25	7/7[c]	—	2/7[c]	7
Total	85	36/50(72%)	13/17(76%)		

[a] Response indicates individual author's definition of stable or better among evaluable patients.

[b] Subjective and objective response are mixed.

[c] Response at 12 weeks.

Flutamide.[49] It has recently been combined with Buserelin, a GnRH analogue, with promising results.[29]

In conclusion, cyproterone acetate is an effective alternative to currently available hormonal therapy and has the advantages of low estrogenic side effects, as noted in the ongoing GnRH analogue trials. Flutamide may have similar response rates, but it also has estrogenic side effects. RU-23909 has not been well characterized as a single agent, but it shows promise in reducing initial side effects associated with GnRH-induced flare.

PROGESTINS

Megestrol acetate has been used in the treatment of benign prostatic hypertrophy and has received a limited trial in the therapy of prostatic carcinoma. Geller et al. treated 20 patients with 160 mg/day PO and documented an objective improvement in bone scan in two of five previously untreated, evaluable patients. Only 1 of 11 previous hormonal failures responded, and there were some patients with stable disease in each group.[50] A potential disadvantage was a rise in plasma testosterone after several months. A more recent trial by the same author used estradiol in doses of 0.5 to 1.5 mg/day to prevent this rise, with success.[51] Whether the addition of low-dose estrogen to this therapy will prove to be less toxic than the standard approach of DES therapy remains to be seen.

Medroxyprogesterone acetate is the other progestin to receive a major trial. Like megestrol, this drug suppresses gonadotropin release and also directly affects the testis and adrenal glands, reducing circulating testosterone levels. Marketed widely outside the United States as an antifertility drug (Depo-Provera, the Upjohn Company), a storm of controversy surrounds that use.[52] In prostate cancer, however, the European Organization for Research in the Treatment of Cancer (EORTC) Urological Group is completing a study comparing medroxyprogesterone acetate to cyproterone acetate or DES for initial therapy. Patients receive medroxyprogesterone (500 mg) IM, three times a week, followed by 100 mg PO, twice daily, as maintenance. The cyproterone dose is 250 mg/day, and the DES dose is 3.0 mg/day. In their most recent update, these investigators concluded that the response rate to this dose of medroxyprogesterone (10 percent) was inferior to that for cyproterone (28 percent) or DES (71 percent).[53] Cardiovascular side effects were highest in the DES arm, reaching 48 percent in patients with previous cardiovascular disease. Further analysis of these data will be necessary before conclusions can be drawn regarding the role of this progestin.

ANTIADRENAL AGENTS

As early as 1945, Huggins performed bilateral adrenalectomies in an attempt to further improve upon the results that could be obtained with orchiectomy.[54] Subsequent reports documented an objective response rate of 36 to 60 percent to this procedure, although a rather high postoperative morbidity and mortality rate was seen.[55] With the improvement in ability to measure low levels of testosterone, it is now evident that these responses were obtained because the adrenals secrete 16 to 217 μg of testosterone a day, and 228 to 294 μg of adrenal androstenedione a day is converted to testosterone.[56] These values represent about 10 percent of the circulating testosterone in non-castrated men.

Aminoglutethimide, originally developed as an anticonvulsant, has been extensively evaluated as an antitumor agent for adrenal, breast, and prostatic cancers. The drug works by inhibiting several important steroidogenic enzymes, including desmolase, which initiates the side chain cleavage that converts cholesterol to pregnenolone. When given alone, there is an increase in pituitary ACTH secretion, which restores steroidogenesis; however, this increase can be successfully blocked by coadministration of physiological doses of cortisol. Using such an approach, "medical adrenalectomy" has been achieved in two studies, the most modern of which documented a 48 percent objective response rate using the NPCP criteria.[56,57] Although the side effects, which may include lethargy, nausea, ataxia or postural hypotension, and skin rash, preclude its use as a first line of therapy, aminoglutethimide has a definite role in achieving response by reducing adrenal androgen production without the risks of surgery.

A second antiadrenal agent, spironolactone, also reduces adrenal androgen biosynthesis by inhibiting a number of enzymes. In the only reported study of its use in treating prostatic carcinoma, subjective responses were seen in three of seven previously orchiectomized men, and a significant reduction in plasma testosterone, androstenedione, and dehydroepiandrosterone was noted.[58] The side effects of spironolactone, gynecomastia, and hyperkalemia are not as frequent or severe as with aminoglutethimide, and this agent deserves a more comprehensive trial.

OTHER AGENTS

A large number of relatively new hormonal agents have received limited trials in the therapy of prostatic carcinoma. Tamoxifen, approved in the United States for palliative therapy of breast carcinoma, binds cytoplasmic estrogen receptors, being transported to the nucleus of target cells and thereby preventing the synthesis of new receptors for both progesterone and estrogen. Based on a few case reports of efficacy of this agent in prostatic carcinoma, Glick et al. completed a phase II study of tamoxifen in 29 patients who had failed previous hormonal therapy. Five (17 percent) achieved a response by NPCP criteria. In addition, two previously untreated patients responded, and there was a subjective response in 10/31 total patients in the trial.[59]

Bromocriptin is an ergot derivative that inhibits prolactin secretion in man. Since there are prolactin receptors on prostatic cells, and since prolactin has potential proandrogenic effects, this drug was administered by the EORTC to 28 patients, 20 of whom were previously untreated. After 16 weeks of treatment, all but two evaluable patients had progressed, and there was a high incidence of vomiting.[60] Jeromin, however, recently combined bromocriptin with estrogen treatment and found that the edema and gynecomastia associated with the estrogen were reduced.[61]

Again, more studies are needed to establish what role, if any, bromocriptin may have in the hormonal management of prostatic cancer.

A third agent, quadrosilan (Cisobitan), is an organo-silicon compound with estrogenic activity. Since it is not related structurally to estrogen, and it does not affect blood coagulation parameters in dogs or rats, it was administered to 54 patients with advanced prostatic carcinoma and compared to a long-acting estrogen compound by Alfthan et al.[62] Using the criteria of the NPCP, Cisobitan produced a partial response or stabilized disease in 50/54 patients, compared to 41/53 patients treated with estrogens. Moreover, cardiovascular deaths occurred in only 4 Cisobitan-treated patients, but 11 estrogen-treated patients. Although these numbers are not statistically significant, this drug may be a useful alternative to estrogen therapy because, like cyproterone acetate and GnRH analogues, it has fewer cardiovascular side effects.

COMBINED HORMONAL MANIPULATION AND CHEMOTHERAPY

Androgen Priming with Cytotoxic Chemotherapy

More than 20 years ago, the possibility of utilizing androgen to stimulate human prostatic cancer cells to divide and thus enhance the cytotoxicity of agents effective against proliferating cells was considered. There were a number of studies in which ^{32}P was given, following a two-week course of testosterone. The outcome of such treatment was unclear; however, many studies reported an increase in the pain of metastatic bone disease, which suggested that there was some biological effect vis-à-vis the tumor cells.[63,64] In reviewing 138 patients in some of these studies, Fowler and Whitmore noted that unfavorable subjective or objective responses occurred in 93 percent of the patients.[65] Among their own 52 androgen-treated patients who did not receive ^{32}P, 87 percent had an unfavorable response.

A single study evaluating chemotherapy after such stimulation has been published by Suarez et al.[66] In this study, 20 orchiectomized patients received 5 mg of fluoxymestrone twice daily along with chemotherapy. Nine of the patients (43 percent) had an objective response, as measured by the NPCP criteria, with a median duration of over nine months.[67]

Estramustine and Prednimustine

A more direct mechanism of combining hormonal therapy with chemotherapy is estramustine phosphate (Fig. 8-4). This compound is a combination of estradiol phosphate and nitrogen mustard. When the phosphate group is removed by the various serum phosphatases, the estrogen component serves as a carrier, with the theoretical advantage of directing toxicity specifically to cells with hormone receptors for estradiol. The drug is also bound by specific prostatic cell proteins, and metabolites include estrogen derivatives that have no alkylating activity. The exact mechanism of action for this drug has never been fully elucidated. Of major impor-

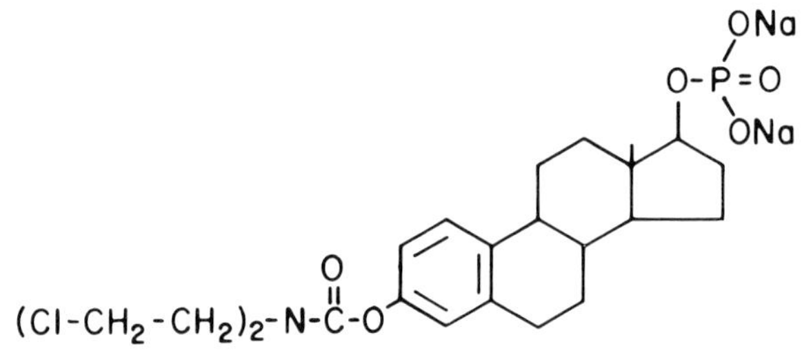

Fig. 8-4. Structure of estramustine phosphate.

tance, however, is its lack of myelosuppressive activity in patients, many of whom have had previous radiation therapy. The dose-limiting toxicity appears to be gastrointestinal. In one of the early studies carried out by the NPCP, 50 patients with stage D prostatic carcinoma were treated with 15 mg/kg daily for periods from 3 to 24 months. A favorable response (objective responders plus stable disease) occurred in 36 percent of 44 evaluable patients. Among these responders were several patients who had previously failed therapy with a variety of estrogenic substances; this again argues against estrocyte being a novel form of estrogen and stresses its rather unique activity in prostatic carcinoma.[67] In a second NPCP study, a 30 percent response rate to estramustine phosphate was again demonstrated in patients who had had extensive pelvic radiation.[68] This latter study, which compared estramustine to streptozotocin or standard therapy, showed that estramustine gave the longest duration of response as well as prolongation of survival among responders compared to non-responders.

Another synthetic steroid structure, prednimustine, was developed by the A.B. Leo Co. Initially called Leo 1031, this drug was shown to be active against chronic lymphocytic leukemia and lymphocytic lymphoma and included responses among patients who had relapsed during therapy with an alkylating agent plus corticosteroid. Again, this suggests a unique site of action.[69] Tried alone and in combination with estramustine in very advanced prostatic cancer patients, prednimustine, as demonstrated by the NPCP, elicited an approximately 35 percent subjective response, and a 13 percent objective response rate in the two groups of patients. Thus far, prednimustine has not been approved for therapy of prostatic carcinoma in the United States, and its ultimate availability remains in doubt.[70]

The most recent trials of the NCPC utilizing the combination of hormonal manipulation plus chemotherapy have involved two major areas. First is the combination of estramustine with other potentially active cytotoxic agents, such as vincristine and *cis*-platinum. No statistically significant benefit for adding estramustine to vincristine was found.[71] The combination of *cis*-platinum and estramustine appeared to have a higher response rate (33 percent) compared to estramustine alone (18 percent) or *cis*-platinum alone (21 percent); however, there was no clear-cut explanation as to the reason for the somewhat lower than reported response rate to estramustine phosphate in this trial.[72]

The NPCP has also moved combined hormonal therapy and chemotherapy to a time that is earlier in the natural history of prostatic carcinoma. In one study, patients with newly diagnosed metastatic cancer were randomized to receive cytoxan plus estramustine versus cytoxan plus DES versus hormonal manipulation alone (DES administration, or orchiectomy). Approximately 80 patients were entered into each group, and although the objective response rates and survival times were similar among groups, there is a suggestion of some improvement in overall survival among the groups receiving chemotherapy compared to those receiving hormonal therapy alone.[73]

In the second trial using chemotherapeutic agents earlier in the treatment of prostatic carcinoma, 188 patients who had been stabilized by orchiectomy or hormone therapy for at least three months were randomized to receive DES, DES plus cytoxan, or DES plus estramustine. Response rates, duration of response, and survival times were not demonstrably different among the groups.

In summary, various combinations of hormonal manipulation with chemotherapy continue to be explored, and in certain trials, the approach has been promising. Nevertheless, such treatment is still best restricted to a controlled trial situation. In particular, the additive risk of testosterone stimulation or the side effects of cytotoxic therapy may well outweigh the modest benefits demonstrated by such trials.[74]

CONCLUSION

The original observations of Huggins and Hodges still remain: Reduction of testosterone favorably benefits the thousands of patients who receive endocrine therapy each year, although the death rate from metastatic prostatic carcinoma remains unchanged. Most of the newer forms of hormonal manipulation mentioned in this chapter are advances only in the sense that they can produce 40-year-old results, but with fewer side effects. The ongoing trials of the NPCP have begun to demonstrate a potential survival benefit for the early addition of cytotoxic chemotherapy to hormonal manipulation in selected patients with advanced disease.[75]

As with many other forms of cancer, there is much work to be done in the fields of understanding etiology, improving detection methods, and applying advances in our understanding of the basic biology of prostatic cancer. In this sense, the development of GnRH analogues is a true advance, since it represents the clinical fruition of more than a decade of excellence in basic science research.

REFERENCES

1. Huggins C, Hodges CV: Studies on prostatic cancer. I. The effect of castration, of estrogen and of androgen injection on serum phosphatases in metastatic carcinoma of the prostate. Cancer Res 1:293, 1941
2. Huggins C, Stevens RE, Jr, Hodges CV: Studies on prostatic cancer. II. The effects of castration on advanced carcinoma of the prostate gland. Arch Surg 43:209, 1941
3. Huggins C, Scott WW, Hodges CV: Studies on prostatic cancer. III. The effects of fever, desoxycorticosterone, and of estrogen on clinical patients with metastatic carcinoma of the prostate. J Urol 46:997, 1941

4. Scott WW, Menon W, Walsh PC: Hormonal therapy of prostatic cancer. Cancer 45:1929, 1980
5. Nesbit RM, Baum WC: Endocrine control of prostatic carcinoma: Clinical and statistical survey of 1818 cases. JAMA 143:1317, 1950
6. Blackard CE, Byar DP, Jordan WP, VACURG: Orchiectomy for advanced prostatic carcinoma: A reevaluation. Urology I:553, 1973
7. Byar DP: VACURG studies of conservative treatment. Scand J Urol Nephrol 55:99, 1980
8. Bailar JC, Byar DP: Estrogen treatment for cancer of the prostate: Early results with three doses of diethylstilbestrol and placebo. Cancer 26:257, 1970
9. Robinson MRG, Thomas BG: Effect of hormonal therapy on plasma testosterone levels in prostatic carcinoma. Br Med J 4:391, 1971
10. Smith PH: Endocrine and cytotoxic therapy. Recent Results Cancer Res 78:154, 1981
11. Schally AV, Arimura A, Baba Y, Nair RMG, Matsuo H, Redding TW, Debeljuk L, White WF: Isolation and properties of the FSH- and LH-releasing hormone. Biochem Biophys Res Commun 43:393, 1971
12. Matsuo H, Nair RMG, Arimura A, Schally AV: Structure of the porcine LH- and FSH-releasing hormone. I. The proposed amino acid sequence. Biochem Biophys Res Commun 43:133, 1971
13. Schally AV, Arimura A, Kastin AJ, Matsuo H, Baba Y, Redding TW, Nair RMG, Debeljuk L: Gonadotropin-releasing hormone: one polypeptide regulates secretion of lutinizing and follicle-stimulating hormones. Science 173:1036, 1971
14. Stewart JM: Personal communication
15. McCunn SM: Physiology and pharmacology of LHRH and somatostatin. Ann Rev Pharmacol Toxicol 22:491, 1982
16. Sumson WK, Snyder G, Fawcett CP, McCunn SM: Chromatographic and biologic analysis of ME and OVLT LHRH. Peptides 1:97, 1980
17. Wildt L, Hausler A, Marshall G, Hutchison JS, Plant TM, Belchetz PE, Knobil E: Frequency and amplitude of gonadotropin-releasing hormone stimulation and gonadotropin secretion in the rhesus monkey. Endocrinology 109:376, 1981
18. Conn PM, Hazem E: Leuteinizing hormone release and gonadotropin-releasing hormone (GnRH) receptor internalization: Independent actions of GnRH. Endocrinology 109:2040, 1982
19. Blum JJ, Conn PM: Gonadotropin-releasing hormone stimulation of luteinizing hormone release: A ligand-receptor-effector model. Proc Natl Acad Sci USA 79:7307, 1982
20. Smith WA, Conn PM: GnRH-mediated desensitization of the pituitary gonadotrope is not calcium dependent. Endocrinology 112:408, 1983
21. Perrin MH, Rivier JE, Vale WW: Radioligand assay for gonadotropin-releasing hormone: Relative potencies of agonists and antagonists. Endocrinology 106:1289, 1980
22. Redding TW, Schally AV: Inhibition of prostate tumor growth in two rat models by chronic administration of D-Trp[6] analogue of luteinizing hormone-releasing hormone. Proc Natl Acad Sci USA 78:6509, 1981
23. Tolis G, Ackman D, Stellos A, Mehta A, Lubric F, Fazekas ATA, Comaru-Shally AM, Shally AV: Tumor growth inhibition in patients with prostatic carcinoma treated with luteinizing hormone-releasing hormone agonists. Proc Natl Acad Sci 79:1650, 1982
24. Ahmed SR, Brooman PJC, Shalet SM, Howell A, Blacklock NJ, Rickards D: Treatment of advanced prostatic cancer with LHRH analogue ICI 118630: Clinical response and hormonal mechanisms. Lancet 2:415, 1983
25. Walker KJ, Nicholson RI, et al: Therapeutic potential of the LHRH agonist, ICI 118630, in the treatment of advanced prostatic carcinoma. Lancet 2:413, 1983

26. Koutsilieris M, Tolis G: Gonadotropin-releasing hormone agonistic analogues in the treatment of advanced prostatic carcinoma. Prostate 4(6):569, 1983
27. Allen JM, O'Shea JP, Mashiter K, Williams G, Bloom SR: Advanced carcinoma of the prostate: treatment with a gonadotrophin-releasing hormone agonist. Br Med J 286:1607, 1983
28. Waxman JH, Wass JAH, et al: Treatment with gonadotrophin-releasing hormone analogue in advanced prostatic cancer. Br Med J 286:1309, 1983
29. Labrie F, Dupont A, et al: New approach in the treatment of prostate cancer: Complete instead of partial withdrawal of androgens. Prostate 4:579, 1983
30. Faure N, Lemay A, et al: Preliminary results on the clinical efficacy and safety of androgen inhibition by an LHRH agonist alone or combined with an antiandrogen in the treatment of prostatic carcinoma. Prostate 4:601, 1983
31. Borgman V, Hardt W, Schmidt-Gollwitzer M, Adenauer H, Nagel R: Sustained suppression of testosterone production by the luteinising-hormone releasing-hormone agonist Buserelin in patients with avanced prostate carcinoma: A new therapeutic approach? Preliminary Communication. Lancet ii:1097, 1982
32. Glode LM, Max D: Leuprolide (D-leu⁶-des gly¹⁰-pro⁹-NH Et-LHRH) in the therapy of advanced prostatic carcinoma. Proc 13th Intl Cong Chemotherapy 242:49, 1983
33. Borgmann V, Nagel R, Al-Abadi H, Schmidt-Gollwitzer M: Treatment of prostatic carcinoma with LHRH analogues. Prostate 4(6):533, 1983
34. Warner B, Worgul TJ, et al: Effect of very high dose D-leucine⁶-gonadotropin-releasing hormone proethylamide on the hypothalamic–pituitary–testicular axis in patients with prostatic cancer. J Clin Invest 71:1842, 1983
35. Dahlen HG, Keller E, Schneider HPG: Linear dose dependent LH release following intranasally sprayed LRH. Horm Metab Res 6:510, 1974
36. Schmidt JD, Scott WW, Gibbonst R, et al: Chemotherapy programs of the national prostatic cancer project. Cancer 45:1937, 1980
37. Hierowski MT, Altamirano P, Redding TW, Schally AV: The presence of LHRH-like receptors in Dunning R3327H prostate tumors. FEBS Lett 154(1):92, 1983
38. Schally AV, Redding TW, Comaru-Schally AM: Inhibition of prostate tumors by agonistic and antagonistic analogs of LH-RH. Prostate 4:545, 1983
39. Jacobi GH, Wenderoth UK: Gonadotropin-releasing hormone analogues for prostate cancer: Untoward side effects of high-dose regimens acquire a therapeutical dimension. Eur Urol 8:129, 1982
40. Hedlund PO, Gustafson H, Sjogren Sven: Cardiovascular complications to treatment of prostate cancer with estramustine phosphate (estracyt) or conventional estrogen. Scand J Urol Nephrol 55:103, 1980
41. Jacobo E, Schmidt JD, Weinstein SH, Flocks RH: Comparison of flutamide (SCH-13521) and diethylstilbestrol in untreated advanced prostatic cancer. Urology 8:231, 1976
42. Stoliar B, Albert DJ: SCH 13521 in the treatment of advanced carcinoma of the prostate. J Urol 111:803, 1974
43. Sogani PC, Whitmore, Jr WF: Experience with flutamide in previously untreated patients with advanced prostatic cancer. J Urol 122:640, 1979
44. Prout, Jr GR, Irwin, Jr RJ, Kliman B, Daly JJ, MacLaughlin RA, Griffin PA: Prostatic cancer and SCH-13521: II. Histological Alterations and the pituitary gonadal axis. J Urol 113:834, 1975
45. Narayana AS, Loening SA, Culp DA: Flutamide in the treatment of metastatic carcinoma of the prostate. Br J Urol 53:152, 1981
46. Geller J, Fishman J, Cantor TL: Effect of cyproterone acetate on clinical, endocrine

and pathological features of benign prostatic hypertrophy. J Steroid Biochem 6:837, 1975

47. Jacobi GH, Altwein JE, Kurth KH, Basting R, Hohenfellner R: Treatment of advanced prostatic cancer with parenteral cyproterone acetate: A phase III randomised trial. Br J Urol 52:208, 1980

48. Giuliani L, Pescatore D, Giberti C, Martorana G, Nata G: Treatment of advanced prostatic carcinoma with cyproterone acetate and orchiectomy—5-year follow-up. Eur Urol 6:145, 1980

49. Raynaud JP, Bonne C, Bouton MM, Lagage L, LaBrie F: Action of a non-steroidal antiandrogen, RU-23909, in peripheral and central tissues. J Steroid Biochem II:93, 1979

50. Geller J, Albert J, Yen SSC: Treatment of advanced cancer of prostate with megestrol acetate. Urology 12(5):537, 1978

51. Geller J, Albert JD: Comparison of various hormonal therapies for prostatic carcinoma. p. 12. Oncology, Highlights of a Symposium held in Monte Carlo, September 21, 1983

52. Rosenfield A, Maine D, Rochat R, Shelton J, Hatcher RA: The food and drug administration and medroxy-progesterone acetate. JAMA 249 (21):2922, 1983

53. Pavone-Macaluso M, Smith PH, Viggiano G, deVoogt H, et al: Updated revue of the studies of the EORTC urological group in prostatic cancer. Proc, 13th Intl Cong Chemo, 242:41, 1983

54. Huggins C, Scott WW: Bilateral adrenalectomy in prostatic cancer. Ann Surg 122:1031, 1965

55. Resnick MI, Grayhack JT: Treatment of stage IV carcinoma of the prostate. Urol Clin NA, 2(1):141, 1975

56. Worgal, TJ, Santen RJ, Samojlik E, Velhuis JD, Lipton A, Harvey HA, Drago JR, Rohner TJ: Clinical and biochemical effect of aminoglutethimide in the treatment of advanced prostatic carcinoma. J Urol 129:51, 1983

57. Robinson MRG, Shearer RJ, Fergusson JD: Adrenal suppression in the treatment of carcinoma of the prostate. Br J Urol 46:555, 1974

58. Walsh PC, Siteri PK: Suppression of plasma adrogens by spironolactone in castrated men with carcinoma of the prostate. J Urol 114, 254, 1975

59. Glick JH, Wein A, Padavic K, Negendank W, Harris D, Brodovsky H: Tamoxifen in refractory metastatic carcinoma of the prostate. Cancer Treat Rt 64(6–7):813, 1980

60. Coune A, Smith P: Clinical trial of 2-bromo-alpha-ergocryptine (NSC-169774) in human prostatic cancer. Cancer Chemotherapy Rt Part 1. 59(1):209, 1975

61. Jeromin L: The serum levels of testosterone and prolactin in patients with prostatic carcinoma treated with various doses of fostrolin and bromocriptin. Int Urol Nephrol 14(I):51, 1982

62. Alfthan O, Andersson L. Esposti PL, Fossa, SD, Gammelgaard PA, Gjores JE, Isacson S, Rasmussen F, Ruutu J, von Schreeb T, Setterberg G, Strandell P, Strindberg B: Cisobitan in treatment of prostatic cancer. Scand J Urol Nephrol 17:37, 1983

63. Cheung A, Driedger AA: Evaluation of radioactive phosphorus in the palliation of metastatic bone lesions from carcinoma of the breast and prostate. Radiology 134:209, 1980

64. Donati RM, Ellis H, Gallagher NI: Testosterone potentiated ^{32}P therapy in prostatic carcinoma. Cancer 19:1088, 1966

65. Fowler, Jr JE, Whitmore, Jr WF: Considerations for the use of testosterone with systemic chemotherapy in prostatic cancer. Cancer 49:1373, 1982

66. Suarez AJ, Lamm DL, Radwin HM, Sarosdy M, Clark G, Osborne CK: Androgen

priming and cytotoxic chemotherapy in advanced prostatic cancer. Cancer Chemotherapy Pharmacol 8:261, 1982

67. Mittelman A, Shukla SK, Murphy GP: Extended therapy of stage D carcinoma of the prostate with oral estramustine phosphate. J Urol 115:409, 1976

68. Murphy GP, Gibbons RP, Johnson DE, Loening SA, Prout GR, Schmidt JD, Bross DS, Ming Chu T, Gaeta JF, Saro J, Scott WW: A comparison of estramustine phosphate and streptozotocin in patients with advanced prostatic carcinoma who have had extensive radiation. J Urol 118:288, 1977

69. Kaufman JH, Hanjura GL, Mittelman A, Aungst CW, Murphy GP: Study of Leo-1031 (NSC-134087) in lymphocytic lymphoma and chronic lymphocytic leukemia. Cancer Treat Rt 60(3):277, 1976

70. Murphy P, Gibbons RP, Johnson DE, Prout GR, Schmidt JD, Soloway MS, Loening A, Chu TM, Gaeta JF, Saroff J, Wajsman Z, Slack N, Scott WW: The use of estramustine versus prednimustine alone in advanced metastatic prostactic cancer patients who have received prior irradiation. J Urol 121:763, 1979

71. Soloway MS, deKernion JB, Gibbons RP, et al: Comparison of estramustine phosphate and vincristine alone or in combination for patients with advanced hormone refractory, previously irradiated carcinoma of the prostate. J Urol 125:664, 1981

72. Soloway MS, Beckley S, Brady MF, Chu TM, et al: A comparison of estramustine phosphate versus *cis*-platinum alone versus estramustine phosphate plus *cis*-platinum in patients with advanced hormone refractory prostate cancer who had had extensive irradiation to the pelvis or lumbosacral area. J Urol 129:56, 1983

73. Murphy GP, Beckley S, Brady MF, et al: Treatment of newly diagnosed metastatic prostate cancer patients with chemotherapy agents in combination with hormones versus hormones alone. Cancer 51:1264, 1983

74. Gibbons RP, Beckley S, Brady MF, Chu TM, et al: The addition of chemotherapy to hormonal therapy for treatment of patients with metastatic carcinoma of the prostate. J Surg Oncol 23:133, 1983

75. Murphy GP, Slack NH, Participating Investigators: Chemotherapy clinical trials of the USA National Prostatic Cancer Project (NPCP). Proc, 13th Intl Cong Chemotherapy 242:18, 1983

9 | Chemotherapy in Prostate Cancer

Frank M. Torti
Bert L. Lum

Cancer of the prostate is the second leading cause of cancer and the third leading cause of cancer-related deaths among American males.[1-3] Only lung and colorectal cancers cause more deaths each year. It was estimated for 1982 that prostate cancer would account for 73,000 new cancer cases and 23,000 deaths.[2] Mortality associated with this disease is seldom observed under age 50, but it increases markedly with age.[4,5] Between 1950 and 1970, the reported incidence of prostate cancer increased from 17 to 21 per 100,000 population; this increase was predominantly observed in American nonwhites and possibly attributable to improvements in the availability of health care, screening, and diagnostic accuracy.[6] During approximately the same time period, the 25-year trend in age-adjusted cancer death rate per 100,000 population showed little change: 21.0 in 1951–1953 versus 22.6 in 1976–1978.[2] However, over a 20-year period, the five-year survival rate of prostate cancer increased from 30 to 59 percent; this probably reflects an increase in the diagnosis of occult lesions that have minimal lethal impact. When metastatic disease is present at diagnosis, the average survival is less than 3 years; this has not changed with time.[7,8]

It is recognized that mortality from prostate cancer seldom occurs before the age of 50, but the incidence of death from the disease increases dramatically with age.[4,5] Death rates from prostatic carcinoma show considerable international geographical variation. The age-adjusted mortality rate in 1974–1975 ranged from 0.1 per 100,000 population in Honduras, to 1 to 2 per 100,000 in Asian countries, and peaked at 22 per 100,000 in Sweden.[9] Whether this difference is due to genetic or environmental factors is speculative, although studies of Polish and Japanese immigrants to the United States suggest that environmental factors play an important role.[10-12]

125

Demographic factors also influence the incidence and mortality of prostate cancer. A striking feature of prostate cancer in the United States is the high incidence in the black population; a 50 percent higher incidence than for whites in areas where blacks make up the majority of the nonwhite population.[4] Data from the SEER program of the National Cancer Institute confirm this trend: the relative five-year survival for blacks is 54 versus 64 percent for the white population.[13] The prostate mortality rates of other ethnic groups in the United States also differ from the national average. For example, rates are lower for American Indians, Chinese-Americans, and Mexican-Americans.[14-16] Studies assessing the influence of socioeconomic class on prostate cancer morality rates have shown little association between lower social or economic status and increased rates in black or white populations.[4,6,17]

To date, no conclusive evidence associates prostate cancer and occupational exposures,[18-20] sexuality,[6,21-24] venereal disease,[17,25] benign prostatic hypertrophy,[26,27] high fat diets,[4,28-30] or viruses.[31-34]

In spite of these careful epidemiological studies, there has been little progress in understanding the etiology or prevention of prostatic cancer. This is in contrast to improved diagnostic methods, the elucidation of the natural history of the disease, and the development and evaluation of surgical techniques, radiation therapy and hormonal and cytotoxic drug therapy.

Prostate cancer therapy is in transition. Improved surgical techniques, new modalities of radiotherapy, and more effective chemotherapy have been introduced. Therapeutic options have increased, but so has the controversy about their appropriate application. This is, in part, due to an elderly population who suffer from other major medical problems that often preclude aggressive therapeutic approaches. Further, the biological spectrum of prostate cancer ranges from a pathological curiosity, with minimal lethal potential, to a rapidly progressive, fatal disease.

Until recently, the number and quality of chemotherapeutic trials in prostate cancer were limited. Few studies prior to 1973 were randomized comparisons, many were anecdotal case reports, and others reported limited numbers of patients from drug-oriented Phase II studies in which few of the specialized examinations required to evaluate patients with prostate cancer were performed. Recently, however, investigations that systematically evaluate the role of cytotoxic agents in prostatic carcinoma have been completed.

RESPONSE CRITERIA IN PROSTATIC CARCINOMA

In most solid tumors, response to chemotherapy is easily quantitated by measuring changes in tumor diameter clinically or radiographically. In prostate cancer, measurable disease in the lung, lymph nodes, and soft tissue is uncommon; bone remains the most common clinically apparent site of metastatic spread and the predominant site of symptomatic disease. The skeletal distribution of metastases makes accurate measurement of response difficult. This creates variability in response criteria and patient eligibility requirements for clinical trials. Further, prostatic carcinoma patients with bone metastasis are frequently excluded from drug-oriented phase II trials because bone is a "non-measurable" disease site.

Quantitation of the Primary Prostatic Tumor Nodule. Sequential digital examination of the prostate gland by the same observer may be a useful measure of disease activity and appears to parallel other measures of response. Occasionally, local response may occur during progression of bone disease.[35] The response of local disease may occur later than response in other disease sites; patients responding to hormonal therapy as evidenced by decreasing acid phosphatase level and bone pain may show little local tumor change at three months, but demonstrate continued improvement in nodule size between three and six months. Anatomical grids displaying the prostate gland in at least two axes are essential for quantitation of local response.

The use of rectal ultrasound in measuring changes in the local tumor have been moderately encouraging. This technique can accurately measure prostate volume and assess stage (periprostatic invasion and/or seminal vesicle involvement). Response to hormonal therapy has been monitored with ultrasonography with good results. However, the utility of this method in determining chemotherapeutic response or progression has been questioned.[36]

Acid Phosphatase. The acid phosphatases are lysosomal enzymes found in glandular epithelium and are present in many body fluids and tissues, including serum, red blood cells, spleen, liver, kidney, and bone, especially in osteoclasts. These enzymes hydrolyze orthophosphoric acid esters in acid environments. Per unit weight, prostatic tissue has 1,000 times the concentration of this enzyme than any other tissue, and malignant prostatic tissue has been demonstrated to have less measurable enzyme activity than normal prostate tissue.[37] The primary role of prostatic acid phosphatases appears to be extracellular; they supply phosphate and catalyze phosphate group activity in spermatozoa.[38] No major metabolic role in prostate cells has been recognized. Prostatic acid phosphatase (PAP) is heterogeneous, with at least two molecular variants (isoenzymes).[39] Most acid phosphatase-containing tissues have two or more isoenzymes.[37,38,40,41] Acid phosphatase level in the serum of healthy volunteers is primarily from enzyme contributed from red blood cells and platelets. Various substrates and enzyme inhibitors have been used to identify and quantitate enzyme activity attributable to the prostate, but prostatic acid phosphatase has not been shown to be more useful than serum acid phosphatase. Although serum acid phosphatase levels may be elevated by hemolysis of red cells and release of platelets during clotting and as a result of a number of malignant and nonmalignant diseases, Murphy et al.[42] found conventional serum acid phosphatase to be as useful as the more specific enzyme assay.

The degree of initial elevation of acid phosphatase has prognostic significance in most series. A comparison of patients with or without metastases, who present with elevated serum acid phosphatase at diagnosis, and patients with normal levels shows that patients with normal serum acid phosphatase levels live longer.[42,43] One exception to this was a study by Ishibe et al.,[44] in which degree of initial elevation of serum acid phosphatase did not correlate with survival following hormonal therapy.

Serum acid phosphatase, when elevated, parallels other measures of response, although imperfectly. Johnson et al.[45] demonstrated normalization of serum acid phosphatase correlated with pain relief and decreased tumor size; in this series, 17 of 91 patients achieved a 50 percent or greater reduction of tumor mass with chemotherapy. Of these 17 responders, 59 percent normalized their serum acid phosphatase levels. As a single-response parameter, the reduction or normalization of serum acid phosphatase level correlates with improved outcome in most series.[44,46,47]

The radioimmunoassay (RIA) method for serum acid phosphatase determinations appears to be a more sensitive diagnostic and screening tool than enzymatic assays, although its lack of specificity has been questioned.[48,49] The clinical utility of the RIA method for measuring response to treatment has been studied in a limited number of patients with encouraging results.[50,51]

Bone Scan. The inability to quantitate easily and accurately the status of disease metastatic to bone is a critical problem in investigative uro-oncology. Most patients with prostate cancer do not commonly have measurable disease by conventional criteria, and most present with bone metastases as the only clinical disease site. Those with measurable disease in soft tissue and other sites may not be characteristic of the general prostate cancer population.[52] Thus, confining clinical trials to this small subset of the population does not obviate the necessity of addressing response to disease in bone.

Bone scintigraphy is the most frequently used clinical procedure in nuclear medicine. The introduction of technetium-99 m radiolabeled phosphate and phosphonate compounds was particularly important in improving the sensitivity of scanning.[53,54] Development of the gamma camera and whole-body scanning devices greatly advanced the clinical utility of the technetium-99 m compounds.

Whole-body imaging is the best method for early detection of tumors metastatic to bone, especially for the osteoblastic lesions in breast and prostatic cancers.[55,56] Radionuclide scans rarely produce false negatives in patients with osseous metastases from prostate tumors. The bone scan is sensitive enough to detect bone lesions in patients with normal radiographic surveys and no elevation in alkaline or prostatic acid phosphatase levels.

Metastases to bone are unevaluable by conventional standards because bone scanning, as conventionally employed, is relatively insensitive to changes in disease activity. Further, almost one-half of the radiographs taken demonstrate increasing osteoblastic changes when the patient is responding unequivocally to treatment, presumably due to healing. These findings have spurred many investigators to recommend repeat scans at three- to six-month intervals.[52,57]

Various approaches to the standardization and quantification of changes on bone scan have been tested recently. In breast cancer, mapping systems in which percent abnormal bone can be estimated appear superior to visual inspection of scans.[52,58] With this system, progression may be identified early, although identification of a response early in treatment remains imperfect. A number of investigators have demonstrated that careful attention to quality-control procedures, including consistent technique and instrumentation, the use of soft tissue background on scans, and consistent counts per information density, improved qualitative judgment of such scans and demonstrated a close correlation with objective evidence of response, stabilization, or progression.[57] Preliminary observations in patients undergoing bone scans, with quantitated measurements of percent urinary excretion of radiolabeled dose administered and bone region (tumor) count rates, suggest that quantifiable and reproducible evidence of response, stabilization, or progression of metastatic bone disease may be possible.[59] Measures of bone turnover, such as that of hydroxypyroline, used in conjunction with other clinical findings, may be helpful in making clinical judgments of tumor response or progression on bone scan.[60] To date, however, there is no conclusive evidence that the extent of bone disease in prostate cancer can be quantitatively determined, nor that changes in the activity of disease can be measured in a way that is consistent and clinically useful.

Prognostic Factors. An additional problem in comparing the efficacy of chemotherapeutic agents in prostatic cancer is to what extent patient and tumor characteristics that influence the natural history of early disease also influence the course of patients undergoing chemotherapy. Although the median survival from diagnosis of metastatic disease is short (12 to 18 months, in most series), a group of patients (approximately 20 percent) survive with metastatic disease for five years or longer.[61] Thus, the biological potential of the individual tumors in the population should be kept in mind when chemotherapeutic trials are designed and assessed. Table 9-1 lists the factors that have been reported to affect response or survival in prostate cancer. Only the Veterans Administration Cooperative Urological Research Group (VACURG) have subjected these variables to multivariate analysis; thus, some factors may not predict an adverse outcome as an independent variable.[61-64] Furthermore, until the quality and duration of tumor response to

Table 9-1. Negative Prognostic Variables Affecting Response and/or Survival in Prostate Cancer

Variables	Group[a]	Therapeutic Modality Response Affected
Demographic		
Age	Duke, VACURG	Chemotherapy
Clinical Findings		
Progression versus presentation with stage D	Duke, VACURG	Hormonal
Urinary obstruction	VACURG	Hormonal, ? chemotherapy
Previous radiation therapy	Duke, ECOG,NPCP	± chemotherapy, ? hormonal
Performance status		Hormonal and chemotherapy
Severity of bone pain	Duke	Chemotherapy, ? hormonal
Weight gain	Duke	Chemotherapy, ? hormonal
Laboratory Findings		
Histological grade	VACURG, NPCP	Hormonal
Initial serum acid phosphatase	VACURG, Duke	Hormonal and chemotherapy
Initial alkaline phosphatase	Duke, VACURG	Chemotherapy, ? hormonal
Anemia	NPCP, VACURG	Hormonal and chemotherapy
Hypoalbumenemia	Duke	Chemotherapy, ? hormonal
Amount of disease on bone scan	Duke, VACURG	Hormonal, ? chemotherapy
Abnormal liver scan	Duke, NPCP	Hormonal and chemotherapy
Positive bone marrow biopsy	NPCP	Hormonal, ? chemotherapy
Pleural effusion	Duke	Chemotherapy, ? hormonal

[a] Duke, Duke Medical Center; ECOG, Eastern Cooperative Oncology Group; NPCP, National Prostatic Cancer Project; VACURG, Veterans Administration Cooperative Urologic Research Group.

therapy in prostatic cancer becomes so great that the prognostic variables are minimized, it is possible that the results of nonrandomized trials may relate more to prognostic factors than to efficacy of the drugs tested.

Partial Response and Stabilization Criteria. In addition to the technical difficulties in assessing response to treatment in prostate cancer, different investigators chose different response parameters in reporting their response data. Table 9-2 highlights the variability among investigators in defining partial response criteria. For example, the magnitude of change in acid phosphatase or alkaline phosphatase levels accepted as a response may dramatically affect the reported response rate. For example, Yagoda et al., at Memorial Sloan-Kettering Cancer Center,[65] found that applying different accepted response definitions could produce a 20 to 30 percent variability in response rate for the same group of patients treated with cisplatin at Memorial Hospital.

Table 9-2. Partial Response Criteria

Response Site	Investigator[a]						
	MSKCC	DUKE	NPCP	ECOG	SWOG	NCI-VA	NCOG
Tumor							
↓50% measurable area	X	X	X	X	X	X	X
↓75% in prostate nodule size	NS	NS	NS	NS	NS	NS	X
Complete resolution of ureteral obstruction, pleural effusion, or diffuse lymphangitic (interstitial) disease	NS	NS	NS	NS	NS	NS	X
Acid phosphatase							
Return to normal		X	X				
50% reduction	X			X	X	X	X
Alkaline phosphatase							
Return to normal		X	X				
50% reduction	NS			X	X	NS	X
Bone							
Recalcification of lytic bone lesions	NS	X	NS	NS	NS	NS	NS
Concomitant radiation for pain constitutes treatment failure	NS	NS	NS	No	Yes	NS	Yes
Functional status							
No significant decrease in weight	NS	X	X	NS	X	X	NS
Performance status must not decrease	NS	NS	NS	No	Yes	NS	Yes

[a] MSKCC, Memorial Sloan-Kettering Cancer Center; Duke, Duke Medical Center; NPCP, National Prostatic Cancer Project; ECOG, Eastern Cooperative Oncology Group; SWOG, Southwest Oncology Group; NCI–VA, National Cancer Institute–Veterans Administration Group; NCOG, Northern California Oncology Group; X, criteria used by investigator; NS, not specified or unknown.

Modified from Torti FM, Carter SK: The chemotherapy of prostatic carcinoma. Ann Intern Med 92:681, 1980.

Another controversial area in definition of response is the inclusion of stabilization of disease by some investigators as an indicator of tumor response. The inclusion of stabilization in response criteria derived from the necessity to measure the progression-free interval for the majority of prostate cancer patients who present without "measurable" disease. Investigators of the National Prostate Cancer Project (NPCP) demonstrated that survival of patients with stable disease was similar to that of partial responders.[35] However, it has been suggested that patients who stabilize may have slower growing tumors, that the apparent delayed progression is a function of an inherently slower growth rate, and that chemotherapy has little or no effect on these patients.[65] Differences in response criteria and the effect of including stabilization categories with response rates must be considered when data from different institutions are compared.

ANIMAL TUMOR MODELS

The search for effective chemotherapy is simplified by the availability of animal or other experimental model systems. These models facilitate the selection of drugs with reasonable therapeutic ratios. Although animal data may not always be directly extrapolated to man, animal models provide an opportunity to develop new therapeutic concepts quickly and at reasonable cost.

No single animal model of prostate cancer entirely parallels human tumors. This is not surprising, given the variable histology, biochemistry, and biological growth potential of human tumors. An ideal experimental animal for human prostatic cancer would develop tumors spontaneously with age, secrete acid phosphatase, have tumors with the same pathological characteristics as human tumors, biotransform testosterone to dihydrotestosterone via 5-alpha reductase, display tumor progression during testosterone administration, show tumor regression upon estrogen administration or castration, have tumors that metastasize to lymph nodes and bone, and in time, evolve into a hormonally unresponsive state.[66,67] More than one animal model is required, depending on which human prostatic cancer is being investigated. The most promising models, to date, appear to be the Dunning rat, Pollard (Wister) rat, and Noble (Nb) rat models. The characteristics of these prostatic tumor models are illustrated in Table 9-3.

Except for the predeliction to osseous metastases, animal tumors provide models for most biological characteristics of human prostate cancer. For example, the Dunning model is a hormonally responsive, well-differentiated adenocarcinoma that metabolizes testosterone via 5-alpha reductase and metastasizes. The Pollard model has characteristics similar to the Dunning model and also displays a highly predictable pattern of metastatic spread. The Nb model develops a variety of metastatic adenocarcinomas with either androgen-dependent or autonomous hormone responsiveness, which may be transplanted into athymic (immunosuppressesd) mice.[66-69]

The chemotherapeutic activity in these model systems is depicted in Tables 9-4 and 9-5. The limited data available thus far from animal tumor models suggest that these models may be used quickly and cost effectively to evaluate the potential

Table 9-3. Prostatic Tumor Models

Model	Animal Species	Histology	Metastatic Sites	Hormone Responsiveness	Other Characteristics
Dunning	Copenhagen-Fisher rats (spontaneous)	R3327 well-differentiated adenocarcinoma	Lymph nodes, lung, liver, peritoneal cavity (no bone)	Hormone responsive, metabolizes testosterone via 5-alpha reductase	Multiple sublines; slow growing; variety of histologies; transplantable; produces acid phosphatase; responds to chemotherapy
Pollard	Wistar rate (spontaneous)	Adenocarcinoma	Lymph nodes, lung, heart, kidneys	Hormone dependent	Predictable metastases; model for testing hormonal and chemotherapy
Noble	Nb (Noble) (hormone induced)	Adenocarcinoma	Lymph nodes, lung, liver, no bone	Hormone dependent and independent	Transplantable to nude mice. Tumors produce acid phosphatase. Androgen dependent, estrogen dependent, and autonomous cell lines reported. Similar in chemotherapeutic responsiveness to man

Table 9-4. Chemotherapeutic Activity in Prostatic Cancer Models

Model/Investigator	Inactive Agents[a]	Active Agents[a]
Pollard		
Pollard et al.[158]		Aspirin; indomethancin; *Corynebacterium parvum;* cyclophosphamide
Dunning		
Heston et al.[159]		ICRF-159
Kadman et al.[160]		ICRF-159
Block et al.[161]	L-asparaginase	Cisplatin
	CCNU	Cyclo
	Actinomycin-D	Cyclo + DES
		Cyclo + DOX; Cyclo + DOX + 5FU; DOX; hydroxyurea; 5FU
Mador et al.[162]	Misonidazole	Cisplatin; estramustine; etoposide (VP-16); vincristine

[a] Statistical significance in activity in relation to control group tumor volume.

[b] *Abbreviations/synonyms,* BCNU, carmustine; CCNU, lomustine; Cyclo, cyclophosphamide; DES, Diethylstilbestrol; DOX, Doxorubicin; 5FU, 5-fluorouracil; ICRF-159, razoxane; MTX, methotrexate.

chemotherapeutic activity of agents in prostatic cancer, that is, drugs found to have antitumor activity in these systems (e.g., cyclophosphamide, BCNU, doxorubicin, 5-fluorouracil, cisplatin, and methotrexate) also show activity in humans. However, agents without activity in these models (e.g., L-asparaginase, actinomycin-D, and CCNU) have had limited or no investigations in humans. Whether the predictions based on these animal models will be equaled or exceeded by in vitro test systems is also under investigation.[70]

GENERAL PRINCIPLES OF METASTATIC CANCER CHEMOTHERAPY

A number of therapeutic principles in the treatment of prostatic cancer are not common to most other neoplastic diseases. The current treatment approach at the multidisciplinary genitourinary oncology clinic at Stanford University Medical Center will be emphasized, so as to illustrate one approach to the standardization of conventional therapy in advanced prostatic disease (Fig. 9-1).

Patient Selection and Therapeutic Considerations. It is well known that the composition of the patient population entering chemotherapy programs influences the response, and thus the interpretation of results of the program. To date, all treatments of metastatic prostate cancer are palliative, and hence, most modalities will be considered for patients during the course of their disease.

Given the narrow risk-benefit margins for many therapeutic decisions, patient philosophy plays an important role in final recommendations. Our general treatment plan takes into account the data from the VACURG, which suggest that most

Table 9-5. Chemotherapeutic Activity in the Noble Prostate Cancer Model

Model/Investigator	Inactive Agents[a]	Active Agents[a]
NOBLE		
Drago et al.[163]: rat, androgen-dependent rat, autonomous	Actinomycin-D	Cyclo[b] >> 5FU > Dox BCNU[b] > cyclo[b] >> 5FU,DOX
Drago et al.[164]:		
2 Pr-129-D-11A, androgen-dependent, mice		5FU
Pr-90, autonomous, athymic mice	DOX	5FU > DOX
Drago et al.[165]:		
102 Pr, autonomous, mice and rats		5FU > Ftorafur
Drago et al.[166]:		
Pr-A.I-1, autonomous, rats	MTX	BCNU > cyclo > DOX
autonomous, mice	MTX	BCNU > cyclo > DOX
Drago et al.[167]:		
Pr-A.I-3, autonomous, rat		Cyclo[b] >> 5FU > MTX > DOX
Drago et al.[168]:		
Pr-90, autonomous, rat		Cyclo,[b] DOX, MTX
Drago et al.[69]:		
2-Pr-129, androgen-dependent, rat androgen-dependent, athymic mice		MTX[b] > DOX[b] >> BCNU[b] > 5FU[b] Cyclo[b] > 5FU
18-Pr, autonomous, rat autonomous, athymic mice		Cyclo[b] > MTX > DOX Cyclo[b] > DOX, 5FU
18-Pr, autonomous, rat	Actinomycin-D	Cyclo > 5FU > BCNU
18-Pr, autonomous, rat		MTX[b] + testosterone > DOX[b] + testosterone

13-Pr-12, autonomous, rat	Vincristine	BCNU > cisplatin > cyclo > 5FU > DTIC
13-Pr-12, autonomous, athymic mice 102-Pr, autonomous, rat and athymic mice	Actinomycin-D	Cyclo[b] > 5FU[b] > MTX > DOX BCNU
Drago et al.[169]:		
Pr-90, autonomous, athymic mice		5Fu > Ftorafur
13-Pr-12, autonomous, athymic mice	DOX	MTX > DOX
13-Pr-12, autonomous, athymic mice (large tumor volume)		MTX > Cyclo[b] Cyclo = MTX > 5FU > BCNU > DOX
Drago et al.[170]:		
A.I.1, autonomous, rat	DOX, DOX + cisplatin	Cyclo[b] > cyclo + cisplatin[b] > cyclo + cisplatin + DOX > cisplatin[c]
Pr A.I.2, autonomous, rat	DOX, Cisplatin, DOX + cisplatin	Cyclo[b] > cyclo + cisplatin > cyclo + cisplatin + DOX[c]
Drago et al.[171]:		
Pr A.I.3, autonomous, rat	Cisplatin, cyclo + cisplatin, DOX, DOX + cisplatin	DOX + cisplatin + cyclo > cyclo[b]
Drago et al.[172]:		
Pr-A.I.III, autonomous, rat	BCNU, DOX, BCNU + DOX, BCNU + 5FU + DOX	Cisplatin + cyclo + DOX > cyclo ≥ cyclo + cisplatin > cisplatin + DOX

[a] Relative activity in relation to statistical significance from control animal tumor volumes. (For drug abbreviations, see Table 9-4.)

[b] Capable of producing complete regression of tumors.

[c] No statistical significance between single agent and combinations.

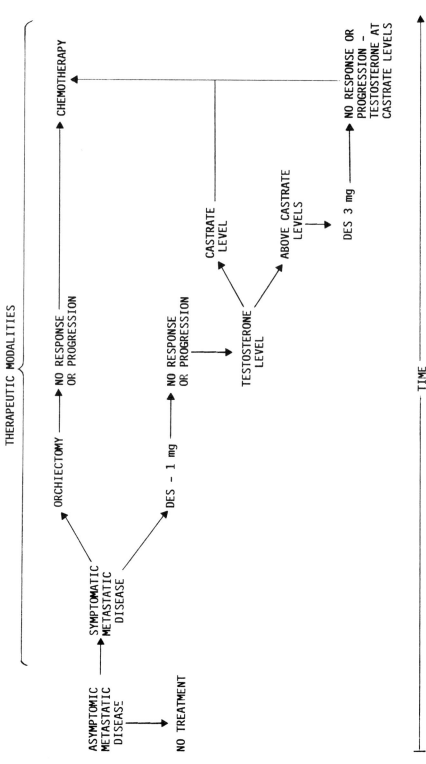

Fig. 9-1. Current treatment approach at Stanford University Medical Center for patients with metastatic prostate cancer to bone.

patients do not benefit by hormonal treatment of asymptomatic disease.[8,26,71] Choice of initial hormonal manipulation, orchiectomy, or estrogenic agents depends upon patient preferences and medical contraindications to estrogenic agents, as each maneuver produces approximately equal results.

The sequence of hormonal and chemotherapeutic maneuvers depends upon anticipated results and morbidity. The initial hormonal manipulation is likely to elicit a response in 60 to 70 percent of symptomatic patients. When estrogenic agents are used, a 1-mg diethylstilbestrol (DES) dose is prescribed, since there is excess morbidity and mortality with 5-mg doses. During DES therapy, serum testosterone and patient compliance is monitored. If castrate serum levels are not achieved, the dose is increased to 3 mg. Patients who have no response or progression at this dose are reassessed to ascertain compliance and testosterone levels. Patients who have no response or progression at castrate serum testosterone levels are next offered chemotherapy. Results are probably superior for chemotherapy in comparison to secondary hormonal maneuvers or other non-chemotherapeutic approaches.[72] Furthermore, prostate cancers may cease to respond to hormones, due to the heterogeneity of the tumor, which after hormone failure, contains mostly hormonally resistant cells.[73]

Palliative radiation therapy is used to delay systemic therapy when possible and is also routinely administered to the breast in low doses (e.g., 900 to 1,200 rads) in three or four daily treatments to reduce gynecomastia from estrogenic agents.[74] Decreasing intervals between effective palliative radiation treatments is a sign of disease progression and indicates a need for systemic therapy. Diffuse bone tenderness also indicates a need for systemic therapy. Patients with diffuse bone tenderness, with one or a few sites of symptomatic bone pain, in our experience, constitute a subset of patients in which a telescoping series of palliative treatments can be predicted; other symptomatic sites develop in such a short time span that systemic treatment is preferred to irradiation.

A number of chemotherapeutic agents have been shown to be active in the treatment of hormone-refractory prostatic carcinoma. In choosing an agent, one must be aware of concomitant disease states in the patient and weigh the potential risks and potential benefits of a particular treatment. For example, in patients with renal insufficiency, cisplatin or methotrexate are contraindicated; in patients with diabetes, streptozocin is contraindicated; in patients with cardiac disease, doxorubicin may be contraindicated; in patients with myelosuppression secondary to radiation therapy or extensive bone marrow involvement, an agent with minimal hematological toxicity is preferred.

Judgments about response should not, in general, be made before 12 weeks of treatment have been completed. Although not well studied, it appears that improvement in painful bone tumors usually occurs within six weeks in patients who have a response. However, many patients may also show short-term variability in painful lesions; and skeletal trauma, strains, etc., may transiently exacerbate pain in existing disease sites. Pain scores should be assessed to determine trends in pain status over a two- to three-month period so response or progression can be tracked. Changes in palpable local tumor are usually evident in three months; however, some patients may show a continued response for at least six months.

CHEMOTHERAPY IN PROSTATIC CARCINOMA: A HISTORICAL REVIEW

Before 1973, cytotoxic chemotherapy in the treatment of prostatic carcinoma was infrequently used and limited to small, nonrandomized comparisons. Many reports evaluated a limited number of patients from drug-oriented phase II studies, in which the patients with prostatic cancer usually were not adequately evaluated. The formation of the National Prostatic Cancer Project (NPCP) as a part of the Organ Site Program for Prostate Cancer, in 1973, marked the beginning of a number of large clinical chemotherapeutic trials, a necessary step in the systematic evaluation of drugs for prostatic cancer. Other national and regional cooperative groups and medical centers also began to place patients on randomized protocols.

In reviewing prostatic cancer chemotherapy trials performed before 1970, Yagoda[75] found over 50 studies in which 32 single agents or combinations were investigated; 18 of these displayed some activity. Nitrogen mustard was the first agent to show activity in prostate cancer patients.[76-78]

In 1959, Weyrauch and Nesbit[79] reported primary tumor regression in three of four patients receiving intraprostatic thio-tepa injections. Diphenylthiocarbazone, which chelates zinc, was the next drug studied. McDonald[80] found subjective improvement in three previously untreated patients. Activity with this drug was also reported by Lo,[81] who found objective improvement in 1 of 10 patients and subjective improvement in 4, and by MacKenzie[82] who reported subjective improvement in 5 of 21 patients. The 1960s were the "modern era" of cytotoxic cancer chemotherapeutic agents. Kofman and Eisenstein,[83] as well as Persky et al.,[84] reported objective as well as subjective activity with mithramycin. Cyclophosphamide was first used in 1965 by Fox: one of four patients had an objective response and two had subjective improvement.[85] In 1968, Flocks and Cheng[86] reported substantial activity with nitrogen mustard in combination with 5-fluorouracil. Table 9-6 lists the results achieved with cytotoxic chemotherapeutic agents prior to 1973.

Table 9-7 lists response rates for patients receiving single agent chemotherapy for metastatic prostatic carcinoma, in more recent studies. This table lists only patients undergoing chemotherapy following failure with at least one hormonal maneuver. Most of these patients had localized radiation therapy to areas of painful

Table 9-6. Cytotoxic Chemotherapeutic Results Achieved Prior to 1973

Agent	No. Treated	No. of Responses (%)
Alanine mustard	29	4 (14)
Cyclophosphamide	34	4 (12)
Diphenylthiocarbazone	39	1 (3)
5-Fluorouracil	39	10 (27)
Methotrexate	24	3 (13)
Mithramycin	21	1 (5)
Vincristine	12	1 (8)

Adapted from Torti FM: Prostatic cancer therapy. p. 58. In Torti FM (ed): Urologic Cancer: Chemotherapeutic Principles and Management RRCR Vol. 85. Springer-Verlag, Berlin/Heidelberg, 1983.

Table 9-7. Overall Response Rates for Single-Agent Chemotherapy of Hormone-Refractory Metastatic Prostatic Carcinoma

Agent	Stabilization included in response		Stabilization not included in response	
	Patients (*N*)	Response (%)	Patients (*N*)	Response (%)
Amsacrine (m-AMSA)	31	7 (23)	19	0 (0)
Cisplatin	101	25 (25)	87	15 (17)
Cyclophosphamide	136	52 (38)		
Dacarbazine (DTIC)	55	15 (27)		
Doxorubicin (adriamycin)	24	20 (84)	179	43 (24)
Estramustine	211	75 (26)	319	56 (18)
Etoposide (VP-16)			5	1 (20)
5-Fluorouracil	62	26 (42)	99	9 (9)
Hexamethylmelamine	14	7 (50)		
Hydroxyurea	33	7 (21)		
Lomustine (CCNU)	29	7 (24)	10	4 (40)
Melaphalan			15	1 (7)
Methotrexate	67	32 (48)		
Prednimustine	62	8 (13)	23	3 (13)
Procarbazine	39	5 (13)		
Semustine (methyl CCNU)	27	8 (30)		
Streptozocin	38	12 (32)		
Vincristine	34	5 (15)		

Modified from Torti FM, Carter SK: The chemotherapy of prostatic cancer. Ann Int Med 92:681, 1980.

osseous metastases prior to chemotherapy. Response rates are divided into those that include and those that exclude disease stabilization in assessment of tumor response to therapy. As discussed earlier, even this division suggests a homogeneity to partial response criteria that does not exist in prostate clinical trials (Table 9-2), nor is there standardization of dose and route of administration in the clinical trial protocols listed in Table 9-12. Nonetheless, cyclophosphamide, doxorubicin, and methotrexate, and perhaps estramustine, darcarbazine, and cisplatin, have activity in metastatic disease. Other agents, such as lomustine (CCNU), semustine (methyl-CCNU), amsacrine (*m*-AMSA), etoposide (VP-16), and hexamethylmelamine, have not been fully evaluated.

Cyclophosphamide. Cyclophosphamide has been tested in randomized trials against a number of single agents and combination chemotherapies. The first NPCP protocol randomized cyclophosphamide (1 g/m^2, IV, every three weeks) against 5-fluorouracil (5-FU) (600 mg/m^2, IV, every week) or standard therapy in hormone-unresponsive patients who had not received significant pelvic radiation therapy. Patients were well matched for prognostic variables (functional status, age, histological grade, etc.). Chemotherapy was superior to standard therapy in terms of objective response, pain relief, and time to progression. Survival in each treatment group was similar.[72]

Cyclophosphamide was the standard of comparison in subsequent NPCP protocols. It was next compared to dacarbazine (DTIC) (200 mg/m^2, IV, days 1 to 5) and procarbazine (100 mg/m^2, PO, days 1 to 22 and 44 to 65). Objective responses for the three agents by NPCP criteria were cyclophosphamide, 26 percent; DTIC, 28 percent; and procarbazine, 13 percent. Two DTIC crossovers to cyclo-

Table 9-8. Cyclophosphamide in Hormone-Refractory Metastatic Prostatic Carcinoma

Drug(s)	Group	No. of Patients	Response (%) Stabilization	Response (%) No Stabilization
Cyclophosphamide alone	See Table 9-7	136	38	
Cyclophosphamide in combination with:				
5-fluorouracil (5FU)	Roswell Park[173]	13	69	
5FU	Mayo[174]	18		11
5FU + methotrexate	Bowman Gray[88]	15	53	
5FU + methotrexate	Memorial Sloan-Kettering[175]	20	35	
Cisplatin + prednisone	Southern Alberta[176]	22	45	
5FU + cisplatin + estramustine	Roswell Park[102]	15		40

phosphamide responded. Toxicity precluded full doses and evaluation of procarbazine. The reason for the somewhat lower response rate to cyclophosphamide in this protocol is unexplained and might, in part, be due to patient selection.[87]

Cyclophosphamide was also compared in hormone-refractory patients to hydroxyurea (3 g/m², PO, every three days) and methyl-CCNU (semustine) (175 mg/m², PO, every six weeks). Cyclophosphamide, in this study, produced a lower objective response rate (35 percent) than in its first evaluation (46 percent), a marginal therapeutic advantage over methyl-CCNU, and a demonstrable advantage over hydroxyurea.

Table 9-8 lists response rates for cyclophosphamide alone and in combination with other chemotherapeutic agents. In nonrandomized trials, cyclophosphamide-containing combination chemotherapy appears to produce higher response rates than rates reported for cyclophosphamide alone. However, in the two randomized trials comparing cyclophosphamide alone to three-drug regimens containing cyclophosphamide, there were no significant differences in response or survival.[87a,88]

Doxorubicin. Although doxorubicin has been studied in a large number of prostatic cancer patients as a single agent and in combination chemotherapy regimens (Tables 9-9 and 9-12), there have been few randomized trials with this agent. A dose–response effect was observed with doxorubicin in prostatic carcinoma: The Southwest Oncology Group (SWOG) reported a 0 percent response rate in 5 good-risk patients receiving 45 mg/m² every three weeks, whereas 5 of 14 patients (36 percent) receiving doses of 60 or 75 mg/m² responded. None of 19 poor-risk patients (i.e., those with hematological suppression or elevated liver function tests) responded at doses of 25 or 50 mg/m².[89]

Table 9-9 lists multiple combination chemotherapeutic regimens that include doxorubicin. Response rates in these studies vary considerably. As with cyclophosphamide, response rates appear to be higher with combination chemotherapy regimens, but there is no definite superiority over single agent therapy. The Eastern Cooperative Oncology Group (ECOG) randomized doxorubicin (60 mg/m², IV, every three weeks) against 5-FU (600 mg/m², IV, every week). In 51 patients treated with 5-FU and 91 treated with doxorubicin, a response and a survival advantage was demonstrated for doxorubicin. Of patients with measurable disease, 25 percent responded to doxorubicin, whereas 7 percent responded to 5-FU.[90] The Mayo Clinic randomized single-agent doxorubicin (60 mg/m², IV, every three to four weeks) against the combination of 5-FU (300 mg/m², IV) plus cyclophosphamide (150 mg/m², IV, daily for five days every five weeks) and found no significant difference (Table 9-12).

Estramustine. Estramustine phosphate is an ester of nitrogen mustard and estradiol. This agent has been studied widely in Europe and to a somewhat lesser extent in the United States, where comparative trials have been primarily performed under the auspices of the NPCP. When used as first hormonal therapy, estramustine produces response rates similar to estrogens alone. At low doses, estramustine reduces serum testosterone.[91] In patients who fail initial hormonal therapy, response rates are variable, ranging from 20 to 50 percent[92-99,101] (Table 9-10).

Protocol 200 of the NPCP compared the nonhematological toxic agents estramustine (600 mg/m², PO, per day) and streptozocin (500 mg/m², IV, for five

Table 9-9. Doxorubicin in Hormone-Refractory Metastatic Prostatic Carcinoma

			Response (%)	
Drug(s)	Group	No. of Patients	Stabilization	No Stabilization
Doxorubicin alone	See Table 9-7	24 + 83	84	23
Doxorubicin in combinatin with:				
Cyclophosphamide	Roswell Park[173]	20	65	
Cyclophosphamide	Wayne State[177]	15	7	
Cyclophosphamide	NCI-VA[178]	22	50	32
Cisplatin	Mt. Sinai[179]	17		53
Cisplatin	Wisconsin[180]	25		24
Cyclophosphamide + 5FU	Western Group[87a]	12	50	
Cyclophosphamide + 5FU	Tennessee[181]	21	81	
Cyclophosphamide + 5FU	Southeastern Group[182]	29	69	
Cyclophosphamide + cisplatin	Wayne State[183]	16	63	
Cyclophosphamide + BCNU	Southeastern Group[184]	27		26
Cyclophosphamide + methotrexate	Boston[185]	12	75	
5FU + mitomycin C	Kasimis[186]	13	54	
5FU + mitomycin C	M. D. Anderson[187]	62		48
5FU + mitomycin C	Arkansas[188]	14	64	

days every six weeks) with standard therapy in hormone-refractory, metastatic stage D patients who had previously received more than 2,000 rads of radiation therapy to the pelvis. The objective response rates for the two agents were similar; 30 percent for estramustine and 32 percent for streptozocin, as compared to 19 percent for standard therapy. In the estramustine group, 7 percent achieved a partial response; in the streptozocin group, there were no partial responders. Re sponse duration was marginally longer for estramustine than for streptozocin (96 versus 81 weeks). Overall survival for the two agents were similar.[100]

Protocol 1100 of the NPCP randomized, hormone-refractory, metastatic prostatic carcinoma patients to single-agent cisplatin (60 mg/m², IV, days 1, 4, 21, 24, then every month), estramustine (600 mg/m², PO, per day), or methotrexate therapy (40 mg/m², day 1, 60 mg/m², day 8, then every week IV). Methotrexate, in this trial, had an objective response rate of 44 percent versus 28 percent each for estramustine and cisplatin. The authors noted that methotrexate response duration appeared longer than that for the other two agents, but this was not statistically

Table 9-10. Estramustine in Hormone-Refractory Metastatic Prostatic Carcinoma

			Response (%)	
Drug(s)	Group	No. of Patients	Stabilization	No Stabilization
Estramustine alone	See Table 9-7	211 + 319	36	18
Estramustine in combination with:				
Prednimustine	NPCP[104]	54	13	
Cisplatin	NPCP[105]	42	33	
Cisplatin + cyclophosphamide + 5FU	Roswell Park[102]	15		40
Cisplatin + methotrexate	Roswell Park[103]	9		44
Lomustine (CCNU)	Roswell Park[103]	21	5	
Vincristine	NPCP[189]	29	24	

significant. Median survival for the three treatment arms was also similar, although methotrexate-treated patients showed better survival rates during the longer follow-up period (45 to 80 weeks).[101]

In a nonrandomized combination chemotherapy trial, Beckley et al.[102] reported a 40 percent complete plus partial response rate in 15 hormone-refractory stage D patients treated with a combination of estramustine (600 mg/m²/day, PO), cyclophosphamide (500 mg/m², IV), 5-FU and cisplatin (50 mg/m², IV), with all intravenous drugs given every three weeks. Madejewicz et al.[103] reported four objective responses in nine patients receiving a combination of estramustine, cisplatin, and methotrexate.

Protocol 400 of the NPCP compared the combination of estramustine (600 mg/m², PO, daily) plus prednimustine (30 mg/m², PO, daily for six or seven days) to prednimustine alone. No advantage was noted with the combination therapy arm. No advantage was found in the NPCP protocol 800 with the addition of vincristine (1 mg/m², IV, every two weeks) to estramustine in hormonally unresponsive, stage D patients who had received extensive radiation therapy. The objective response rates were 26 percent for estramustine alone (4 percent partial responses), 24 percent for the combination (no partial responses), and 15 percent (3 percent partial responses) for vincristine.[104]

The NPCP protocol 1200 randomized hormone-refractory, previously irradiated, stage D patients to estramustine (600 mg/m², PO, daily), cisplatin (60 mg/m², IV, days 1 and 21, then every month), or a combination of the two agents. No complete or partial responses were observed in any treatment arm. The objective response rates were 33 percent for the combination of estramustine plus platinum, 21 percent for cisplatin alone, and 18 percent for estramustine. The differences between estramustine and the combination were not statistically significant, in terms of objective response, response duration, or survival.[105]

Cisplatin. Cisplatin has been utilized in hormone-refractory prostatic carcinoma with variable results. The therapeutic value of this agent should be carefully assessed and weighed against its toxicity, which includes, most notably, nephrotoxicity, ototoxicity, and gastrointestinal toxicity.

Early results with this agent were reported by Merrin,[106] with objective responses found in 13 of 45 patients (29 percent) and disease stabilization in an additional 6 patients. Cisplatin was administered at a 1 mg/kg, IV, dose for six weeks, then every three weeks until relapse. Yagoda et al.[65] treated only those patients with measurable tumor nodules and found a 12 percent (3 of 25) objective response rate. Depending upon the response criteria used, the same patients could be considered to have a response rate from 4 to 23 percent. The dose schedule employed by Yagoda was a 50 to 75 mg/m², IV, dose every three weeks. The ECOG utilized a lower dosage of cisplatin as compared to previous studies, 50 mg/kg every three weeks; no responses were noted in 18 hormone-refractory metastatic prostatic cancer patients.

The experience of the NPCP with cisplatin includes two studies previously discussed in detail. Some activity, but no advantage over estramustine, methotrexate, prednimustine, or the combination of estramustine plus prednimustine, has been demonstrated. Other combinations of agents with cisplatin have produced responses

Table 9-11. Cisplatin in Hormone-Refractory Metastatic Prostatic Carcinoma

Drug(s)	Group	No. of Patients	Response (%)	
			Stabilization	No Stabilization
Cisplatin alone	See Table 9-7	101 + 87	25	17
Cisplatin in combination with:				
Doxorubicin	Mt. Sinai[179]	17		53
Doxorubicin	Wisconsin[180]	25		24
Doxorubicin + cyclophosphamide	Wayne State[183]	16	63	
Cyclophosphamide + prednisone	Southern Alberta[176]	22	45	
Estramustine	NPCP[105]	42	33	
Cyclophosphamide + 5FU + estramustine	Roswell Park[102]	15		40
Estramustine + methotrexate	Roswell Park[103]	9		44

Table 9-12. Randomized Trials of Single Agents versus Combination Chemotherapy in Hormone-Refractory Metastatic Prostatic Carcinoma

Treatment A	Treatment B	Treatment C	Group	Conclusions
Doxorubicin	5FU + Cyclophosphamide		Mayo[174]	No difference
5-Fluorouracil	Cyclophosphamide + 5FU + doxorubicin		Southeastern Oncology Group[182]	No difference
Cyclophosphamide	Cyclophosphamide + 5FU + doxorubicin		Western Group[87]	No difference
Cyclophosphamide	Cyclophosphamide + 5FU + methotrexate		Bowman Gray[88]	No difference
Prednimustine	Prednimustine + estramustine		NPCP[104]	No difference
Lomustine	Cyclophosphamide + 5FU + methotrexate		Memorial Sloan-Kettering[175]	No survival difference
Estramustine	Vincristine	Estramustine + vincristine	NPCP[189]	No difference
Estramustine	Cisplatin	Estramustine + cisplatin	NPCP[105]	Ongoing study, no statistical difference

in the range of 45 to 63 percent (including stabilization) or 24 to 53 percent (using response criteria excluding stabilization) (Table 9-11).

Studies of cisplatin thus far have shown variable response rates. The therapeutic utility of cisplatin in advanced hormone-refractory prostatic carcinoma is still uncertain, since few randomized comparisons of this agent to other active cytotoxic chemotherapeutic agents have been completed (Table 9-12).

NEW APPROACHES TO CHEMOTHERAPY FOR PROSTATIC CARCINOMA

Adjuvant Chemotherapy

Adjuvant chemotherapy, the administration of cytotoxic agents following such definitive therapy as radiation and/or surgery, is frequently used in the treatment of breast cancer, Wilms' tumor, Ewings sarcoma, rhadbomyosarcoma, and osteosarcoma. Investigations of adjuvant chemotherapy of prostatic carcinoma have been limited.

DeVere White et al.,[107] at Boston University, found that 37 of 112 patients had positive lymph nodes at lymphadenectomy (stage D1). These 37 patients received prostatic radiation. Twelve patients also received adjuvant chemotherapy consisting of cyclophosphamide 750 mg/m^2, IV, plus doxorubicin 50 mg/m^2, IV, every three weeks. In the 12 patients receiving chemotherapy, 4 (33 percent) had disease progression as compared to 12 of 25 (48 percent) of the untreated group. Median time to progression was 15 months in the chemotherapy group versus 11.6 months in the untreated group.

The NPCP is also studying the role of adjuvant chemotherapy. In protocol 900, patients are randomized to cyclophosphamide, estramustine, or to no treatment following total prostatectomy/cryosurgery plus lymph node dissection or lymphography and needle biopsy. In NPCP protocol 1000, patients received definitive radiation therapy before randomization to cyclophosphamide or estramustine.[108] Results of these trials are not yet available.

Chemohormonal Therapy

The concomitant administration of hormonal agents plus chemotherapy in patients as first treatment for advanced disease is based on two observations: (1) Chemotherapy is usually more effective when administered early in the course of the patient's disease and (2) prostate tumors are probably heterogeneous, with both hormone-sensitive and -insensitive cells. Thus, combined chemotherapy and hormonal therapy would have activity against both cell populations. To date, limited data are available on the use of chemohormonal therapy in previously untreated metastatic prostatic carcinoma.

Merrin reported on 34 patients treated with orchiectomy plus DES plus cisplatin.[109] A partial objective response rate was noted in 22 of 34 patients (65 percent), stabilization in 6 (18 percent), and subjective responses in another 5 (15 percent). The length of the objective responses was 9.3 months (range, 3 to 29 months). Compared to other studies in hormone-refractory patients, the authors felt that early therapy appeared to provide some benefit; the objective responses rate was better with early therapy, 64 versus 29 percent, and the mean response was longer with early therapy, 9.3 months versus 6 months.

Beckley et al.,[102] at Roswell Park, also reported results with combined therapy in stage D patients with no prior therapy. The treatment regimen used was a combination of oral estramustine (600 mg/m² daily) plus cisplatin (50 mg/m²), 5-FU (500 mg/m²), and cyclophosphamide (500 mg/m²), all given intravenously every three weeks. All ten previously untreated patients responded to therapy, with 70 percent of patients achieving partial responses and 30 percent stabilizations; in a hormone-refractory group of 15 patients receiving the same treatment, 40 percent achieved a complete or partial response, and 6 percent disease stabilization.

Benson et al.[110] randomized 153 previously untreated patients to DES (3 mg/day) or estramustine (15 mg/kg daily). At the first objective evaluation, 33 percent (26 of 79) DES patients and 24 percent (18 of 74) estramustine patients had progressive disease. The median time to progression was 868 days for estramustine versus 515 for DES. In a similar study reported by Smith,[110b] 21 percent of estramustine patients as compared to 12 percent of a DES-treated group had progressive disease.

Servadio et al.[111] reported on 24 patients with stage D disease treated with a combination of orchiectomy, DES (3 mg/day), cyclophosphamide (10 mg/kg), and 5-FU (10 mg/kg) given every three weeks intravenously. Of these patients (20 of 24), 83 percent had a partial response in the prostate; another 17 percent had a less than partial response locally; and 79 percent had a partial disappearance or stabilization of disease on bone scan. Two complete responders on bone scan had disease recurrence in bone three to three and one-half years later, and in 83 percent, elevated acid phosphatases returned to normal. All patients presenting with urinary obstruction had resolution of symptoms. They concluded that survival of 63.5 percent at five years is encouraging, compared to the reported survival rates for patients receiving hormonal therapy alone.

Ihde et al., in 1981,[112] reported on an early chemotherapy regimen consisting of cisplatin, doxorubicin, and cyclophosphamide in 17 patients who had no prior hormonal therapy. Partial responses were achieved in 41 percent and disease stabilization in 29 percent. The median response duration in partial responders was eight months.

The NPCP protocol 500 randomized 301 previously untreated, stage D patients who received DES (3 mg/day or orchiectomy, DES (3 mg/day DES, PO), plus cyclophosphamide (1 g/m², IV, every three weeks), or cyclophosphamide plus estramustine (600 mg/m² daily PO). Objective complete plus partial responses were noted in 41 percent of the DES/orchiectomy-treated patients, 34 percent of the DES plus cyclophosphamide group, and 25 percent of the estramustine plus cyclophosphamide group. Disease stabilization was 40 percent, 55 percent, and 57 percent, respectively. There were no significant differences in response, response duration, or survival among the three arms. The authors felt that the addition of chemotherapy to hormonal therapy increased both overall survival and response in patients initially presenting with painful bone lesions.[113]

Although many of the studies utilizing chemohormonal therapy in previously untreated, stage D patients with prostatic carcinoma have produced encouraging results, the largest randomized study to date (NPCP protocol 500) showed no advantage of chemohormonal therapy over hormonal therapy. Further study of other chemohormonal combinations on an investigational basis is warranted. Given the excellent symptomatic response with conventional hormonal therapy, it is still questionable whether chemohormonal therapy or chemotherapy alone has a role in treating asymptomatic, stage D prostatic cancer.

Intraarterial Chemotherapy

Intraarterial (IA) infusion chemotherapy has been studied in patients with localized tumors in the belief that this technique will increase drug delivery to the infused area at a higher drug concentration than achievable by intravenous administration, and simultaneously decrease the amount of drug reaching the systemic circulation, thus enhancing tumor cell kill and minimizing systemic toxicities.[114,115] Limited clinical data exist to demonstrate any substantial benefits for IA chemotherapy over the traditional IV route.[114] Recently, encouraging results have been achieved with continuous IA infusions in metastatic colon cancer to the liver.[116] In urologic malignancies, intraarterial chemotherapy has had promising results in the treatment of bladder cancer. In Japan, IA chemotherapy with doxorubicin has produced complete response rates of 54 percent of bladder cancer patients in studies with limited numbers of patients.[117-119] In the United States, combined IA and IV drug administration in bladder cancer led to overall response rates from 50 to 58 percent, with complete responses in 37 to 40 percent of patients.[120-122]

Drug penetration into the prostate, a common problem in the treatment of chronic bacterial prostatitis, is less important in acute prostatitis, as increased vascular permeability allows adequate drug penetration.[123] Little is known about the clinical importance and penetratability of antineoplastic agents into normal or malignant prostatic tissue. In animal models, doxorubicin and methotrexate penetrate prostatic tissue, whereas mitomycin-C does not. In these models, a four-fold increase in prostatic drug concentration was noted for doxorubicin when given IA as compared to IV.[124] Few data are available for human prostatic drug levels. Ono et al.,[125] in Japan, determined doxorubicin tissue levels following a 60-mg IV dose: 4.66 mcg/g in the prostate, 13.35 mcg/g in the renal cortex, 12.71 mcg/g in the renal medulla, 7.5 mcg/g in bladder tumor, 7.27 mcg/g in lymph nodes, 3.25 mcg/g in bladder mucosa, 3.03 mcg/g in the urethral wall, and 2.66 mcg/g in the bladder wall.

There are only a few reports of carefully evaluated IA chemotherapy in prostatic carcinoma. Nevin and Hoffman[126] treated hormone-refractory patients with IA 5-FU alone, or with doxorubicin or bleomycin. In five patients who failed estrogen and radiation therapy and who later received IA chemotherapy, three had survival times of 40 months or longer. In 16 patients with hormone-refractory tumors receiving IA chemotherapy followed by radiation therapy, 8 had a complete response in local tumor.

Kato et al. reported treating nine hormone-refractory patients with IA transcatheter embolization with ethylcellulose microencapsulated mitomycin-C. A partial response was noted in six of eight evaluable cases.[127]

The results of these IA studies are encouraging in terms of the potential for control or local tumor in the prostate and, perhaps, local lymph nodes. Further investigation of IA chemotherapy for localized disease (stages B2 to D1) is warranted.

Androgen Priming

The limited effectiveness of chemotherapy in prostatic carcinoma might be partially explained on a tumor-cell kinetics basis. Prostatic tumors are frequently indolent and often progress slowly; the doubling time may be as long as 30 days, which reflects a long cell generation time, small growth fraction, and a slow cellular death rate. This small growth fraction may be further reduced by the large tumor volume extant when chemotherapy is considered, which traditionally is after hormonal failure and/or palliative radiation therapy.[128] Tumors with small growth fractions are relatively resistant to cell cycle phase-specific cytotoxic agents; thus, cell kill could theoretically be enhanced by increasing tumor cell replication or by synchronizing tumor cells into a phase of the cell cycle during which a particular drug is active.[129-131]

Experimental evidence in animal models suggests that testosterone rapidly increases prostatic DNA synthesis to at least pre-castrate levels.[73,132] However, symptomatology from androgen stimulation, that is, bone pain, anorexia, and elevated acid phosphatase levels, may reflect an increased metabolic activity of tumor cells rather than sudden proliferation.[133]

Androgen priming is not new to prostatic cancer therapy; it has been used before in radioactive phosphorous (^{32}P) therapy.[134-140] Overall, in studies reviewed by Fowler and Whitmore, approximately 90 percent of patients experience unfavorable subjective and/or objective responses, with the majority experiencing bone pain. In one study, a serious irreversible morbidity was reported in 7 percent of patients, five of whom later died.[141]

The use of androgen priming with chemotherapy has been limited to a study at the University of Texas,[142] in which 21 patients (18 hormone-refractory) were treated with the androgen fluoxymesterone (5 mg, PO, twice daily, days 1 to 4) and cyclophosphamide (600 mg/m², IV) and methotrexate (40 mg/m², IV), both on day 3. Of these patients, 43 percent responded to therapy; this included one (5 percent) complete response, three (14 percent) partial responses, and disease stabilization in five (24 percent). Possible androgen-related toxicities included one case of acute psychosis, one case of spinal cord compression, and increased bone pain in 50 percent of patients. The overall response rate in this study is quite similar to that of cyclophosphamide alone or in combination with other agents (Tables 9-8 and 9-12). The authors suggested that cell kinetic studies be performed to better define the effects of androgen administration before further clinical studies were undertaken.

Biological Response Modifiers

The few animal studies of prostatic cancer that have been performed have produced conflicting results in the evaluation of immunotherapy. In one study, *Corynebacterium parvum* immunotherapy was shown to be beneficial; in another study, specific immunotherapy with irradiated tumor cells was not beneficial; but some slight benefit was shown with to the interferon-inducer pyran copolymer.[143,144]

Specific active immunotherapy utilizing transurethral cryodestruction of the prostate to induce antibody production against prostatic antigens was reported by Soanes et al.[145] In their study, three patients had tumor regression, which included an improved bone scan in one patient and a decrease in soft tissue disease in two patients. Gursel et al. found little objective evidence of disease regression in 11 patients receiving transperineal cryotherapy. Of 10 patients, only 1 had an improved bone scan, and 8 experienced pain relief.[146]

Nonspecific immunotherapy with BCG has been studied by a few investigators in prostatic cancer. Merrin et al. injected BCG intraprostatically in seven stage D patients. Five of the seven had objective responses, defined as a 50 percent reduction in tumor size. However, no change was noted in measurable metastatic disease. One patient receiving an intratumoral injection to a metastatic lesion showed tumor necrosis. The clinical condition improved in one patient, stabilized in two, and progressed in four.[147]

Robinson et al. reported two trials utilizing intraprostatic BCG injections. The first trial consisted of six hormone-refractory patients; four experienced improvement of urinary obstruction and general medical status, but there was no postmortem evidence of tumor necrosis.[148] In the second trial, eight hormone-refractory patients were treated with intraprostatic BCG injections; all patients developed treatment-related complications of gastrointestinal bleeding, fever, and granulomas in organs.

Guinan et al.[149] randomized 42 stage D patients to BCG plus conventional therapy or conventional therapy alone. There were no significant differences between groups in regards to age, treatment with hormones, tumor grade, hemoglobin, performance status, or acid phosphatase levels. There was a significantly longer survival in the BCG-treated group (38 weeks versus 28 weeks; $p < 0.05$), as well as a significantly reduced infection rate.

Although promising initial results in other urologic tumors have been obtained with interferon, no systematic study in prostatic cancer has been reported.[150,151]

Immunotherapy for carcinoma of the prostate has not been fully evaluated in well-designed phase I, II, and III studies. Results obtained thus far provide little evidence of a substantial therapeutic benefit. Well-controlled trials should be performed to identify the activity of biological response modifiers in low- and high-tumor volume prostatic cancers.

Retinoids

Retinoids are a family of molecules that are made up of the natural and synthetic analogues of retinol (vitamin A). This class of compounds are important in the control of cellular differentiation and cellular proliferation. In experimental animal models, retinoids have shown the ability to suppress or reverse the carcinogenic process. In in vitro systems, the ability to suppress development of malignant phenotypes and to act on fully transformed, invasive, neoplastic cells to suppress proliferation and terminal differentiation of cells to a more benign, non-neoplastic phenotype has been demonstrated.[152] One cell type affected by retinoids is the epithelial cell in such organs as the bronchi and trachea, stomach, intestine, uterus, kidney, bladder, testis, pancreatic duct, and skin.

In animal bladder cancer models, retinoids significantly inhibit pre-neoplastic and neoplastic bladder lesions.[153] In prostatic cancer, in vitro cell culture experimentation has shown that retinoids can arrest or reverse the progression of carcinogen-induced lesions in prostatic epithelium.[154,155]

Systematic study of retinoids in human prostatic carcinoma have not been reported. One patient with prostatic cancer in a phase I trial of retinol had a short (2-month) response in terms of reduced bone pain and lowered acid phosphatase levels.[156]

Retinoids appear to be a promising avenue of study in the chemoprevention or treatment of low stage prostatic carcinoma. Because as the etiology and predisposing factors of prostatic carcinoma remain unclear, identification of patients for chemoprevention trials will be difficult.

CONCLUSIONS

When compared to other solid tumors, the quality and quantity of data available on the chemotherapy of prostatic carcinoma are limited. The prostate cancer population tends to make a poor patient population for the study of chemotherapy; these patients are usually elderly, they have been treated previously with one or more hormonal therapies, they are usually anemic, and they often are not ambulatory. Thus, clinical trials in this group are difficult, and dramatic responses unusual. Measurable disease is infrequently present and consequently judgments on efficacy are difficult. This has prompted some investigators to avoid studying this disease and has led others to express undue pessimism or optimism about the role of cytotoxic chemotherapy. Nonetheless, the problem of patients with poorly controlled bone pain refractory to hormonal therapy is compelling.

Modest advances have been made recently in our understanding of some of the epidemiological and biological determinants of prostatic cancer and in the identification of a number of active drugs for palliation of advanced disease. These agents include cisplatin, cyclophosphamide, dacarbazine, doxorubicin, estramustine, and methotrexate. A number of other drugs with promising activity require verification in larger numbers of patients. As yet, there is no convincing evidence for the superiority of combination chemotherapy over single agents in response rate, response duration, or survival. Investigations with chemohormonal therapy or chemotherapy prior to hormonal therapy have thus far shown no demonstrable differences from hormonal treatment (DES/orchiectomy) alone. Further study of these approaches is warranted to define the role of chemohormonal therapy in early stage D disease.

Further evaluation of the therapeutic value of biological response modifiers is needed, as well as tests of the activity of newer approaches, such as intraarterial chemotherapy, adjuvant chemotherapy, and chemotherapy or chemoprevention with retinoids.

The role of chemotherapy in prostatic carcinoma is still not clearly defined; we feel that cytotoxic chemotherapy is still experimental in this disease. Patients should be encouraged to enter clinical trials that will further define the use and timing of chemotherapeutic agents in prostatic carcinoma.

REFERENCES

1. Enstrom, JE, Auston DF: Interpreting cancer survival rates. Science 195:847, 1977
2. Cancer Facts and Figures 1982. American Cancer Society, New York, 1981
3. Third National Cancer Survey: Advanced three year report (DHEW Publication No. NIH 74 637) National Institutes of Health, Bethesda, Maryland, 1974
4. Blair A, Fraumeni JF: Geographic patterns of prostate cancer in the United States, J Natl Cancer Inst 61:1379, 1978
5. Franks LM: Etiology, epidemiology and pathology of prostatic cancer. Cancer 32:1092, 1973
6. Ernster VL, Selvin S, Sacks ST, Austin DF, Brown SM, Winkelstein W: Prostatic cancer: Mortality and incidence rates by race and social class. Am J Epidemiol 107:311, 1978
7. Nesbit RM, Plumb RT: Prostatic carcinoma: A follow-up on 795 patients treated prior to the endocrine era and a comparison of survival rates between these and patients treated by endocrine therapy. Surgery 20:263, 1946
8. Veterans Administration Cooperative Urological Research Group: Treatment and survival of patients with cancer of the prostate. Surg Gynecol Obstet 124:1011, 1967
9. Silverberg E: Cancer statistics 1980. CA 30:23, 1980
10. Staszewski J, Haenszel W: Cancer mortality among Polish-born in the United States. J Natl Cancer Inst 35:219, 1965
11. Haenszel W, Kurihara M: Studies of Japanese immigrants. I. Mortality from cancer and other diseases among Japanese in the U.S. J Natl Cancer Inst 40:43, 1968
12. Dunn JE: Cancer epidemiology in populations of the United States—with emphasis on Hawaii and California—and Japan. Cancer Res 35:3240, 1975
13. Ries LG, Pollack ES, Young JL: Cancer patient survival: Surveillance, epidemiology, and end results program, 1973–79. J Natl Cancer Inst 70:693, 1983
14. Creagen ET, Fraumeni JF: Cancer mortality among American Indians, 1950–1967. J Natl Cancer Inst 49:959, 1972
15. Menck HR, Henderson BE, Pike MC, Mack T, Martin SP, SooHoo J: Cancer incidence in the Mexican–American. J Natl Cancer Inst 55:531, 1975
16. Fraumeni JF, Mason TJ: Cancer mortality among Chinese–Americans, 1950–1969, J Natl Cancer Inst 52:659, 1974

17. Wynder EL, Mabuchi K, Whitmore WF: Epidemiology of cancer of the prostate. Cancer 28:344, 1971
18. Lemen RA, Lee JS, Wagoner JK, Blejer HP: Cancer mortality among cadmium production workers. Ann NY Acad Sci 217:273, 1976
19. Kolonel L, Winkelstein W: Cadmium and prostatic carcinoma. Lancet ii; 556, 1977
20. Ross RK, McCurtis JW, Henderson BE, Menck HR, Mack TM, Martin SP: Descriptive epidemiology of testicular and prostatic cancer in Los Angeles. Br J Cancer 39:284, 1979
21. Greenwald P, Damon A, Kirmss V, Polan AK: Physical and demographic features of men before developing cancer of the prostate. J Natl Cancer Inst 53:341, 1974
22. Greenwald P, Kirmss V, Burnett WS: Prostate cancer epidemiology: Widowerhood and cancer in spouses. J Natl Cancer Inst 62:1131, 1979
23. Hutchinson GB: Epidemiology of prostatic cancer. Semin Oncol 3:151, 1976
24. Rotkin ID: Studies in the epidemiology of prostate cancer: Expanded sampling. Cancer Treat Rt 61:173, 1977
25. Heshmat MY, Kovi J, Herson J, Jones GW, Jackson MA: Epidemiologic association between gonorrhea and prostatic carcinoma. Urology 6:457, 1975
26. Greenwald P, Kirmss V, Polan AK, Dick VS: Cancer of the prostate among men with benign prostatic hyperplasia. J Natl Cancer Inst 53:335, 1974
27. Armenian HK, Lilienfeld AB, Diamond EL, Bross IDJ: Relation between benign prostatic hyperplasia and cancer of the prostate. Lancet ii:115, 1974
28. Graham S, Haughey B, Marshall J, Priore R, Byers T, Rzepka T, Mettlin C, Pontes JE: Diet in the epidemiology of carcinoma of the prostate gland. J Natl Cancer Inst 70:687, 1983
29. Reddy BS, Cohen LA, McCoy GD, Hill P, Weisburger JH, Wynder EL: Nutrition and its relationship to cancer. Adv Cancer Res 32:237, 1980
30. Cole P, Cramer D: Diet and cancer of endocrine target organs. Cancer 40:434, 1977
31. Rapp F, Geder L, Murasko D, Lausch R, Ladda R, Huang ES, Webber M: Long-term persistence of cytomegalovirus genome in cultured human cells of prostatic orign. J Virol 16:982, 1975
32. Sanford EJ, Geder L, Laychock A, Rohner TJ, Rapp F: Evidence for the association of cytomegalovirus with carcinoma of the prostate. J Urol 118:789, 1977
33. Geder L, Rapp F: Herpes virus and prostate carcinogenesis. Arch Androl 4:71, 1980
34. Domochowski L, Ohtsuki Y, Seman G, et al: Search for oncogenic viruses in human prostate cancer. Cancer Treat Rpt 61:119, 1977
35. Slack MH, Mittleman A, Brady MF, Murphy GP: The importance of the stable category for chemotherapy treated patients with advanced and relapsing prostate cancer. Cancer 46:2393, 1980
36. Resnick MI: Noninvasive techniques in evaluating patients with carcinoma of the prostate. Urology (suppl) 18:25, 1981
37. Yam LT: Clinical significance of the human acid phosphatases: A review. Am J Med 56:604, 1974
38. Bodansky O: Acid phosphatase. Adv Clin Chem 15:43, 1972
39. Smith JK, Lolutby LK: The heterogeneity of prostatic acid phosphatase. Biochem Biophys Acta 151:607, 1968
40. Foti AG, Herschman H, Cooper JF: Isoenzymes of acid phosphatase in normal and cancerous human prostatic tissue. Cancer Res 37:4120, 1977
41. Lam KW, Li O, Li CY, Yam LT: Biochemical properties of human prostatic acid phosphatase. Clin Chem 19:483, 1973
42. Murphy GP, Reynoso G, Kenny GM, Gaeta JF: Comparison of total and prostatic

fraction serum acid phosphatase levels in patients with differentiated and undifferentiated prostatic carcinoma. Cancer 23:1309, 1969

43. Nesbit RM, Baum WC, Mich AA: Serum phosphatase determination in diagnosis of prostatic cancer. A review of 1150 cases. JAMA 145:1321, 1951

44. Ishibe T, Usui T, Nihira H: Prognostic usefulness of serum acid phosphatase levels in carcinoma of the prostate. J Urol 112:237, 1974

45. Johnson DE, Scott WW, Gibbons RP, Prout GR, Schmidt JD, Murphy GP: Clinical significance of serum acid phosphatase levels in advanced prostatic carcinoma. Urology 8:123, 1976

46. Byar DP: Treatment of prostatic cancer: studies by the Veterans Administration Cooperative Urological Research Group (VACURG) Bull NY Acad Med 48:751, 1972

47. Citrin DL, Elson P, DeWys WD: Treatment of metastatic prostate cancer—an analysis of response criteria in patients with measurable soft tissue disease. Proc Am Soc Clin Oncol 2:142, 1983

48. Bruce AW, Mahan DE: The role of prostatic acid phosphatase in the investigation and treatment of adenocarcinoma of the prostate. Ann NY Acad Sci 390:110, 1982

49. Mahan DE, Doctor BP: A radioimmune assay for human prostatic acid phosphatase levels in prostatic disease. Clin Biochem 12:10, 1979

50. Vihko P, Lukkarinen O, Kontturi M, Vihko R: Effectiveness of radioimmunoassay of human prostate-specific acid phosphatase in the diagnosis and follow-up of therapy in prostatic carcinoma. Cancer Res 41:1180, 1981

51. Moon TD, Vessella RL, Eickhoff M, Lange PH: Acid phosphatase for monitoring prostatic carcinoma. Comparison of radioimmunoassay and enzymatic techniques. Urology 22:16, 1983

52. Citrin DL, Hougen C, Zweibel W, Schlise S, Pruitt B, Ershler W, Davis TE, Harberg J, Cohen AI: The use of serial bone scans in assessing response of bone metastases to systemic treatment. Cancer 47:680, 1981

53. Subramaniam G, McAfee JG, Bell EG, Blair RJ, O'Mara RE: 99m-TC labeled polyphosphates a skeletal imaging agent. Radiology 102:701, 1972

54. Yano Y, McRae J, VanDyke DC, Anger HO: Technetium-99m-labeled stannous ethane-1-hydroxy-1, 1-diphosphonate: a new bone scanning agent. J Nucl Med 14:73, 1973

55. Pistenma DA, McDougall IR, Kriss JP: Screening for bone metastasis. Are scans necessary? JAMA 231:46, 1975

56. Shafer RB, Reinke DB: Contribution of the bone scan, serum acid and alkaline phosphatase, and the radiographic bone survey to the management of newly diagnosed carcinoma of the prostate. Clin Nucl Med 2:200, 1977

57. Pollen JJ, Gerber K, Ashburn WL, Schmidt JD: Nuclear bone imaging in metastatic cancer of the prostate. Cancer 47:2585, 1981

58. Galasko CSB, Doyle FM: The response to therapy of skeletal metastases from mammary cancer: assessment of scintigraphy. Br J Surg 59:85, 1972

59. Martin B, Goodwin D, Shortliffe L, Torti FM: Measurement of response or progression of bone metastases in prostate cancer using a method for quantitative bone scanning. Proc Am Soc Clin Oncol 2:136, 1983

60. Mooppan MMV, Wax SH, Kim H, Wang JC, Tobin MS: Urinary hydroxypyroline excretion as a marker of osseous metastasis in carcinoma of the prostate. J Urol 123:694, 1980

61. Bayard S, Greenberg R, Showalter D, Byar D: Comparison of treatments for prostatic cancer using an exponential-type life model relating survival to concomitant information. Cancer Chemotherapy Rt 58:845, 1974

62. Byar DP: VACURG studies on prostatic cancer and its treatment. p. 241. In Tannenbaum M (ed): Urologic Pathology: The Prostate, Lea & Febiger, Philadelphia, 1977
63. Byar DP: Survival of patients with incidentally found microscopic cancer of the prostate: Results of a clinical trial of conservative treatment. J Urol 108:903, 1972
64. Byar DP: The Veterans Administration Cooperative Urological Research Group's studies of cancer of the prostate. Cancer 32:1126, 1973
65. Yagoda A, Watson RC, Natale RB, Barzell W, Sogani P, Grabstald H, Whitmore WF: A critical analysis of response criteria in patients with prostatic cancer treated with cis-diamminedichloride platinum II. Cancer 44:1553, 1979
66. Coffey DS, Isaacs JT: Requirements for an idealized animal model of prostatic cancer. Prog Clin Biol Res 37:379, 1980
67. Sandberg AA, Gaunt R: Model systems for studies of prostatic cancer. Semin Oncology 3:177, 1976
68. Javadpour N (ed): Recent Advances in Urologic Cancer. p. 123. Williams & Wilkins, Baltimore, 1982
69. Drago JR, Goldman LB, Gershwin ME: Chemotherapeutic and hormonal considerations of the Nb rat prostatic adenocarcinoma model. Prog Clin Biol Res 37:325, 1980
70. Sarosdy MF, Lamm DL, Radwin HM, von Hoff DD: Clonogenic assay and in vitro chemosensitivity testing of human urologic malignancies. Cancer 50:1332, 1982
71. Veterans Administration Cooperative Urological Research Group: Carcinoma of the prostate: treatment comparisons. J Urol 98:516, 1967
72. Scott WW, Gibbons RP, Johnson DE, Prout GR, Jr., Schmidt JD, Saroff J, Murphy GP: The continued evaluation of the effects of chemotherapy in patients with advanced carcinoma of the prostate. J Urol 116:211, 1976
73. Isaacs JT: Hormonally responsive versus unresponsive progression of prostatic cancer to antiandrogen therapy as studied with the Dunning R-3327-AT and -G rat adenocarcinomas. Cancer Res 42:5010, 1982
74. Gagnon JF, Moss WT, Stevens KR: Pre-estrogen breast irradiation for patients with carcinoma of the prostate: A critical review. J Urol 121:182, 1979
75. Yagoda A: Non-hormonal cytotoxic agents in the treatment of prostatic adenocarcinoma. Cancer 32:1131, 1973
76. Berger M, Buu-Hoi NP: Treatment of prostatic cancer with alpha-bromo-alpha,BB-triphenylethylene (Y59). Lancet ii:172, 1947
77. Karnofsky DA, Abelman WH, Crarer LF, Burchenal JH: The use of nitrogen mustard in the palliative treatment of carcinoma. Cancer 1:634, 1949
78. Ariel IM, Kanter L: Nitrogen mustard therapy: Clinical studies on the effects of methyl-bis-(beta chloroethyl)amine hydrochloride upon various types of neoplastic disease. Am J Surg 77:509, 1949
79. Weyrauch HM, Nesbet JD: Use of triethylene thio-phosphoramide (thio-TEPA) in the treatment of advanced carcinoma of the prostate. J Urol 81:185, 1959
80. McDonald DF: Effect of diphenyl-thiocarbazone on prostates of animals and in human prostatic cancer. J Urol 83:458, 1960
81. Lo MC: Clinical application of diphenylthiocarbazone (dithizone) in carcinoma of the prostate. Canad Med Assoc J 82:1203, 1960
82. MacKenzie AR, Bhisitkul IP, Whitmore WF, Jr: The treatment of metastatic prostate cancer with dithizone (diphenylthio-carbazone). Invest Urol 1:229, 1963
83. Kofman S, Eisenstein R: Mithramycin in the treatment of disseminated cancer. Cancer Chemother Rt 32:77, 1963

84. Persky L, Guerrier K, Rabin R, Albert DJ: Mithramycin and metastatic carcinoma of the prostate. J Urol 104:884, 1970

85. Fox M: The effect of cyclophosphamide on some urinary tract tumors. Br J Urol 37:399, 1965

86. Flocks RH, Cheng S-F: Combination therapy for prostatic carcinoma with special emphasis on the role of chemotherapy. J Iowa Med Soc 58:125, 1968

87. Schmidt JD, Scott WW, Gibbons RP, Johnson DE, Prout GR, Leoning SA, Soloway MS, Chu TM, Gaeta JF, Slack NH, Saroff J, Murphy GP: Comparison of procarbazine, imidazol-carboxamide and cyclophosphamide in relapsing patients with advanced carcinoma of the prostate. J Urol 121:185, 1979

87a. Chlebowski RT, Hestorff R, Sardoff L, Weiner J, Bateman JR: Cyclophosphamide (NSC-26271) versus the combination of adriamycin NSC-123127), 5-fluorouracil (NSC-19893) and cyclophosphamide in the treatment of metastatic prostatic cancer. A randomized trial. Cancer 42:2546, 1978

88. Muss HB, Howard V, Richards F, White DR, Jackson DV, Cooper MR, Stuart JJ, Resnick MI, Brodkin R, Spurr CL: Cyclophosphamide versus cyclophosphamide, methotrexate, and 5-fluorouracil in advanced prostate cancer. Cancer 47:1949, 1981

89. O'Bryan RM, Baker LH, Gottlieb, et al: Dose response evaluation of adriamycin in human neoplasia. Cancer 39:1940, 1977

90. DeWys, WD, Begg CB, Brodovsky H, et al: A comparative trial of adriamycin and 5-fluorouracil in advanced prostatic cancer: Prognostic factors and response. Prostate 4:1, 1983

91. Fritjofsson A, Norlen BJ, Hogberg R, Rajalakshmi M, Cckan SZ, Diczfalusy E: Hormonal effects of different doses of estramustine phosphate (Estracyt) in patients with prostatic carcinoma. Scand J Urol Nephrol 15:37, 1981

92. Andersson L, Edsmyr F, Jonsson G, Konyves I: Estramustine phosphate therapy in carcinoma of the prostate. Rec Res Cancer Res 60:73, 1977

93. Fossa SD, Miller A: Treatment of advanced carcinoma of the prostate with estramustine phosphate. J Urol 115:406, 1976

94. Lindberg B: Treatment of rapidly progressing prostatic carcinoma with estracyt. J Urol 108:303, 1972

95. Nilsson T, Jonsson G: Clinical results with estramustine phosphate (NSC-89199): A comparison of the intravenous and oral preparations. Cancer Chemotherapy Rt 59:229, 1975

96. Mittelman A, Shukla SK, Welvaart K, Murphy GP: Oral estramustine phosphate (NSC-89199) in the treatment of advanced (stage D) carcinoma of the prostate. Cancer Chemotherapy Rt 59:219, 1975

97. Mittelman A, Shukla, Murphy GP: Extended therapy of stage D carcinoma of the prostate with oral estramustine phosphate. J Urol 115:409, 1976

98. Nagel R, Kollin SP: Treatment of advanced carcinoma of the prostate with estracyt. p. 267. In Marberger H (ed): Prostatic Disease, Liss, New York, 1976

99. Nagel R, Kollin CP: Treatment of advanced carcinoma of the prostate with estramustine phosphate. Br J Urol 49:73, 1977

100. Murphy GP, Gibbons KP, Johnson DE, Leoning SA, Prout GR, Schmidt JD, Bross DS, Chu TM, Gaeta JF, Saroff J, Scott WW: A comparison of estramustine phosphate and streptozotocin in patients with advanced prostatic carcinoma who have had extensive irradiation. J Urol 118:288, 1977

101. Loening SA, Beckley S, Brady MF, Chut M, DeKernion JB, Dhauwala C, Gaeta JF, Gibbons RP, McKiel CF, McLeod DG, Pontes JE, Prout GR, Scardino PT, Schlegel JV, Schmidt JD, Scott WW, Slack NH, Soloway MS, Murphy GP: Comparison

of estramustine phosphate, methotrexate, and cisplatinum in patients with advanced, hormone refractory prostate cancer. J Urol 129:1001, 1983

102. Beckley S, Wajsman Z, Maeso E, Pontes E, Murphy G: Estramustine phosphate with multiple cytotoxic agents in treatment of advanced prostatic cancer. Urology 18:592, 1981

103. Madejewicz S, Catane R, Mittelman A, Wajsman Z, Murphy GP: Chemotherapy of advanced hormonally resistant prostatic carcinoma. Oncology 37:53, 1980

104. Murphy GP, Gibbons RP, Johnson DE, Prout GR, Schmidt JD, Soloway MS, Leoning SA, Chu TM, et al: The use of estramustine and prednimustine versus prednimustine alone in advanced metastatic prostate cancer patients who have received prior irradiation. J Urol 121:763, 1979

105. Soloway MS, Beckley S, Brady MF, Chu TM, deKernion JB, Dhabuwala C, Gaeta JF, Gibbons RP, Loening SA, McKiel AF, McLeod DG, Pontes JE, Prout GR, et al: A comparison of estramustine phosphate versus cisplatinum alone versus estramustine phosphate plus cisplatinum in patients with advanced hormone refractory prostate cancer who had extensive irradiation to the pelvis or lumbosacral area. J Urol 129:56, 1983

106. Merrin CE: Treatment of previously untreated (by hormonal manipulation) stage D adenocarcinoma of the prostate with combined orchiectomy, estrogen, and cisdiamine-dichlorophatinum. Urology 15:123, 1980

107. de Vere White R, Paulson DF, Glenn JF: The clinical spectum of prostate cancer. J Urol 117:323, 1977

108. Loening S, Narayana A: Adjuvant chemotherapy to definitive treatment of prostate cancer. Prostate 1:321, 1980

109. Merrin C: Treatment of advanced carcinoma of the prostate (stage D) with infusion of *cis*-diamminedichlorophatinum II (NSC-119875): A pilot study. J Urol 119:522, 1978

110. Benson RC, Gill GM, Cummings KB: A randomized double blind cross-over trial of diethylstilbestrol (DES) and estramustine phosphate (Emcyt) for D prostatic carcinoma. Presented at the American Urological Association 77th Annual Meeting, Kansas City, 1982

110b. Smith PH: Endocrine and cytotoxic therapy. Rec Res Cancer Res 78:154, 1981

111. Servadio C, Mukamel E, Lurie H, Nissenkorn I: Early combined hormonal and chemotherapy for metastatic prostatic carcinoma. Urology 21:493, 1983

112. Ihde DC, Bunn PA, Cohen MH, Eddy JL, Dunnick NR, Bensimon H, Javadpour N, Minna JD: Combination chemotherapy as initial treatment for stage D-2 prostatic cancer: Response rate and results of subsequent hormonal therapy. Proc Am Assoc Cancer Res 22:163, 1981

113. Murphy GP, Beckley S, Brady MF, Chu TM, DeKernion JB, Dhabuwala C, Gaeta JF, Gibbins RP, Leoning SA, McKiel CF, McLeod DG, Pontes JE, Prout GR, Scardino PT, Schlegel JU, Schmidt JD, Scott WW, Slack NH, Soloway MS: Treatment of new diagnosed metastatic prostate cancer patients with chemotherapy agents in combination with hormones versus hormones alone. Cancer 51:1264, 1983

114. Chen HS, Gross JF: Intra-arterial infusion of anticancer drugs: Theoretical aspects of drug delivery and review of responses. Cancer Treat Rt 64:31, 1980

115. Eckman WW, Patlak CS, Fenstermacher JD: A critical evaluation of the principles governing the advantages of intra-arterial infusions. J Pharmacokinet Biopharm 2:257, 1974

116. Ensminger W, Niederhuber J, Gyves J, Thrall J, Cozzi E, Doan K: Effective control

of liver metastases from colon cancer with an implanted system for hepatic arterial chemotherapy. Proc Am Soc Clin Oncol 1:94, 1982

117. Iguchi M, Matsuura T, Minami K, Kurita T: Evaluation of superselective intra-arterial administration therapy with adriamycin against bladder cancer. Presented at the First Conference on Treatment of Urinary Tract Tumors with Adriamycin. Tokyo, Japan, May 12, 1979

118. Uyama T, Moriwaki S: Treatment of cancers of the urinary organ by intra-arterial infusion of Adriamycin. Presented at the First Conference on Treatment of Urinary Tract Tumors with Adriamycin, Tokyo, Japan, May 1979

119. Kanoh S, Umeyama T, Nemoto S, Ishikawa S, Nemoto R, Rinsho K, Yazaki T, Koiso K, Takahashi S, Kitagawa R: Long term intra-arterial infusion chemotherapy with adriamycin for advanced bladder cancer. Cancer Chemother Pharmacol 11(suppl):S51, 1983

120. Logothetis CJ, Samuels ML: Combined intra-arterial and intravenous chemotherapy with cytoxan, adriamycin and cisplatin (CISCA) for the unresectable urothelial tumors. Proc Am Soc Clin Oncol 2:136, 1983

121. Logothetis CJ, Samuels ML, Wallace S, Chuang V, Trindade A, Grant C, Haynie TP, Johnson DE: Management of pelvic complications of malignant urothelial tumors with combined intra-arterial and IV chemotherapy. Cancer Treat Rep 66:1501, 1982

122. Wallace S, Chuang VP, Samuels M, Johnson D: Transcatheter intra-arterial infusion of chemotherapy in advanced bladder cancer. Cancer 49:640, 1982

123. Ristuccia AM, Cunha BA: Current concepts in antimicrobial therapy of prostatis. Urology 20:338, 1982

124. Schmidbauer CP, Porpaczy P, Georgopoulos A, Rameis H, Endler TA: Pharmacokinetics of antitumor drugs in renal and prostatic interstitial fluid after intravenous and intra-arterial application—an experimental model. Proceedings of the 13th International Cancer Congress, Seattle, Washington, September 1982 (Abstract)

125. Ono H, Nakano H, Hiromoto N, Nihira H: Fundamental and clinical studies of adriamycin on urinary tract cancer. I. Studies on concentration of Adriamycin in serum, urinary tract tissues, and tumor tissues. Presented at the First Conference on Treatment of Urinary Tract Tumors with Adriamycin. Tokyo, Japan, 1979, p. 77

126. Nevin JE, Hoffman AA: Use of arterial infusion of 5-fluorouracil either alone or in combination with supervoltage radiation as a treatment for carcinoma of the prostate and bladder. Am J Surg 130:544, 1975

127. Kato T, Mori H, Abe R, Shindo M, Nemoto R: Transcatheter microembolization for hormone resistant prostatic carcinoma. Presented at the American Urological Association 77th Annual Meeting, May 1982, Kansas City, Missouri

128. Schmidt JD: Chemotherapy of prostatic cancer. Urol Clin North America 2:185, 1975

129. Drewinko B, Patchen M, Yang LY, Barlogie B: Differential killing efficacy of twenty antitumor drugs on proliferating and non-proliferating human tumor cells. Cancer Res 41:2328, 1981

130. Valeriote F, Van Putten L: Proliferative dependent cytotoxicity of anticancer agents: a review. Cancer Res 53:2619, 1975

131. DeWys WD: A quantitative model for the study of the growth and treatment of a tumor and its metastases with correlation between proliferative state and sensitivity to cyclophosphamide. Cancer Res 32:367, 1972

132. Sufrin G, Coffey DS: A new model for studying the effect of drugs on prostatic growth. I. Antiandrogens and DNA synthesis. Invest Urol 11:45, 1973

133. Robson MC, Schirmer HKA, Scott WW: The effect of varying dosages of testosterone on the prostate gland of the rat. Invest Urol 3:10, 1965

134. Donati RM, Ellis H, Gallagher NI: Testosterone potentiated P-32 therapy in prostatic carcinoma. Cancer 19:1088, 1966

135. Edland RW: Testosterone potentiated radiophosphorous therapy of osseous metastases in prostate cancer. Am J Roent Rad Ther Nucl Med 120:678, 1974

136. Johnson DE, Haynie TP: Phosphorous-32 for intractable pain in carcinoma of the prostate. Urology 9:137, 1977

137. Joshi DP, Seery WH, Goldberg LG, Goldman L: Evaluation of phosphorous-32 for intractable pain secondary to prostatic carcinoma metastases. JAMA 193:151, 1965

138. Morales A, Connolly JG, Burr RC, Bruce AW: The use of radioactive phosphorous to treat bone pain in metastatic carcinoma of the prostate. Canad Med Assoc J 103:372, 1970

139. Morin LJ, Stevens JD: Radioactive phosphorous in the treatment of metastasis to bone from carcinoma of the prostate. J Urol 97:130, 1967

140. Parsons RL, Campbell JL, Thomley MW: Experiences with P-32 in the treatment of metastatic carcinoma of the prostate: A follow-up report. J Urol 88:812, 1962

141. Fowler JE Jr, Whitmore WF Jr.: Considerations for the use of testosterone with systemic chemotherapy in prostatic cancer. Cancer 49:1373, 1982

142. Suarez AJ, Lamm DL, Radwin HM, Sarosdy M, Clark G, Osborne CK: Androgen priming and cytotoxic chemotherapy in advanced prostatic cancer. Cancer Chemother Pharmacol 8:261, 1982

143. Pollard M, Chang CF, Burleson GR: Investigations on prostate adenocarcinomas in rats. Cancer Treat Rt 61:153, 1977

144. Weissman RM, Coffey DS, Scott WW: Cell kinetic studies of prostatic cancer: Adjuvant therapy in animal models. Oncology 34:133, 1977

145. Soanes WA, Ablin RJ, Gouder MJ: Remission of metastatic lesions following cryosurgery in prostatic cancer. J Urol 104:154, 1970

146. Gursel EO, Roberts M, Veenema RJ: Regression of prostatic cancer following sequential cryotherapy in the prostate. J Urol 108:928, 1972

147. Merrin C, Han T, Klein E, Wajsman Z, Murphy GP: Immunotherapy of prostatic carcinoma with *Bacillus Calmette-Guerin.* Cancer Treat Rt 59:157, 1975

148. Robinson MRG, Rigby CC, Pugh RCB, Dumonde DC: Adjuvant immunotherapy with BCG in carcinoma of the prostate. Br J Urol 49:221, 1977

149. Guinan P, Toronchi E, Shaw M, Crispin R, Sharifi R: *Bacillus Calmette-Guerin* (BCG) adjuvant therapy in stage D prostate cancer. Urology 20:401, 1982

150. Ikic D, Nola P, Maricic Z, Smudj K, Oresic V, Knezevic M, Rode B, Jusic D, Soos E: Application of human leukocyte interferon in patients with urinary bladder papillomatosis, breast cancer and melanoma. Lancet i:1022, 1981

151. Quesada JR, Swanson DA, Trindale A, Gutterman JV: Renal cell carcinoma: Antitumor effects of leukocyte interferon. Cancer Res 43:940, 1983

152. Sporn MB, Roberts AB: Role of retinoids in differentiation and carcinogenesis. Cancer Res 43:3034, 1983

153. Lum BL: Intravesical chemotherapy of supeficial bladder cancer. p. 3. In Torti FM (ed): Urologic Cancer: Chemotherapeutic Principles and Management. (RRCR Vol. 85). Springer-Verlag, Berlin/Heidelberg, 1983

154. Chopra DP, Wilkoff LJ: Inhibition and reversal of carcinogen-induced lesions in mouse prostate in vitro by all trans-retinoic acid. Proc Am Assoc Cancer Res 16:35, 1975

155. Lasnitzki I: The influence of A hypervitaminosis on the effect of 20-methyl cholanthrene on mouse prostate glands grown in vitro. Br J Cancer 9:434, 1955

156. Goodman GE, Alberts DS, Meyskeus F, Peng YM, Beadry J, Leigh S, Chang SY:

Pharmacokinetics and phase I trial of retinol in cancer patients. Proc Am Assoc Cancer Res 23:129, 1983

157. Torti FM, Carter SK: The chemotherapy of prostatic carcinoma. Ann Int Med 92:681, 1980

158. Pollard M, Luckert PH: Chemotherapy of metastatic prostate adenocarcinomas in germ free rats. I. Effects of cyclophosphamide (NSC-26271). Cancer Treat Rt 60:619, 1976

159. Heston WDW, Kadmon D, Fair WR: Effect of high dose diethylstilbestrol and ICRF-159 on the growth and metastases of the R3327 MAT-LYLU prostate derived tumor. Cancer Lett 13:139, 1981

160. Kadmon D, Heston WDW, Fair WR: Effect of surgery and adjuvant chemotherapy on the R-3327 MAT-LYLU tumor. Prostate 2:299, 1981

161. Block NL, Camuzzi F, Denefrio J, Troner M, Claflin A, Stover B, Politano VA: Chemotherapy of the transplantable adenocarcinoma (R-3327) of the Copenhagen rat. Oncology 34:110, 1977

162. Mador D, Richie B, Meeker B, Moore R, Elliot FG, McPhee MS, Chapman JD, Lakey H: Response of the Dunning R3327H prostatic adenocarcinoma to radiation and various chemotherapeutic drugs. Cancer Treat Rt 66:1837, 1982

163. Drago JR, Gershwin ME, Goldman LB: Prostate adenocarcinoma model: Nb rat chemotherapy. Surg Forum 30:558, 1979

164. Drago JR, Maurer RE, Gershwin ME, Eckels D, Palmer JM: The effect of 5-fluorouracil and adriamycin on heterotransplantation of Noble rat prostatic tumors in congenitally athymic (nude) mice. Cancer 44:424, 1979

165. Drago JR, Maurer RE, Goldman LB, Gershwin ME: Immunobiology and therapeutic manipulation of heterotransplanted Nb rat prostatic adenocarcinoma. Cancer Chemother Pharmacol 3:167, 1979

166. Drago JR, Goldman LB, Gershwin ME: Chemotherapy and radiation of Nb rat prostatic adenocarcinoma: Nb Pr-A.I-1. J Surg Res 28:492, 1980

167. Drago JR, Goldman L, Gershwin ME: Evaluation of chemotherapeutic responsiveness in Nb rat prostate cancer model. Invest Urol 18:80, 1980

168. Drago JR, Goldman LB: Evaluation of nonhormonal cytotoxic chemotherapy in the Nb rat (Pr-90) prostatic carcinoma. Cancer 45:757, 1980

169. Drago JR, Gershwin ME: Heterotransplantation of Nb rat prostatic adenocarcinomas into congenitally athymic nude mice: Chemotherapy of autonomous tumors. Cancer 47:55, 1981

170. Drago JR, Worgul T, Gershwin ME: Combination chemotherapy in a prostate tumor model: Nb rat prostatic adenocarcinoma model. J Surg Oncol 16:353, 1981

171. Drago JR, Worgul T: Treatment of Nb-Pr-A.I.-3 (autonomous) tumor with combination chemotherapy. Cancer Chemother Pharmacol 5:163, 1981

172. Drago JR: Chemotherapeutic treatment of the Nb rat adenocarcinoma androgen-insensitive tumor. J Surg Oncol 21:264, 1982

173. Merrin C, Etra W, Wajsman Z, Baumgartner G, Murphy G: Chemotherapy of advanced carcinoma of the prostate with 5-fluorouracil, cyclophosphamide and adriamycin. J Urol 115:86, 1976

174. Eagan RT, Hahn RG, Myers RP: Adriamycin (NSC-123127) versus 5-floruouracil (NSC-19893) and cyclophosphamide (NSC-26271) in the treatment of metastatic prostate cancer. Cancer Treat Rt 60:115, 1976

175. Herr HW: Cyclophosphamide, methotrexate, and 5-fluorouracil combination chemotherapy versus chloroethyl-cyclohexy-nitrosourea in the treatment of metastatic prostatic cancer. J Urol 127:462, 1982

176. Berry J, MacDonald RN: Cisplatin, cyclophosphamide, and prednisone therapy for stage D prostatic cancer. Cancer Treat Rt 66:1403, 1982

177. Izbicki RM, Amer MH, Al-Sarraf M: Combination of adriamycin and cyclophosphamide in the treatment of metastatic prostatic carcinoma: A phase II study. Cancer Treat Rt 63:999, 1979

178. Ihde DC, Bunn PA, Cohen MH, Eddy JL, Dunnick NR, Bensimon H, Javadpour N, Minna JD: Combination chemotherapy as initial treatment for stage D-2 prostatic cancer: Response rate and results of subsequent hormonal therapy. Proc Am Assoc Cancer Res 22:163, 1981

179. Perloff M, Ohnuma T, Holland JF, Kennedy BJ, Mills RC: Adriamycin and diamminedichloroplatinum in advanced prostatic carcinoma. Proc Am Soc Clin Oncol 18:333, 1977

180. Citrin DL, Hogan TF: A phase II evaluation of adriamycin and cisplatinum in hormone resistant prostate cancer. Cancer 50:201, 1982

181. Soloway MS, Shippel RM, Ikard M: Cyclophosphamide, doxorubicin hydrochloride and 5-fluorouracil in advanced carcinoma of the prostate. J Urol 122:637, 1979

182. Smalley RV, Bartolucci AA, Hernstreet G, Hester M: A phase II evaluation of a 3-drug combination of cyclophosphamide, doxorubicin, and 5-fluorouracil and of 5-fluorouracil in patients with advanced bladder carcinoma or stage D prostatic carcinoma. J Urol 125:191, 1981

183. Al-Sarraf M: Combination of cytoxan, adriamycin and cisplatinum (CAP) in patients with advanced prostatic cancer. Proc Am Assoc Cancer Res 21:198, 1980

184. Presant CA, VanAmburg A, Klahr C, Metter GE: Chemotherapy of advanced prostate cancer with adriamycin, BCNU, and cyclophosphamide. Cancer 46:2389, 1980

185. Straus MJ, Ambinder JM, Engelking C, Billet D: Treatment of advanced prostate cancer with cyclophosphamide, adriamycin and methotrexate. Proc Am Soc Clin Oncol 1:115, 1982

186. Kasimis BS, Moran EM, Miller JB, Forbes KA, Chalfin SA, Kaneshiro CA, Poblet MT: Treatment of hormone resistant metastatic carcinoma of the prostate with 5-FU, adriamycin, and mitomycin-C (FAM). Proc Am Soc Clin Oncol 1:107, 1982

187. Logothetis CJ, Samuels ML, von Eschenback AC, Trindade A, Ogden S, Grant C, Johnson DE: Doxorubicin, mitomycin-C, and 5-fluorouracil (DMF) in the treatment of metastatic hormonal refractory adenocarcinomas of the prostate, with a note on the staging of metastatic prostate cancer. J Clin Oncol 1:368, 1983

188. Hsu S-D, Babaian RJ: 5-fluorouracil, adriamycin, mitomycin-C (FAM) in the treatment of hormonal-resistant stage D adenocarcinoma of the prostate. Proc Am Soc Clin Oncol 2:133, 1983

189. Soloway MS, deKernion JB, Gibbons RP, Johnson DE, Leoning SA, Pontes JE, Prout GR, Schmidt JD, et al: Comparison of estramustine phosphate and vincristine alone or in combination for patients with advanced hormone refractory, previously irradiated carcinoma of the prostate. J Urol 125:763, 1981

190. Torti, FM: Prostatic cancer chemotherapy. p. 58. In Torti FM (ed): Urologic Cancer: Chemotherapeutic Principles and Management. (RRCR Vol. 85). Springer-Verlag, Berlin/Heidelburg, 1983

10 | Intravesical Chemotherapy in Superficial Bladder Cancer

Mark S. Soloway

Approximately 70 to 85 percent of individuals with bladder cancer will have their initial tumor confined to the mucosa or lamina propria, stages Ta or T1, utilizing the TNM system. Although relatively few of these patients will subsequently have tumors that invade muscle and thus require either radiation therapy or cystectomy, approximately 50 percent will develop a subsequent tumor, despite apparently adequate endoscopic removal at their initial tumor episode. This provides the rationale for intravesical therapy.

Most drugs that are suitable for intravesical instillation are initially evaluated for efficacy by determining whether they eradicate biopsy-documented tumors, that is, treatment. Once this has been established, most of these agents are incorporated into an adjuvant or prophylaxis role, for example, regular intravesical instillations at some time following endoscopic removal of all visible tumor.

Before reviewing the various drugs used for intravesical chemotherapy, it is important to outline the steps the urologist takes in the evaluation and endoscopic resection of a patient with bladder cancer (Table 10-1).

Table 10-1. Key Factors in the Evaluation of
Bladder Cancer

Urinary cytology
Endoscopic appearance of normal and abnormal
 urothelium
Mucosal biopsies—selected-site and/or random
Stage and grade of tumor
Bimanual examination
Status of upper urinary tract

ENDOSCOPIC EVALUATION OF SUPERFICIAL BLADDER CANCER

Although the diagnosis of bladder cancer may be made during an office or an outpatient cystoscopy under topical anesthesia, definitive evaluation, with endoscopic resection of the tumor, should be performed when complete bladder relaxation can be assured. This not only allows the urologist to adequately remove the tumor and take as many biopsies as he thinks necessary, but makes possible a thorough visualization of all areas of the bladder. It is my personal preference, when possible, to utilize a block or spinal anesthetic, since this allows maximum relaxation of the bladder. In addition, it is readily tolerated in elderly patients. Many of these procedures can be performed in the outpatient surgery suite.

Endoscopic equipment has improved greatly over the last 10 years. Fiberoptic bundles and improved lens systems provide excellent visualization of all areas of the bladder. A ureteroscope has been developed that allows visualization of the entire ureter and a part of the renal collecting system. Endoscopic photography has also been simplified. I use an Olympus endoscopic system, with an Olympus camera and light source, to photograph abnormal areas of the bladder for documentation before and after tumor resection. This provides a permanent record of the initial lesion. Photographs of endoscopic findings should become part of the patient's permanent hospital record.

At the time of the initial endoscopic resection, it is my practice to send the urine obtained following passage of the cystoscope for cytological analysis. A bladder-washing specimen, secured by barbotage with saline through the cystoscope, is also obtained and the fluid is mixed with the cystoscopic urine. The millipore filter technique, utilized at our center, provides superb cytological specimens. The yield of tumor cells by performing both the cystoscopic urine and the bladder washing is improved, as has been documented at our institution.[1]

The location, appearance (papillary or sessile), size, and number of all tumors should be carefully noted on a bladder diagram at the time of endoscopy. This bladder diagram is critical for protocol studies but should also be a part of the patient's record for reference during subsequent endoscopic sessions.

During the patient's initial assessment, a decision regarding the need for cold-cup mucosal biopsies should be made. If a patient has more than one tumor or if the tumor does not appear to be papillary and low grade, the likelihood of severe atypia or carcinoma in situ (CIS) in other areas of the bladder is greater, even though the mucosa appears normal. Thus, since this may alter the urologist's treatment plan, biopsies probably should be performed. Specimens are often taken from selected sites, notably lateral to each ureteral orifice, the posterior midline, and the dome. In addition, any raised, granular, or erythematous region should be biopsied. Importantly, a biopsy from the prostatic urethra should be considered in patients with a positive cytology, but lacking an obvious tumor, and in patients with CIS or tumors located near the bladder neck.

Wolf and Hojgaard[2] recently confirmed the predictive value of selected mucosal biopsies (SMB) in patients with T1 or T2 bladder cancer. Seven selected-site mucosal biopsies were obtained in 53 patients. Eleven of these patients subsequently had recurrences at the same site as the original tumor and thus these were felt to be true recurrences. The remaining patients had selected mucosal biopsies, with no recurrence of the initial lesion.

Of 15 patients who had moderate or severe urothelial dysplasia or CIS in the selected mucosal biopsies, 13 (87 percent) had new occurrences during the follow-up period. On the other hand, of 27 patients with negative mucosal biopsies, only 7 (26 percent) had new occurrences. Thus, the presence of urothelial dysplasia or CIS was predictive of new occurrence. Most of these new occurrences appeared within six months of diagnosis of the initial tumor.

Of these 20 patients, 9 who had new occurrences had Ta lesions and 11 had tumors that invaded the lamina propria or muscle. Of the 11 patients who had invasive lesions, 8 had CIS in the selected mucosal biopsies, which confirms the predictive value in noting CIS in a selected mucosal biopsy.

The predictive value of severe dysplasia, or CIS, has previously been documented by Jones and Schade[3] and Murphy et al.[4-5] Thus, the incorporation of intravesical chemotherapy or another adjuvant therapy might be particularly indicated in those patients with abnormal SMB.

The bimanual examination is also an integral part of the endoscopic assessment. This should be performed both before and after endoscopic tumor resection. If a mass or induration is palpated and does not disappear following endoscopic resection, an invasive tumor should be suspected.

The resection itself can be facilitated by the use of a continuous flow resectoscope. This keeps the bladder at an approximately one-third capacity and, with suprapubic pressure, these tumors can be radily resected. This is particularly helpful for tumors located in the posterior wall or dome where the bladder is thinner and perforation is more likely to occur. A patient's initial tumor is usually removed in its entirety. This usually includes mucosa and lamina propria. If muscle invasion is suspected, muscle must be biopsied for pathology studies. If the tumor is clearly low grade and exophytic, however, it is unnecessary to resect into the muscle and, in fact, simple fulguration of the tumor is usually adequate.

The urologist should attempt to resect all visible tumor even when it is believed that further surgical intervention will be required. Often the gross appearance is more ominous than the true pathological stage. Tumors adjacent to the ureteral orifice can be resected safely. Intraveneous methylene blue or indigo carmine is helpful in identifying the ureteral orifice when tumor covers one or both orifices.

In the older age group, reflux related to resection of the orifice is not a critical concern.

A point of controversy concerns the resection of an enlarged prostate while a bladder tumor is being resected. Although there is no evidence that subsequent tumor is increased either in the bladder or the prostatic urethra when these procedures are done at the same time, compared to when they are performed as two procedures, a 20 percent "recurrence" rate in the prostatic urethra or bladder neck has been reported.[6-7] Thus, these studies do not eliminate the possibility that some of these recurrences result from seeding as a result of resecting the prostate when potentially viable tumor cells are present. Implantation of a high-grade tumor into the prostatic urethra is potentially lethal. Thus, it is my feeling that when there is a possibility that the bladder lesion may be of high grade, both procedures should not be done at the same time.

Following the initial endoscopic resection, monitoring of patients can probably be individualized. Urinary cytology is inexpensive and can be obtained every three months. If an experienced cytopathologist is available, a high-grade tumor should be identified by cytology with an accuracy of 95 percent.[8] The likelihood of a grade II tumor being identified is approximately 75 percent. Thus, if a voided and/or cystoscopic urine or bladder washing fails to reveal tumor cells, the clinician can be reasonably confident that a high-grade tumor is not present. Since the purpose of intensive endoscopic monitoring following initial tumor resection is to detect potentially lethal new tumors as soon as possible, I retrospectively reviewed the course of 25 patients with an initial grade I, stage Ta lesion to determine whether cytology could achieve this goal.

The patients, 22 men and 3 women, mean age 64, were monitored for an average of 64 months (range 6 to 144 months). Cystoscopy and cytology were performed every three months for two years and then every six months. A total of 250 cystoscopic and 182 cytological studies were reviewed, and 140 of the endoscopies included mucosal biopsies. Cytoscopy was normal in 140 (56 percent) of the sessions.

Six (25 percent) patients had a subsequent tumor of a higher grade or stage. Cytology performed at the time of recurrence was positive in four patients (67 percent): two grade II and two grade III tumors. Two patients had a grade II, noninvasive transitional cell carcinoma (TCC) with negative cytology. Subsequent tumors in these two patients have been grade I. All the 25 patients are alive.

Given the patient inconvenience and expense of cystoscopy compared to cytology, this retrospective review suggests that, when an experienced cytopathologist is available, patients with grade I, noninvasive TCC may be monitored primarily by urinary cytology, with less frequent endoscopy. A prospective study must be performed to confirm this.

Evaluation of the upper urinary tract by excretory urography or occasionally retrograde ureteropyelography is performed infrequently, usually every one to three years. Urinary cytology is helpful in monitoring the upper urinary tract.

Stage, grade, and multicentricity are all important factors that must be considered in determining the optimal therapy for a given patient. Individuals with tumors that have invaded the lamina propria (stage T1 or A) or those whose tumors that have invaded muscle (T2 or B) are at greater risk of dying from bladder cancer than those whose tumor is confined to the mucosa. Once the tumor has invaded the muscle, it is no longer considered superficial. The importance of invasion into lamina propria was underscored by Anderström et al.[9] Only 3 of 78 patients with a Ta lesion, independent of grade, died of bladder cancer, in contrast to 24 of 99 with a T1 lesion. A surveillance study performed by the national Bladder Cancer Collaborative Group analyzed the likelihood of subsequent invasion into muscle in a group of patients presenting initially with superficial disease.[10] Only 4 percent of those with Ta tumors progressed, in contrast to 30 percent whose initial tumor had invaded the lamina propria. Grade is also an important factor, but probably less than stage. Patients presenting with higher-grade tumors tend to have a higher recurrence rate and a greater likelihood of subsequent invasion.[11,12]

It has been suggested that patients with multiple tumors have a higher incidence of recurrence and muscle invasion than those with unifocal tumors. Lerman et al.[13] found a recurrence rate of 31 percent in patients with a solitary papillary tumor, compared to 66 percent in patients with multiple lesions. Lutzeyer at al.[14] indicated an overall recurrence rate of 64 percent with a three-year follow-up in 315 patients. The chance of recurrence was 46 percent for patients with an initial solitary tumor, compared to 73 percent for patients with multiple tumors.

Although the risk of death from bladder cancer when it presents as superficial disease is quite low, the majority of patients will have a subsequent tumor following initial endoscopic resection. Theoretically, these subsequent tumors might be divided into two categories: true *recurrences* of the initial tumor and new *occurrences*. At this time, we cannot differentiate between these two and thus the term "recurrence" is often utilized. It might be helpful to review the etiologies for this high incidence of subsequent tumor or recurrences, since this leads to the rationale for intensive intravesical chemotherapy.

NEW OCCURRENCES

A great deal of evidence supports the contention that the majority of subsequent tumors arise as a result of carcinogens that continue to affect the remaining urothelium following resection of the initial tumor(s). Melicow[15] was one of the early proponents of the concept that subsequent tumors arise from preneoplastic or in situ areas. Progressive growth of these lesions leads to new occurrences. Evidence supporting this concept comes from the analysis of cystectomy specimens removed for invasive cancer.[16,17] Approximately 80 percent of such bladders reveal carcinoma or CIS in areas distant from the obvious invasive lesion.

The results from selected-site or random mucosal biopsies from regions of the bladder that appear endoscopically normal also highlight the high incidence of epithelial hyperplasia, dysplasia, CIS, and even carcinoma.[2,4,5,18] In a study from this institution, we found that 46 percent of such specimens had atypia, 14 percent CIS, and 16 percent carcinoma.[4] Once again, all of these regions appeared normal, endoscopically.

TUMOR IMPLANTATION OR SEEDING

Circumstantial evidence indicates that some of the subsequent tumors may, in fact, be due to implantation or seeding from the original tumor. Experimental studies in animals have shown that there is preferential implantation of transitional cells on the cauterized urothelial surface.[19,20] Implantation of transitional tumor cells that are transurethrally placed into the murine bladder will only rarely implant on normal mucosa. However, if the bladder has been traumatized by the same type of cautery that is used in the surgical suite, implantation occurs in 50 percent. In man, tumor cells regularly exfoliate form transitional carcinoma, and thus, it is not unreasonable to assume that the urothelial surface traumatized by instrumentation or tumor resection provides a fertile surface for these cells to implant and grow.

Albarran and Imbert,[21] in 1903, were the first to comment that implantation was a factor in the high recurrence rate. Hollands[22] later observed that there was a high incidence of tumors in the posterior urethra and bladder neck following surgical resection of a bladder tumor, in contrast to the rarity of this site as a location of initial bladder tumors.

One of the more convincing pieces of evidence indicting endoscopic resection as a factor in the high incidence of subsequent tumors is the different location of recurrences compared to primary tumors. The dome and posterior wall are unusual sites for initial tumors; however, they are quite commonly the site of subsequent tumors. Most recently this was reported by Heney et al.,[23] who observed that initial tumors were located in the dome in 5.2 percent of cases, but subsequent tumors were present at this site in 29 percent of patients.

Falor and Wars[24] observed the same marker chromosomes in subsequent tumors compared to a patient's initial tumor. This leads one to suspect that the tumors were monoclonal.

Independent of the etiology for the high incidence of subsequent tumors, the fact that each patient has a 50 to 80 percent chance of developing another lesion, despite complete endoscopic resection of the first tumor, mitigates against transurethral resection as the sole management for patients with superficial bladder cancer. It seems worthwhile to consider additional therapy, for example, topical therapy, initiated shortly after surgical resection.[25] Drugs instilled into the bladder would affect the entire urothelial surface and inhibit the growth of preneoplastic lesions, to eradicate viable tumor cells remaining in contact with the urothelium following tumor resection. Depending upon the likelihood of recurrence, the urologist must decide whether intravesical chemotherapy should be utilized, whether it should be intensive intravesical chemotherapy, whether a maintenance schedule is appropriate, and which drug should be given.

A few principles are common to all the chemotherapeutic agents used by the intravesical route. Toxicity can be divided into systemic and local (Table 10-2).

Systemic side effects are myelosuppression and allergic reactions. One of the major advantages of the intravesical route is that a high concentration of drug can be obtained with relatively little absorption. Factors influencing the amount

Table 10-2. Side Effects of Intravesical
Chemotherapy

Myelosuppression (only thio-tepa)
Bladder irritative symptoms
Reduction in bladder capacity
Vesico-ureteral reflux due to alteration in anatomy
  of the ureteral orifice
Allergic reactions
Hematuria

of drug absorbed include the molecular weight of the drug, the concentration of the drug, the pH and volume of the solution, the length of contact, and the status of the urothelial surface.

The influence of pH has only recently been explored. Eksborg et al.[26] suggest that doxorubicin be kept at a pH below 8 by a phosphate buffer to minimize absorption.

Hellsten et al.[27] examined the influence of instilled volume on drug absorption in a rat model. The authors varied the concentration of doxorubicin from 1 to 4 mg/ml. Plasma doxorubicin concentrations were examined 1 hour after intravesical instillation. At higher intravesical concentrations, volume was a factor in the amount absorbed. When the instillate was placed in a 0.2 ml volume, plasma concentrations were 13 and 19 ng/ml, compared to 79 and 75 ng/ml for the 3 and 4 mg/ml concentrations with an instillate volume of 0.4 ml.

The usual contact times have been 2 hours, since this seems to be a reasonable time to request an individual to retain a solution in the bladder. A relative state of dehydration will obviously allow retention of the initial concentration for a longer period of time.

One of the most important factors affecting both absorption and local toxicity, for example, frequency, dysuria, and suprapubic pressure, is the status of the urothelium when treatment is initiated. Extensive resection of the mucosal surface prior to instillation of a drug will certainly enhance absorption. Other mucosal alterations increasing the amount of drug absorbed are cystitis and tumor. Allowing some healing to take place after surgery may diminish absorption; however, if implantation of viable tumor cells is a factor in recurrences, this delay may not be desirable. Good judgment usually can dictate when therapy should be initiated. If the drug is of low molecular weight, e.g., thio-tepa, then one should probably reduce the dose or delay starting treatment if an extensive resection has been performed. On the otherhand, drugs such as mitomycin and doxorubicin are absorbed minimally and can be instilled soon after resection of a small tumor.

THIO-TEPA

Until the last few years, thio-tepa (N,N′,N″-triethylene thiophosphoramide) was the only agent used for intravesical chemotherapy in the United States. The only other drug being used for intravesical instillation elsewhere was ethoglucid (in Great Britain and Canada). Thio-tepa is an alkylating agent chemically related to nitrogen mustard. Following formation of ethylenimine radicals, there is alkylation of purine and pyrimidine bases with cross-linking between DNA, RNA, and proteins. The usual dose is 30 to 60 mg, with a concentration of 1 mg/ml. The schedule varies among investigators and cooperative groups; however, the one more commonly employed is weekly for four weeks, followed by monthly instillation for approximately one year. The standard contact time is 2 hours, but varies from 30 to 120 minutes. The patient is generally requested to rotate while the drug is within the bladder, in order to bring it into contact with as much of the mucosal surface as possible.

The major side effect of this low molecular weight (189) agent is myelosuppression. A leukocyte and platelet count should be performed before each instillation, and should be normal before therapy is instituted.

The efficacy of thio-tepa when used as definitive treatment for patients with multi-focal superficial cancer was established many years ago.[28] The overall response rate, which includes both complete responses (CR) and partial responses (PR) ranges from 47 to 79 percent.[25] These studies established the efficacy of this agent and its ability to eradicate superficial tumors.

Most of the recent studies have concentrated on the prophylactic use of thio-tepa following eradication of all tumor. The dosage, administration schedule, and timing of the first dose following endoscopic resection vary widely among studies. The quantity of the drug absorbed from the bladder depends upon many factors, but importantly, the intactness of the epithelium as well as the dose and contact time are important variables. Up to 60 percent of thio-tepa may be absorbed when the drug is instilled immediately following resection of a large tumor. Until recently, the fear of absorption has prevented urologists from initiating drug therapy until two to four weeks after surgery.

Burnand et al.[29] were among the first groups to employ a high dose of thio-tepa immediately following endoscopic resection. They used a dose of 90 mg for 30 minutes. Patients receiving thio-tepa had a reduced incidence of subsequent tumor compared to patients who did not. Of 19 treated patients, 8 remained free of tumor, compared to only 1 of 31 patients in the control group. Surprisingly, leukopenia was not a problem.

Gavrell at al.[30] employed a regimen of 30 mg twice daily for three days beginning on the day of surgery. Other patients received the initial dose and continued thio-tepa weekly for six weeks, then at monthly intervals for one year, and then every three months thereafter. Prior to initiation of this intravesical chemotherapeutic regimen, the patients averaged one recurrence every 9.5 months. Following prophylactic thio-tepa, the group receiving the multidose therapy within the first week averaged one recurrence every 33 months, whereas the second group averaged one recurrence every 41 months. Only 2 of 22 patients become leukopenic. Thus, once again, these authors demonstrated the safety and efficacy of early initiation of intravesical therapy with this drug.

The National Bladder Cancer Collaborative Group A performed one of the few multi-institutional studies evaluating thio-tepa.[31] Importantly, this was a dose–response study in which 30-mg doses were compared with 60-mg doses. Therapy was initiated one month following endoscopic resection of all evident tumor. Patients who received thio-tepa had a statistically significant reduction in subsequent tumor incidence. Of the patients who received the drug, 66 percent were free of tumor at one year compared to only 40 percent of the controls ($P = 0.02$). There was no difference between those who received 30 or 60 mg.

A multi-institutional trial was also performed in Europe to evaluate the effect of topical therapy on the disease-free interval following transurethral resection of superficial bladder tumors.[32] Patients received thio-tepa, 30 mg/30 ml or VM-26 (an epipodophyllotoxin), 50 mg/30 ml, or no therapy. Once again, therapy was not initiated until one month after endoscopic resection. Treatment was continued weekly for 4 weeks and then monthly for 11 months. The incidence of subsequent tumors was 49.3 percent in the group receiving thio-tepa, compared to 62 percent in the group receiving VM-26. The control group had a tumor incidence of 52.2 percent. Thus although there was no significant difference among the groups in regard to recurrence rate, analysis of the number of tumors per 100 patient months indicated a significant benefit for those receiving thio-tepa. A Veterans Administration Cooperative Study in the United States comparing prophylactic thio-tepa or vitamin B6 to a control group showed similar benefits of thio-tepa.[33]

Another study, this one performed by England et al.,[34] used early, multiple-dose thio-tepa initiated soon after endoscopic resection of all visible tumor. Forty-five patients entered this trial, and most had a long history of prior bladder cancer. The dose was 30 mg/50 mg of saline instilled for a 2-hour duration on postoperative days 1, 3, and 5. If myelosuppression occurred, the dose was reduced. If tumor was present at the first three-month endoscopy, this tumor was resected, and thio-tepa continued. Patients were judged to have responded if the bladder became tumor-free or if the number of subsequent tumors was reduced to a small fraction of the patient's prior tumor pattern. The authors emphasized that most patients had numerous tumors at each endoscopy prior to initiation of thio-tepa. Using as a criterion of response a significant reduction in tumor pattern, 17 of 21 (81 percent) with Ta lesions and 14 of 24 (63 percent) with T1 tumors responded. The overall response rate was 71 percent. In the entire group, seven patients died of bladder cancer. One of these patients had a primary in the renal pelvis. Thus, the death rate in the entire population was 16 percent. Despite initiation of thio-tepa within 24 hours and with an intensive regimen, there was no evidence of significant toxicity.

Since myelosuppression has been a major factor in delaying the initiation of thio-tepa after endoscopic resection, and since there is widespread disagreement on the likelihood of leukopenia among several reports, I reviewed our own experience.[35] The occurrence of myelosuppression in 670 consecutive instillations was analyzed, 50 of which were given within 48 hours of transurethral resection. We found that 3.9 percent of the instillations (26/670) were associated with some degree of myelosuppression, and 18 percent of the patients experienced myelosuppression at some time. Some of these individuals, it should be emphasized, had received the drug for up to seven years. Importantly, no patient experienced myelosuppression with the initial dose of thio-tepa, and in no case was myelosuppression associated with sepsis or bleeding.

In the National Bladder Group study, 11 percent of the 93 patients in the prophylaxis part of the study exhibited some toxicity.[31] Urinary tract irritative symptoms were the most common reported problem and were somewhat higher in patients receiving 60 mg compared to those receiving 30 mg. Leukopenia and thrombocytopenia were uncommon.

Thio-tepa absorption has been studied. Jones and Swinney calculated that approximately 33 percent of an administered dose was absorbed.[36] Pavone-Macaluso[37] reported that up to 73 percent of the drug was absorbed if instilled within one week of an extensive transurethral resection. A survey of the literature indicates that the incidence of myelosuppression varies from 2 to 25 percent.[38] Although it is rarely fatal, there are isolated reports of profound and prolonged suppression. Urinary tract irritative symptoms are clearly the most common side effect of thio-tepa, as with other intravesically instilled agents. Usually this is not due to a bacterial infection, but rather is a chemical cystitis.

Mukamel et al.[39] evaluated the incidence of vesicoureteral reflux that might be related to thio-tepa administration. In a group of patients with prior transurethral resection of bladder tumors, approximately 43 percent had unilateral reflux. This was compared to a group of 61 patients treated by transurethral resection plus thio-tepa. Twenty-five (41 percent) of the patients had reflux. They reviewed the location of the tumors in both of these groups to determine whether reflux might have been related to the site of tumor resection. In approximately 50 percent of the ureters involved with reflux, there was no tumor at the site of the ureteral orifice; thus, reflux was attributed to intravesical chemotherapy.

EPODYL

Epodyl (Ethoglucid), a diepoxide alkylating drug, has been used in both Great Britain and Canada for intravesical chemotherapy. The molecular weight of Epodyl is 252, which is higher than thio-tepa (189). This probably accounts for the lower incidence of myelosuppression.

Epodyl has not been compared to thio-tepa in a randomized study, and thus we can only review the few reports of the efficacy of this agent, for treatment as well as for prophylaxis.

The standard dose of Epodyl is 100 ml of a 1 percent solution. The treatment schedule varies, but is usually weekly for 8 to 12 weeks, and then either every other week or monthly. Such a schedule was used by Colleen et al.[40] in 39 patients with low-grade tumors. Of these patients, 23 had no tumor at six months following Ethoglucid treatment. Unfortunately, 25 percent of these patients had to discontinue the drug due to irritative symptoms.

Neilsen and Thybo[41] reported a 43 percent response rate in 44 patients with superficial bladder cancer. This figure includes both CR and PR. Robinson et al. treated 51 patients and noted a 33 percent CR and 39 percent PR rate. Only two patients had myelosuppression.

Riddle[42] probably has had the most experience with Epodyl in intravesical chemotherapy of bladder cancer. They treated 139 patients who were not amenable to clearing of their bladder endoscopically. Of importance, his long-term follow-up data indicated that the five-year survival rate for patients whose tumors were confined to the mucosa (Ta) was 73 percent. This contrasts to a 49 percent rate for those with invasion into the lamina propria (T1). Of the patients with initial CIS, 26 percent were tumor free at five years, as were 13 percent with T1 tumors. The incidence of side effects was 16 percent. Riddle emphasized that failure to respond within 12 months, particularly with progression in tumor grade as well as progression from CIS to invasion, were poor prognostic signs and recommended that such patients be seriously considered for cystectomy.

Kurth et al.[43] reported a very interesting randomized trial using Epodyl. Patients received either no adjuvant treatment following endoscopic resection of tumors or a single dose of Epodyl. Between 1973 and 1979, 130 patients with Ta tumors were treated with Epodyl; 60 patients received Ethoglucid, and the remainder served as controls. This was a prophylaxis study and the dose used was 1.13 g dissolved in 100 ml of water; the retention time was one hour. Treatment was given the day following tumor resection.

There was no difference in the time to the first recurrence between the groups of patients being treated for their first tumor, but the recurrence rate per 100 patient months was 1.46 for the group treated with Ethoglucid compared to 4.22 for those not receiving any drug. This difference is significant ($p < 0.01$). For those with a history of tumor, the values were 4.43 for those receiving chemotherapy, compared to 7.17 for those not receiving the drug. Of particular importance, none of the patients who received Ethoglucid had an increase in stage with subsequent tumors, compared to 12 of 70 having transurethral resection (TUR) alone. This difference is also highly significant.

Ethoglucid is not commercially available in the United States, but is available in Europe in 1-ml vials. Due to this limited availability, and the fact that some of the drug is absorbed, the number of studies utilizing this drug will probably continue to be limited.

MITOMYCIN C

Mitomycin C (MMC), an antitumor antibiotic derived from *Streptomyces caespitosus,* is believed to inhibit DNA synthesis. The drug does not require metabolic activation and, thus, topical application is appropriate.

Probably the first trial of MMC as an intravesical chemotherapeutic agent was performed by Mishina et al.[44] in Japan. They used a dose of 20 mg/20 ml sterile water three times a week. They reported a CR rate of 44 percent, with a PR rate of 32 percent in a total of 50 patients.

The only dose–response study was performed by Bracken et al.[45] A total of 43 patients with stage ta or T1 tumors received MMC in a dose of 20 to 60 mg in an equal volume of water weekly for eight weeks. Response was evaluated by endoscopy at week 12. The overall response rate for the entire study was 84 percent. This includes 49 percent, CR; 30 percent, PR; and 5 percent, "improved." Although there were insufficient numbers of patients in each dose category to make a categorical statement as to the optimal dose, the response rate did appear to be higher when the dose exceeded 25 mg.

Following this study, a dose of 40 mg/treatment has been generally advocated in the United States; however, many other doses have been used, and it must be stressed that an optimal dose and schedule has yet to be determined.

I have treated 57 patients utilizing this eight-week treatment regimen. The first six patients received 30 mg; the remainder, 40 mg at each instillation. All patients had Ta or T1 bladder cancer and were biopsied to document the stage and grade of the lesion. This treatment regimen was thus therapeutic, *not* prophylactic. Most of the patients had failed thio-tepa and were considered candidates for cystectomy prior to initiation of MMC therapy. The ages ranged from 58 to 97, for 39 men and 18 women.

Initial evaluation of these patients included a bimanual examination, cystoscopic urine and bladder washing for cytology, and a bladder diagram. In no instance was a solitary lesion completely excised at the time of the first biopsy, but it should be stressed that very few patients had only one lesion: 16 patients had grade I lesions; 21, grade II; 8, grade III; and 12, multifocal CIS (also grade III).

All patients were instructed to limit fluids for approximately 10 hours prior to the intravesical instillation of MMC. The instillation time was 2 hours. Four weeks following the last of the eight weekly treatments, endoscopy, including cytology, was performed.

Complete response required the absence of visible or microscopic bladder cancer and the absence of tumor cells in the urine cytology. All patients with initial CIS had selected-site as well as mucosal biopsies from suspicious areas. A PR required a greater than 50 percent decrease in the size of all tumors, with no new neoplasm. Patients with a positive cytology, but negative biopsies and negative endoscopy were considered partial responders.

The majority of patients achieving a CR and some of the patients with an excellent PR were continued on a monthly maintenance schedule of MMC (40 mg/40 ml).

The overall response rate for the 57 patients was 77 percent. The CR rate was 37 percent (21/57). Analysis of response by tumor grade indicates that 11 of the 12 patients with multifocal CIS had a CR (5) or a PR (6). Of the patients with grade III tumors, 7 of 8 responded, compared to 10 of 16 with grade I lesions.

Of the 32 patients with tumors confined to the mucosa (Ta), 31 percent had a CR, and 38 percent had a PR. This is very similar to those patients with CIS or T1 lesions.

Thirty patients developed tumors while on thio-tepa, and thus were true thio-tepa failures, although 13 percent (4/30) of these patients had a CR with MMC. An additional 57 percent had a PR, and 30 percent failed. These figures are in contrast to the 14 patients who had MMC as first-line treatment, with 64 percent having CR, and 14 percent a PR. Thus, the overall response rate is similar for thio-tepa failures and newly treated patients. However, as might be expected, the probability of a CR was quite different.

The long-term follow-up is of great importance in evaluating the effectiveness of intravesical chemotherapy.[46] I have analyzed the data on these 57 patients for up to 45 months. In general, those individuals who had a CR, independent of whether they had stage Ta or T1 lesions, greatly benefited from MMC. Of the 10 patients with initial stage Ta lesions, only 1 required a cystectomy (for recurrent CIS). Of the others, 4 have had endoscopic fulguration or resection of low-grade "recurrence." Five patients had only multifocal CIS and achieved a CR. One of these five subsequently developed an invasive tumor, which required a cystectomy. He eventually died with metastases. The other four have remained tumor free and, with the exception of one patient, have been cytology negative. Of the six patients with T1 lesions who had a CR to MMC, none have required more than a transurethral fulguration for a noninvasive papillary tumor. No cystectomies or radiation therapy have been required with a follow-up of over three years.

In contrast to those patients who have had a CR at the first three-month evaluation, those who have had a PR have more frequently required subsequent therapy, either cystectomy or radiation. Of 12 patients with stage Ta lesions, 3 have required a cystectomy and 1 had radiation therapy for progressive disease. Of the six patients who had a PR with initial CIS, one required a cystectomy, but the follow-up is not over two years in three of the patients. Five patients with stage T1 lesions had a PR, two have had a cystectomy, and one had radiation therapy. Thus, there appears to be a clear separation based upon the initial response to MMC.

Toxicity related to MMC has been limited to one man who developed a generalized rash and three individuals who had a palmer and/or genital rash. It is unclear whether these rashes are due to absorption, with a generalized allergic response, or due to a contact dermatitis. The localized rashes often respond to topical steroids. Thorough washing of the genitalia and hands after treatment and the first several voidings has been helpful. Myelosuppression has not occurred. We no longer perform routine white or platelet counts in monitoring this group of patients.

It is important to mention that the endoscopic appearance of the bladder following MMC and many other of the intravesical agents is quite variable and may mimic a neoplasm. Although the urothelium may be entirely normal, previous tumors or biopsy sites may appear necrotic and white. This highlights the importance of urinary cytology in monitoring these patients. One area that must be constantly monitored is the prostatic urethra. Although urinary cytology should be helpful in diagnosing a high-grade neoplasm of the prostatic urethra, a cold-cup biopsy should be considered if there is any alteration in the prostatic urothelial mucosa or if the cytology is positive, but the bladder looks absolutely normal.

Prout et al.[47] have also reported on their results with therapeutic MMC. They treated 28 patients with superficial bladder cancer, using a regimen identical to the one described above. Their overall CR rate was 50 percent: 31 percent (5/16) in those who had failed prior thio-tepa and 75 percent in the remainder of the patients.

Lockhart et al.[48] recently reviewed their experience in 25 men with MMC used as prophylaxis following transurethral resection. Mitomycin C, 20 or 40 mg/20 ml water, was begun two weeks after resection and continued weekly for eight weeks. If a subsequent endoscopy was negative, the patient was maintained on monthly instillations of the same dose.

Thirteen (52 percent) of the patients have remained tumor free, with an average follow-up of 17 months (3 to 36 months). The other 12 patients (48 percent) developed recurrences while on therapy. Their average time to recurrence was approximately eight months.

Of interest, nine of the patients had recurrences in the prostatic urethra. They were treated by transurethral resection, radiation therapy, or radical surgery. Only 8 of the 12 patients who developed recurrences are currently free of tumor.

Huland and Otto[49] has also used MMC prophylactically following endoscopic resection of fulguration of tumor in patients with Ta or T1 tumors. He re-cystoscoped the patients to ensure that there was no visible tumor and that cytology was negative before randomizing them to either no further intravesical therapy or MMC. Mitomycin (20 mg per dose) was not initiated until three or four weeks after surgery to allow healing. In his initial study, there were 31 patients in the control group and 28 in the MMC group. After approximately two years, the MMC group was doing so much better that the control group was eliminated, and all patients received prophylactic MMC following TUR. He has now evaluated his results with a 30-month follow-up on all patients. A total of 48 patients thus were treated with MMC. The average age and the percent of patients with first or second tumor was virtually identical for both the control and the MMC-treated groups.

In the control group, 48 percent had T1 tumors; in the MMC-treated group, 46 percent. In the control group, 19 percent had grade III lesions; in the MMC-treated group, 10 percent. However, if one combines grade II and III, there were 29 percent in the control group and 29 percent in the MMC-treated group.

With an average follow-up of 30 months, the recurrence rate in the control group was 51.6 percent, in the MMC group, an extremely low 10.1 percent. Only one of the patients in the MMC group has had a progression in stage, compared to 8 of the 16 recurrences in the control group. No patient in the MMC group had an increase in grade; four recurrences in the control group were a higher grade. Calculation of the recurrences per 100 patient months indicates that it is 0.46 for the MMC group and 3.6 for the control group.

None of the patients in the prophylactic MMC group have died of bladder cancer, compared to five in the control group.

Wajsman et al.[50] examined the MMC absorption in eight patients. All had multiple superficial tumors and two had had prior radiation therapy. In two, the drug was instilled within 48 hours of resection. Small quantities of MMC were detected in most patients, but the plasma concentrations did not correlate with the quantity of MMC recovered in the urine. There was no myelosuppression. The maximum amount of MMC noted in any of the plasma samples was 36.4 ng/ml, which is much less than the microgram per millimeter amounts obtained after intravenous injection.

Van Oosterom et al.[51] analyzed the serum levels of MMC using high performance liquid chromatography (HPLC) in 15 patients after a 60-mg intravesical dose. The instillation time was one hour. They found that the level of absorption was quite low, varying from 0.1 to 1.1 percent of the administered dose. The highest plasma concentration was approximately 30 ng/ml, but most of the patients had levels far below this.

There has only been one reported case of bladder contraction related to MMC.[52] The individual was a 68-year-old man with a four-year history of low-grade, noninvasive transitional cell carcinoma prior to beginning a course of MMC. Prior to initiation of MMC, he had had multiple transurethral resections, as well as thio-tepa. On initiation of MMC, his bladder capacity was 400 ml. He received 40 mg MMC for 8 consecutive weeks and then monthly therapy with the same dose for 18 months. Eventually, the patient's bladder capacity diminished to 77 cc, and urinary diversion and cystectomy was required. There was no tumor in the bladder.

DOXORUBICIN HYDROCHLORIDE

Doxorubicin hydrochloride (adriamycin) another compound effective in a wide variety of neoplasms, has been recently investigated for activity as an intravesical agent. The dose and treatment schedule has been less standardized than for either thio-tepa or MMC. Most studies have utilized doxorubicin prophylactically following transurethral resection of all evident tumor, and not to treat evaluable lesions.

The majority of studies evaluating doxorubicin for intravesical therapy have been done in Europe or Japan. When used for definitive treatment, its efficacy is roughly comparable to that for thio-tepa. Approximately one-third of patients achieve a complete remission, whereas an additional one-third have a greater than 50 percent reduction in the amount of tumor.

Niijima[53] evaluated 80 patients given either 30, 50, or 60 mg doxorubicin on three consecutive days with total response rates (CR + PR) of 56, 72, and 74 percent, respectively. Multiple tumors responded better than solitary lesions. Niijima also reported the results of a Japanese cooperative group investigating intravesical doxorubicin, with 194 patients treated three times per week at the doses mentioned above. Those receiving the 50- and 60-mg dose appeared to do better than those who received only 30 mg. The response rates for all the patients were 20 percent CR, 37 percent PR, and 43 percent failed.

Pavone-Macaluso[54] also looked at several doses of doxorubicin for definitive treatment of superficial bladder cancer. His dose range was 10 to 40 mg. Although there were no CR, 12 to 33 percent of the patients had a PR.

Schulman et al.[55] reported on a study of doxorubicin used prophylactically following endoscopic resection. The dose was 50 mg/50 ml and was instilled within 24 hours following transurethral resection of either stage Ta or T1 tumors. The drug was given twice the first week, weekly for four weeks, and then bimonthly for one year. Side effects, primarily irritative symptoms, were observed in 25 percent of the patients.

Garnick et al.[56] reported their experience with the prophylactic use of intravesical doxorubicin in 27 patients who had rapidly recurrent superficial transitional cell carcinoma (TCC) of the urinary bladder. The mean duration of disease on entry into this protocol was 5.5 years, with a range of 3 months to 18 years. Of the 27 patients, 11 failed prior thio-tepa, although failure was not precisely defined.

At entry, 2 patients had CIS, 7 had stage Ta, and 16 had stage T1 tumors. Two patients had stage T1 tumors, with concomitant CIS. Six of the patients had grade III and three, grade IV lesions. The others were grades I–II.

The doxorubicin dose used by this group was 60 mg/50 ml of normal saline, with a retention time of one hour. Some of the patients had the dose escalated to 90 mg. Therapy was initiated one week after complete transurethral resection of all obvious disease, with subsequent doses given every 3 weeks for a total of eight doses, every 6 weeks for two doses and finally every 12 weeks for two doses. This resulted in a total of 12 instillations over 57 weeks.

Response was evaluated by comparing the patient's prior tumor history to that after initiation of doxorubicin. In the 2 years prior to initiation of this agent, there were 118 endoscopies and 90 (76 percent) had tumor. Following doxorubicin, there were 88 endoscopies and only 16 (18 percent) revealed tumor. This difference is statistically significant.

Of the treated patients, 55 have maintained a CR at last report. This includes a negative cytology. But 26 percent developed a "recurrence," three with invasion, and an additional 11 percent developed a positive cytology. The median duration of response in all the patients was 9 months, with a range of 3 to 21 months.

Some irritative symptoms occurred in 30 percent of the patients, and 41 percent had hematuria. Serum levels of doxorubicin were analyzed using HPLC, and only one patient had a detectable level. No patient had myelosuppression.

Abrams et al.[57] conducted a randomized trial of single-dose doxorubicin, 50 mg/50 ml of saline, compared to no treatment in patients with superficial bladder cancer. All tumors were Ta or T1 and had been entirely resected. Although random biopsies were not performed, no patient with identifiable CIS was included in this study. Therapy was initiated on the day following resection, with an instillation time of only 30 minutes.

There were 28 patients in the control group, and 29 patients received doxorubicin. Their on-study characteristics were similar. Most of the patients had a several-year history of superficial bladder cancer.

Of patients receiving chemotherapy, 72 percent, compared to 39 percent of the controls, had a decrease in the number of subsequent tumors. Of the 29 patients receiving doxorubicin, 21 were felt to have "responded," compared to 11 of 28 in the control group. Recurrence was seen in 6 of the patients in the treated group during the monitoring period, compared to 3 of 28 of the control patients. The incidence of side effects was extremely low.

Jakse et al.[58] used intravesical doxorubicin to treat patients with superficial bladder cancer, notably CIS. His treatment schedule has been doxorubicin, 40 mg or 80 mg, diluted in 20 or 40 ml of saline, respectively. The solutions were instilled biweekly, when the 40-mg dose was used, or monthly when the 80-mg dose was used. Instillation time was two hours. This schedule was continued for one year and, during the subsequent year, the intervals were lengthened to one or two months.

Jakse divided his patients into three categories. There were 14 patients with primary CIS and no prior or concurrent bladder cancer. All were symptomatic. Interestingly, of the 14 patients, 5 were females. Two of these patients were treated with intravesical MMC (40 mg/40 ml), with the same treatment schedule as indicated above for doxorubicin. Of the 14 patients, 10 (71 percent) had a CR. In two patients not responding to doxorubicin, subsequent therapy with MMC resulted in a CR. In 2 of these 12 patients, CIS of the prostatic urethra developed later and was transurethrally resected, with no evidence of subsequent tumor. Only one of the patients in this group with primary CIS died of bladder cancer. The average follow-up of the entire group was 29 months (range 6 to 69 months).

Seventeen patients were indicated to have secondary CIS. In a group of patients who had an initial resection of a superficial bladder cancer, 17 had secondary CIS found on follow-up cytology or a bladder biopsy. Three had prior radiation therapy. Only two in this group were women. All patients were treated with doxorubicin with a follow-up averaging 42 months.

Of the 17 patients in this group, 13 (76 percent) were thought to have a good response to therapy. One had transurethral resection of CIS in the prostatic urethra and is without disease at 42 months. Of the four patients who failed, one had a radical cystectomy and the three others had transurethral resection of their tumor. There were two deaths, one of which was due to bladder cancer.

A third group of 15 patients had CIS detected at the time of transurethral resection of a superficial tumor in another area of the bladder. Only one of these patients was a female. Twelve received doxorubicin and three were treated with MMC. Follow-up averaged 28 months. Of the 15 patients, 11 (73 percent) had a CR. None died of bladder cancer. Three of the seven patients who initially responded had subsequent areas of CIS after six to nine months and were successfully retreated with either doxorubicin or MMC.

Of importance, only 1 of the 46 patients died with a locally progressing bladder tumor not controlled by conservative measures. The mean follow-up in the entire group was 33 months. Other aspects of interest in this study are the four patients with prostatic involvement. Three either refused or were unfit for cystectomy, and thus were treated by transurethral resection of the prostate. All are alive without evidence of tumor 20 to 56 months later.

Long-term follow-up on intravesical therapy is important. Of the 22 patients treated for two years, 10 (45 percent) with a CR have had subsequent CIS or papillary tumors after 6 to 30 months.

Kurth et al.[43] recently reviewed the current status of the European Organization for Research in the Treatment of Cancer (EORTC) trials for superficial bladder cancer. In 1979, the EORTC urologic group compared three drugs used for prophylaxis after transurethral resection. As of February 1983, 323 patients had been randomized to recieve either thio-tepa, doxorubicin, or cisplatin.

After a mean follow-up of 13 months, the recurrence rate per 100 patient months (4.78) was not significantly different between the three arms. The mean time between recurrences was approximately 21 months in each arm.

Of the patients receiving thio-tepa, 5 percent had toxicity severe enough to require cessation of treatment; this occurred in 9 percent of those receiving doxorubicin. The incidence of side effects was 15 percent in the cisplatin group, and this arm was dropped. Some platinum-treated patients had an anaphylactic reaction.

A concurrent trial performed by a different group of European investigators compared prophylaxis with doxorubicin or Epodyl to a control group. Once again, all patients had either primary or recurrent superficial bladder cancer stages Ta or T1. The TUR alone group had a recurrence rate of 9.17, compared to 2.91 in the group receiving intravesical chemotherapy. This difference was highly significant ($P < 0.001$). The mean interval between tumors was 34.3 months for the groups receiving intravesical therapy, compared to 10.9 months for the control group. When the authors compared doxorubicin and Epodyl, no difference was noted.

Doxorubicin can be dissolved in either normal saline or sterile water for intravesical use. Following reconstitution, the solution is stable for 24 hours at room temperature, and 48 hours when refrigerated.

The molecular weight of doxorubicin is 580, and thus absorption is quite low. It has been found that very little of this drug is absorbed. Leukopenia has not been reported. Most of the side effects are related to irritative bladder symptoms, in up to 25 percent of patients. Some patients will require discontinuation of therapy because of this chemical cystitis.

BACILLUS CALMETTE-GUERIN

The basis for the use of *Bacillus Calmette-Guerin* (BCG) in the treatment of superficial bladder cancer rests on the theory that there are tumor antigens on the surface of bladder tumor cells and that contact between BCG and these antigens may induce a more pronounced host response to the tumor. In experimental tumor systems, BDG injection directly into a tumor has effectively eliminated the tumor, and this technique is more efficacious than "immunization" at a distant site. It thus seemed appropriate to instill BCG directly into the bladder. It should be stressed, however, that, to date, there is no conclusive evidence that intravesical (with or without intradermal) BCG actually works through an immunological mechanism, as opposed to a nonspecific, intense inflammatory response.

Morales[59] and Morales et al.[60] were probably the first to utilize this concept, treating nine patients utilizing the Pasteur strain of BCG. The dose was 120 mg dissolved in 50 cc of normal saline, and patients also received 5 mg intradermally. This combined treatment was continued weekly for six weeks. Morales compared the patient's prior tumor history to that following BCG therapy. He noted a dramatic reduction in subsequent tumor incidence, with 22 recurrences in 77 months before initiation of BCG, compared to only 1 recurrence in 41 combined patient months in the 12-month period after BCG. Side effects consisted of local irritative symptoms, fever, and malaise.

Two prospective randomized studies have been performed in an effort to repeat Morales' findings. The same strain of BCG was utilized. This strain comes from the Institute Armand Frappier in Quebec, Canada. Once again, both the intravesical and intradermal routes were utilized. One of these (Camacho et al.[61]) was a prophylaxis study. Fifty-one patients with a history of prior superficial bladder cancer were randomized to receive either transurethral resection of their tumor alone or transurethral resection followed by BCG, two weeks after surgery.

The control group had 2.97 tumors per patient-month prior to surgery and 2.37 following endoscopic resection of tumor. Patients receiving BCG had 3.6 tumors per patient-month pretreatment, and 0.75 posttreatment. The difference between the two patient arms was significant ($P = 0.001$). Side effects were similar to those described by Morales.

Lamm et al.[62,63] performed the other randomized study, utilizing the same BCG regimen. The control group had a tumor incidence following transurethral resection of 52 percent (14/27), compared to 20 percent (6/30) in the BCG-treated group. This difference was highly significant. Lamm indicated that the treatment and control group had approximately the same mean tumor grade and number of prior tumor recurrences before entering the study. Once again, all tumor was endoscopically resected in both groups before initiation of BCG or no treatment.

Side effects associated with BCG were not insignificant in Lamm's analysis. Virtually all the patients developed irritative symptoms, 40 percent had hematuria, and 20 percent fever lasting approximately 24 hours.

Lamm stressed that purified protein derivative (PPD) skin reactivity was an excellent predictor of response to BCG. Of 51 patients who received BCG, 35 had a negative PPD response prior to treatment and 22 (63 percent) converted following therapy. Only one of this group developed a subsequent tumor. On the other hand, patients who were already skin test-positive prior to BCG, or who did not convert, had a 31 percent incidence of subsequent tumor.

Lamm noted a 64 percent success rate in patients who had failed prior intravesical chemotherapy. In a separate analysis of those patients who had CIS, there was a 64 percent (9/14) CR rate, with a mean follow-up of 15 months.

One of the few studies that failed to indicate a beneficial effect with the use of intravesical BCG was reported by Flamm and Grof.[64] These investigators used either 60 or 120 mg of intravesical BCG in either a single dose as prophylaxis following transurethral resection, or in two doses one week apart. In 45 patients treated with BCG, with a follow-up of two to five years, 36 percent had a persistent tumor, and 59 percent a recurrence. This study suffers from the fact that it was not a randomized trial and, more importantly, that the patients had a limited number of instillations of BCG.

Utilizing the Tice strain of BCG, Brosman[65] performed a prospective randomized study in which patients received either thio-tepa (60 mg/60 ml) or intravesical BCG ($5 \pm 3 \times 10^8$ colony-forming units or approximately 60 mg/60 ml). The instillation time for each regimen was two hours. It is important to mention that Brosman did not use intradermal therapy, as did some of the other workers. Instillation of BCG was continued weekly for six weeks, every other week for three months, and then monthly for a total of two years.

In Brosman's study, 27 patients received BCG, and 22 thio-tepa. An additional 12 patients who failed thio-tepa were later placed on BCG. None of 19 patients who received thio-tepa had a recurrence within 24 months, compared to none of the 39 BCG-treated patients. This study, thus, provides some information is contrary to that of the report by Lamm; BCG was efficacious without concomitant intradermal injections. In addition, BCG appeared to be more effective than thio-tepa. Almost all of Brosman's patients receiving BCG had fever and malaise. Four patients had pulmonary infections thought to be related to BCG. They were treated with Isoniazide (INH).

Some reports on the use of intravesical BCG have concentrated on the treatment of CIS. Morales[66] treated seven patients, all of whom had CIS-associated, noninvasive papillary tumors. As indicated BCG was given both intravesically and intradermally. Eight weeks following the last immunization, endoscopic evaluation, with appropriate biopsies, was performed. Five of the seven treated patients were tumor free, with a negative cytology. Follow-up ranged from 12 to 33 months, with a mean of 22 months.

Herr et al.[67] has also reported on the use of intravesical BCG (no intradermal therapy) for CIS. Of 17 patients, 11 (65 percent) had complete eradication of tumor, with a mean follow-up of 18 months.

One very interesting recent report by Netto and Lemos[68] utilized oral BCG. The Moreau-RJ strain was used. The BCG was given in a liquid form, with each dose containing 100 mg (equivalent to 2×10^9 viable bacilli). Patients received doses of either 800, 400, or 200 mg three times weekly, depending upon whether skin tests showed no, moderate, or marked reactions. Treatment was continued indefinitely, but skin testing was done every three months, and the dose of BCG was "adjusted" according to the skin test response.

The authors indicated that they randomized their population into three groups. The first group consisted of 22 patients treated by transurethral resection alone, the second group of 17 patients was treated with thio-tepa following transurethral resection, and the third group was treated with BCG in the dose indicated. The average follow-up for the three groups was approximately three years.

The group receiving thio-tepa had a rather unique schedule. The dose was 60 mg/60 ml beginning two days following endoscopic resection and continued daily for seven days, then monthly for three months, and then every third month for one year. The patients were monitored with leukocyte and platelet counts.

The group treated by transurethral resection alone had a recurrence rate of 80 percent (16/20); those treated with the intensive thio-tepa regimen had a recurrence rate of 43 percent (6/14); and those treated with oral BCG had a dramatic 6 percent recurrence rate (1/16). It should be noted that all tumor recurrences were superficial, with no muscle invasion. None of the patients had side effects during the study.

It is difficult for this author to understand the lack of symptoms, particularly in those receiving this intensive regimen of thio-tepa. The small number of patients indicates that this study requires confirmation.

A number of strains of BCG have been produced, although some are not readily available. The strains that have received the most interest include the Tice strain, made by the Research Foundation in Chicago, and the Pasteur strain, from the Institute Armond Frappier in Canada. The Glaxo strain produced in England, as well as by Eli Lilly Company in Indianapolis, has been reported in animal studies not to be as effective as the other strains.[69] The Tice product is a freeze-dried preparation containing $5 \pm 3 \times 10^8$ colony-forming units per ampule. On reconstitution, the mycobacterium are alive and require refrigeration at a temperature of 5 °C or lower. Apparently no preventative measures are required handling the agents, since the risk of infection to personnel is quite small; however, the usual precautions in handling any bacterial product should be taken.

The differences in the different substrains of BCG regarding their clinical activity has also been demonstrated in the clinic. In a recent study of patients receiving adjuvant treatment with BCG after surgical resection of a melanoma, those who received lyophilized Tice BCG had a more favorable clinical course than did those who received fresh, frozen Pasteur BCG.[70] Different batches of the Tice strain of BCG have been shown to have different degrees of activity, as monitored by several parameters in vitro as well as in vivo. In particular, Bennett et al.[71] found that the efficacy of different batches of this strain of BCG in protecting mice against circulating tumor cells correlated with the clinical course of patients receiving these individual batches of BCG in a study in which the BCG was given intrapleurally as adjuvant therapy in surgically resected lung cancer. The authors stress that the variability in the antitumor activity among the preparations of BCG was not surprising, when it is realized that BCG is a living organism and thus subject to the genetic changes inherent in rapidly dividing organisms. In addition, BCG is not standardized for its antitumor activity, but rather for vaccination against tuberculosis. In the production of BCG, there are several sequences in which variations between individual batches might arise. It thus may be important in the future to utilize a test, such as protection against circulating tumor cells, to ensure that the individual batches are of equal efficacy.

SYSTEMIC CHEMOTHERAPY FOR SUPERFICIAL BLADDER CANCER

Intravesical chemotherapy has been the standard modality for bathing the entire urothelium of the bladder. There is potential, albeit minimal morbidity to repeated catheterization for administration of these drugs. Many of the agents produce a chemical cystitis, with associated irritative bladder symptoms. Some produce allergic reactions, either a contact dermititis or a generalized rash. The primary advantage of the intravesical route is the high concentration of drug that can be delivered with minimal absorption and, thus, a low incidence of systemic toxicity, e.g., myelosuppression.

It might be possible for some agents to be given by the systemic route and achieve a relatively high concentration in the urine. This would avoid repeated catheterization. Although the concentration of a given drug would be much less than could be achieved by direct intravesical instillation, the contact time would be longer. The potential systemic side effects would be dose dependent. Several

Table 10-3. Systemic Therapy for Superficial
Bladder Cancer

Methotrexate
Cyclophosphamide
Cisplatin
Pyridoxine (B6)
Retinoids

parenterally administered drugs have recently had a limited trial for use in superficial bladder cancer (Table 10-3).

METHOTREXATE

Methotrexate, a folate antagonist, is well absorbed when given orally, with 90 percent of the dose excreted in the urine within 24 hours. It has been shown to be active in patients with advanced bladder cancer.[72,73]

Hall et al.[74] treated 16 patients with multiple, recurrent stage T1 transitional cell carcinoma with 50 mg of methotrexate orally weekly for 18 months after transurethral resection of all evident tumor. In 11 of these patients, the frequency and number of subsequent tumors was reduced. In three, the drug did not alter the recurrence pattern. Two patients progressed and required cystectomy. In an attempt to quantitate the response, Hall noted that 2 of 61 endoscopic examinations in the 16 patients prior to methotrexate failed to reveal tumor, compared to 21 of 65 endoscopies following therapy. The number of tumors found at each endoscopic examination was 10.3 pre-methotrexate, compared to 4.4 post-methotrexate. Systemic toxicity was minimal. Two patients had mild mucositis, but this did not require alteration of treatment. Only 3 of 1,200 doese were deferred because of thrombocytopenia. No patient had significant leukopenia.

CYCLOPHOSPHAMIDE

Intraveneous cyclophosphamide (Cytoxan) has a rather pronounced effect on the urothelium of the bladder. Following a large dose of cyclophosphamide, epithelial denudation occurs, followed by subsequent epithelial hyperplasia. The cytological architecture of the cells is altered. These alterations include nuclear vesicles, with chromatin clumping. Cytoplasmic vacuolization is also a prominent feature. This effect of cyclophosphamide on the urinary bladder has lead to its consideration for use as treatment for bladder cancer.

England et al.[75] initiated a limited trial in 15 patients with multifocal CIS, who received cyclophosphamide in a dose of 1 g/m^2 every three weeks for six months. Seven of the patients had primary carcinoma *in situ* and eight had prior tumors (seven T1 and one T2). Five patients had prior radiation therapy.

At the initial three-month evaluation, 12 patients had a negative biopsy and cytology. The irritative symptoms associated with CIS had improved dramatically, and 5 of these 12 complete responders had no evidence of disease from 6 to 15 months after therapy was discontinued. Three patients recurred after six to nine months following discontinuation of cyclophosphamide. Two had a CR when the drug was reinitiated.

This preliminary report might prompt others to consider this agent for the treatment of patients with high-grade, superficial bladder cancer in the hope of obtaining a CR, but because of the known carcinogenicity of cyclophosphamide for the urothelium, prolonged use would seem ill-advised.[76]

Adolphs and Bastian[77] used a combination of intravenous cyclophosphamide (700 mg/m^2), in addition to the Connaught strain of BCG (120 mg in 50 cc normal saline). Cyclophosphamide was instituted two weeks after transurethral resection of all obvious superficial bladder cancer, and two weeks after that, BCG was initiated; BCG by skin scarification was also given with the first intravesical dose. Intravesical and percutaneous BCG was repeated five times at weekly intervals.

Of 90 patients receiving this combination, 8 developed a recurrence, with a median duration time of 13.3 months. In a matched control group of 65 patients, 32 (49 percent) had a subsequent tumor over a four-year follow-up. In this nonrandomized study, it is difficult to determine which of the agents, BCG or cyclophosphamide, was the effective modality.

CIS-DIAMMINEDICHLOROPLATINUM

Cis-diamminedichloroplatinum (cisplatin, DDP) is probably the most effective single agent for advanced bladder cancer.[78,79] For this reason, Needles et al.[80] performed a trial of systemic DDP in superficial bladder cancer.

Fifteen patients received DDP at a dose of 1.25 mg/kg on a monthly basis. All patients had tumor during the year prior to treatment, and it was felt that they were at great risk of subsequent tumor. Of these patients, 2 had no tumor when treatment was started and 13 had measurable disease. Six had CIS, two had a T1 lesion, and seven had both CIS and a T1 lesion.

Fourteen patients were evaluable for response. Four (28 percent), had no visible tumor at the 4- to 12-week follow-up. One of these patients continued to receive DDP, but subsequent tumor was seen and a cystectomy was required at week 32. A second responder continued DDP for 5 months and had no evidence of disease at 18 months. The other responders had a cystectomy at 6 to 35 months. Thus, the long-term benefit in the few patients who did respond was limited.

To further emphasize both the advanced nature of disease in this group of patients, as well as the lack of efficacy of systemic DDP, 10 of the 14 adequately treated cases (71 percent) underwent a cystectomy at a median of 7 months after initiation of DDP. Although some of these patients did have a decrease in the overall number of tumors, and some had a CR at the first endoscopic evaluation, most had a persistently positive urinary cytology.

This is the only report of the use of systemic DDP for superficial bladder cancer. The population treated was clearly at high risk for recurrence and the drug was relatively ineffective.

PYRIDOXINE

The rationale for exploring the use of pyridoxine (vitamin B_6) for patients with superficial bladder cancer is based upon evidence that tryptophan metabolites may have a role in the etiology of bladder tumors. Much of this information is derived from animal studies in which pellets containing tryptophan metabolites, upon implantation into the urinary bladder of rodents, produce transitional cell carcinoma.[81] Following these studies, the excretion of a variety of these tryptophan metabolites was determined in both normal subjects as well as individuals with bladder cancer. In approximately 50 percent of the latter group, the level of these metabolites was significantly higher than in the control population.[82] A subsequent study indicated that pyridoxine in a dose of 25 mg daily decreased these levels of tryptophan metabolites to normal.[83]

The first prospective randomized study of pyridoxine as prophylaxis for patients with superficial cancer was reported by Byar and Blackard[33] for the Veterans Administration Cooperative Group, with 121 patients from 10 VA Hospitals randomized to three treatment groups. One group received 25 mg daily of pyridoxine; the other groups were randomized to receive either a placebo or intravesical thiotepa in the usual dose of 60 mg weekly for four weeks and then monthly. All patients had "stage I" bladder cancer, which was completely resected prior to entering the study.

The placebo group had a recurrence rate of 60.4, compared to 46.9 for those receiving pyridoxine and 47.4 for those receiving intravesical thio-tepa. Differences between these groups were not significant. However, when the number of tumors per 100 patient months was analyzed, there was a significant reduction in the recurrence rate in the group receiving thio-tepa. For the group receiving pyridoxine, there was a significant reduction in the incidence of subsequent tumor if patients who had had a recurrence within the first 10 months were excluded. Thus, there was a suggestion that long-term treatment with pyridoxine may have a beneficial effect on the carcinogenic process.

VITAMIN A ANALOGUES

Chemoprevention is a term coined to indicate the attempt to reverse the progression of premalignant cells to cancer by noncytoxic therapy. One class of compounds that has been suggested for chemoprevention is the retinoids. These agents can regulate maturation and cell differentiation in epithelial tissues, including the urinary bladder, and in rodent models, analogues of vitamin A delayed the carcinogenic process.[84,85] Cohen et al.[86] reported that vitamin A deficiency accelerated tumor induction by the urothelial carcinogen FANFT.

In a phase I–II study, the National Bladder Cancer Collaborative Group A initiated a trial of one of these analogues, *cis*-retinoic acid, in patients with frequent bladder tumors.[87] The drug was initiated after transurethral resection, and thus, it was used to prevent subsequent tumors. This trial was discontinued after 22 patients were accessioned because of drug toxicity and lack of efficacy. Of the 18 evaluable patients, 15 (83 percent) developed a "recurrence" within 12 months.

Studer et al.[88] investigated the efficacy of an aromatic retinoid as prophylaxis for patients with superficial bladder cancer. The compound etretinate has been shown to inhibit rat bladder carcinogenesis. The randomized, double-blind, multi-center trial was performed in Switzerland. Eighty-six patients were entered into the study and almost all had a prior history of bladder cancer, stages Ta or T1. Patients received either 25 or 50 mg of etretinate, or a placebo. During the study, almost all of the patients receiving the higher dose of etretinate had the dose reduced to 25 mg because of side effects (e.g., dryness of the skin, lips, and mucous membranes).

As of Studer's report at the 1983 American Urologic Association meeting, 25 of the patients had been followed for at least two years, with 40 patients still in the study. Nine patients in the placebo group and two in the etretinate group were withdrawn because of tumor progression.

During the first year, there was a slight reduction in the number of endoscopic resections required per patient for those receiving the test drug compared to placebo—0.7 versus 1.0, respectively. This difference, of course, is not significant. There was also a small reduction in the number of tumors per endoscopic session in the group receiving etretinate compared to the placebo—3.8 versus 4.3.

Thus, this study can be contrasted to the National Bladder Clinical Collaborative Group study utilizing *cis*-retinoic acid in which the study was stopped because of complications and lack of efficacy. Here, with a different retinoic acid, there is a suggestion that the test compound may have some beneficial effect. Certainly, many more patients will need to be evaluated and follow-up will need to be extended.

SUMMARY

The urologist now has to decide not only whether intravesical chemotherapy following resection or biopsy of a superficial bladder tumor should be initiated, he must also select which agent to use and, in some cases the appropriate dose, since it may not have been established in clinical trials. Other factors include the schedule and the number of treatments. Because of its established efficacy and low cost, thio-tepa would still seem to be the drug of choice for initial management. Most likely, it would be used prophylectically following endoscopic resection of all evident superficial bladder cancer. The urologist must decide whether to initiate thio-tepa after resecting an initial solitary tumor or whether to reserve the drug for patients who have already demonstrated that they will develop a subsequent tumor. My personal preference is to give all patients intravesical chemotherapy within 24 hours following transurethral resection of a bladder tumor. If I believe, depending upon tumor grade, stage, or multiplicity, or the results of the selected mucosal biopsies, that the chance of subsequent tumor is quite high, then I will continue thio-tepa for three more weekly treatments, followed by monthly instillations for a total of one year. If the patient remains tumor free, then the drug will be discontinued.

If a patient develops a subsequent tumor on regular thio-tepa therapy, then he is a "thio-tepa failure" and one of the other agents should be used, either as treatment if the tumors are such that they cannot easily be resected or as an adjuvant following resection of all obvious disease.

When carcinoma in situ is found in biopsies from erythematous, granular mucosa or from selected mucosal biopsies of normal-appearing urothelium, then it is likely that all disease has not been eradicated. Cytology will confirm this. Mitomycin C, doxorubicin, and BCG have all been used in these circumstances and are variably effective. Prospective randomized trials comparing these agents have not been performed; thus, no one drug is clearly superior. The two antitumor drugs are more expensive than BCG, but BCG has a somewhat higher incidence of both local and systemic side effects. None of these three drugs has been approved by the Food and Drug Administration for intravesical use. There is ample literature, however, to support their efficacy in the treatment of superficial bladder cancer.

ACKNOWLEDGMENTS

This work was supported by PHS grants CA 15934 and CA 18643 awarded by the National Cancer Institute and the Veterans Administration Medical Research Service.

REFERENCES

1. Murphy WM, Crabtree WN, Jukkola AF, Soloway MS: Diagnostic value of urine versus bladder washing in patients with bladder cancer. J Urol 126:320, 1981
2. Wolf H, Hojgaard K.: Urothelial dysplasia concomitant with bladder tumors as a determinate factor for future new occurrences. Lancet i:134, 1983
3. Schade ROK, Swinney J.: The association of urothelial abnormalities with neoplasia: A 10-year follow-up. J Urol 129:1125, 1983
4. Soloway MS, Murphy WM, Rao MK, Cox CE: Serial multiple-site biopsies in patients with bladder cancer. J Urol 120:57, 1978
5. Murphy WM, Nagy GK, Rao MK, Soloway MS, Pariji GC, Cox CE, Friedell GH: "Normal" urothelium in patients with bladder cancer. Cancer 44:1050, 1979
6. Green LF, Yalowitz PA: The advisability of concomitant transurethral excision of vesical neoplasm and prostatic hyperplasia. J Urol 107:445, 1972
7. Laor E, Grabstald H, Whitmore WF: The influence of simultaneous resection of bladder tumors and prostate on the occurrence of prostatic urethral tumors. J Urol 126:171, 1981
8. Murphy WM, Soloway MS, Jukkola AF, Crabtree WN, Ford KS: Urinary cytology and bladder cancer. The cellular features of transitional cell neoplasms. Cancer 53:1555, 1984
9. Anderström C, Johansson S, Nilsson S: The significance of lamina propria invasion on the prognosis of patients with bladder tumors. J Urol 124:23, 1980
10. Cutler SJ, Heney NM, Friedell GHL: Longitudinal study of patients with bladder cancer: Factors associated with disease recurrence and progression. p. 35. In Bonney

WW, Prout GR, Jr (eds): AUA Monographs, Bladder Cancer. Williams & Wilkins, Baltimore, 1982

11. Barnes RW, Dick AL, Hadley HL, Johnston OL: Survival following transurethral resection of bladder carcinoma. Cancer Res 37:2895, 1977

12. Loening S, Narayana A, Yoder L, Slymen D, Penick G, Culp D: Analysis of bladder tumor recurrence in 178 patients. Urology 16:137, 1980

13. Lerman RI, Hutter RVP, Whitmore WF: Papilloma of the urinary bladder. Cancer 25:333, 1970

14. Lutzeyer W, Rübben H, Dahm H: Prognostic parameters in superficial bladder cancer: An analysis of 315 cases. J Urol 127:250, 1982

15. Melicow MM: Histological study of vesical urothelium intervening between gross neoplasms in total cystectomy. J Urol 68:261, 1952

16. Soto EA, Friedell GH, Tiltman AJ: Bladder cancer as seen in giant histologic sections. Cancer 39:447, 1977

17. Farrow GM, Utz DC, Rife CC: Morphological and clinical observations of patients with early bladder cancer treated with total cystectomy. Cancer Res 36:2495, 1976

18. Cooper TP, Wheelis RF, Correa RJ, Gibbons RP, Mason JT, Cummings KB: Random mucosal biopsies in the evaluation of patients with carcinoma of the bladder. J Urol 117:46, 1977

19. Soloway MS, Masters S: Urothelial susceptibility to tumor cell implantation-influence of cauterization. Cancer 46:1158, 1980

20. Soloway MS, Nissenkorn I, McCallum L: Urothelial susceptibility to tumor cell implantation: Comparison of cauterization with *N*-methyl-n-nitrosourea. Urol (in press)

21. Albarran J, Imbert L: Les tumeurs du rein. p. 452. Masson et Cie, Paris, 1903

22. Hollands FG: The results of diathermy treatment of villous papilloma of the bladder. Br J Urol 22:342, 1950

23. Heney, NM, Nocks BN, Daly JJ, Prout GR, Jr., Newall, JB, Griffin PP, Perrone TL, Szyfelbein WA: Ta and T1 bladder cancer: Location, recurrence and progression. Br J Urol 54:152, 1982

24. Falor WH, Ward RM: Prognosis in early carcinoma of the bladder based on chromosomal analysis. J Urol 119:44, 1978

25. Soloway MS: Rationale for intensive intravesical chemotherapy for superficial bladder cancer. J Urol 123:461, 1980

26. Eksorg S, Nilsson S, Edsmyr F: Intravesical instillation of adriamycin: A model for standardization of the chemotherapy. Eur Urol 6:218, 1980

27. Hellsten S., Axelsson B, Eksborg S: Absorption of adriamycin after intravesical administration. Experimental studies in the rat. Presented at the 13th International Congress of Chemotherapy. Aug 28, 1983, Vienna

28. Veenema RJ, Dean AL, Roberts M, Fingerhut B, Chowdury BK, Tarassoly H: Bladder carcinoma treated by direct instillation of thiotepa. J Urol 88:60, 1962

29. Burnand KG, Boyd PJR, Mayo ME, Shuttleworth KED, Lloyd-Davies RW: Intravesical thiotepa as an adjuvant to cystodiathermy in the treatment of transitional cell bladder cancer. Br J Urol 48:55, 1976

30. Gavrell GJ, Lewis RW, Meehan WL, Leblanc GA: Intravesical thiotepa in the immediate postoperative period in patients with recurrent transitional cell carcinoma of the bladder. J Urol 121:410, 1978

31. Koontz WW, Prout GR, Smith W, Frable WJ, Minnis JE: The use of intravesical thiotepa in the management of non-invasive carcinoma of the bladder. J Urol 125:307, 1981

32. Schulman C, Sylvester R, Robinson M, et al: Adjuvant therapy of T1 bladder carcinoma:

Preliminary results of an EORTC randomized study. p. 338. In Bonadonna G, Mathe G, Salmon SE (eds); Recent Results in Cancer Research. Vol. 68. Springer-Verlag, Berlin 1979

33. Byar D, Blackard C: Comparisons of placebo, pyridoxine, and topical thio-tepa in preventing recurrence of stage I bladder cancer. Urology 10:556, 1977

34. England HR, Flynn JT, Paris AMI, Blandy JP: Early multiple-dose adjuvant thiotepa in the control of multiple and rapid T1 tumour neogenesis. Brit J Urol 53:588, 1981

35. Soloway MS, Ford K: Thio-tepa induced myelosuppression: Review of 670 bladder instillations. J Urol 130:889, 1983

36. Jones HC, Swinney J: Thiotepa in the treatment of tumors of the bladder. Lancet ii:615, 1961

37. Pavone-Macaluso M, Gebbia N, Biondo F, Bertitolini S, Caramia G, Rizzo FP: Permeability of the bladder mucosa to thiotepa, adriamycin, and daunomycin in men and rabbits. Urol Res 4:9, 1976

38. Hollister D, Jr, Coleman M: Hematologic effects of intravesicular thio-tepa therapy for bladder carcinoma. JAMA 244:2065, 1980

39. Mukamel E, Glanz I, Nissenkorn I, Cytron S, Servadio C: Unanticipated vesicoureteral reflux: A possible sequela of long-term thio-tepa instillations to the bladder. J Urol 127:245, 1982

40. Colleen S, Ek A, Hellsten S, Lindholm CE: Intracavitary Epodyl for multiple, noninvasive highly differentiated bladder tumors. Scand J Urol Nephrol 14:43, 1980

41. Neilsen HV, Thybo E: Epodyl treatment of bladder tumors. Scand J Urol Nephrol 13:59, 1979

41a. Robinson MRG, Shetty MB, Richards B, Bastable J, Glashan RW, Smith PH: Intravesical epodyl in the management of bladder tumors. J Urol 118:972, 1977

42. Riddle PR: The management of superficial bladder tumors with intravesical epodyl. Br J Urol 45:84, 1973

43. Kurth KH, Schulman C, Pavone-Macaluso M, Robinson M, de Pauw M, Sylvester R: Current status of the EORTC protocols for superficial bladder cancer. Proc 13th International Congress of Chemotherapy, August, 1983, Vienna

44. Mishina T, Ota K, Murata S, Ooe H, Yasuyuki M, Takahashi T: Mitomycin-C bladder instillation therapy for bladder tumors. J Urol 114:217, 1975

45. Bracken RB, Johnson DE, Von Eschenback AC, Swanson DA, DeFuria D, Crooke S: Role of intravesical mitomycin-C in management of superficial bladder tumors. Urol 16:11, 1980

46. Soloway MS, Ford KS: Subsequent tumor analysis of 36 patients who have received intravesical mitomycin C for superficial bladder cancer. J Urol 130:74, 1983

47. Prout GR, Griffin PP, Nocks BN, DeFuria MD, Daly JJ: Intravesical therapy of low stage bladder carcinoma with mitomycin C: Comparison of results in untreated and previously treated patients. J Urol 127:1096, 1982

48. Lockhart JL, Chaikin L, Bondhus MJ, Politano VA: Prostatic recurrences in the management of superficial bladder tumors. J Urol 130:256, 1983

49. Huland H, Otto U: Mitomycin instillation to prevent recurrence of superficial bladder carcinoma. Eur Urol 9:84, 1983

50. Wajsman Z, Dhafir RA, Pfesser M, McDonald S, Block AM, Dragone N, Pontes JE: Studies of mitomycin C absorption after intravesical treatment of superficial bladder tumors. J Urol (in press)

51. Van Oosterom AT, de Bruijan EA, Dan DN, Hartigh J, Van Oort WJ, Pinedo HM, Jaden UR: The pharmokinetics of intravenous, intrahepatic, and intravesical administra-

tion of mitomycin C. In Aktuelle Ronkologie. Eb. g. Nagel Zuchschwerdt-Verlag. 1984 (In press)

52. Wajsman Z, McGill W, Englander L, Huben RP, Pontes JE: Severely contracted bladder following intravesical mitomycin-C therapy. J Urol 130:340, 1983

53. Niijima T: Intravesical therapy with adriamycin and new trends in the diagnostics and therapy of superficial bladder tumors. p. 36. In WHO, Diagnostics and treatment of superficial urinary bladder tumors. Collaborating center for research and treatment of urinary bladder cancer, Stockholm, 1978

54. Pavone-Macaluso M, Caramia G: Adriamycin and daunomycin in the treatment of vesical and prostatic neoplasias: preliminary results. p. 180. In Carter SK, DiMarco A, Ghione M, Krakoff IH, Mathe G (eds): International Symposium on Adriamycin. Springer-Verlag, Berlin/Heidelberg/New York, 1972

55. Schulman CC, Denis LJ, Oosterlinck W, Desy W, Chantrie M, Vancangh PJ: Early adjuvant adriamycin in superficial bladder cancer. Presented at American Urological Association Meeting, Boston, 1981

56. Garnick MB, Schade D, Israel M, Maxwell B, Richie JP: Intravesical doxorubicin for prophylaxis in the management of recurrent superficial bladder carcinoma J Urol 131:239, 1984

57. Abrams PH, Choa RG, Gaches CGC, Ashken MH, Green NA: A controlled trial of single dose intravesical adriamycin in superficial bladder tumors. Br J Urol 53:585, 1981

58. Jakse G, Hofstadter F, Marberger H: Intracavitary doxorubicin hydrochloride therapy for carcinoma in situ of the bladder. J Urol 125:185, 1981

59. Morales A: Adjuvant immunotherapy in superficial bladder cancer. Natl Cancer Inst Monogr 49:315, 1978

60. Morales A, Edinger D, Bruce AW: Intracavitary *bacillus Calmette-Guerin* in the treatment of superficial bladder tumors. J Urol 116:180, 1976

61. Camacho F, Pinsky C, Kerr D, Whitmore W, Oettgen H: Treatment of superficial bladder cancer with intravesical BCG. Proc Am Soc Clin Oncol 21:359, 1980

62. Lamm DL, Thor DE, Winters WD, Stogdill VD, Radwin HM: BCG immunotherapy of bladder cancer: Inhibition of tumor recurrence and associated immune responses. Cancer 48:82, 1981

63. Lamm DL, Thor DE, Stogdill VD, Radwin HM: Bladder cancer immunotherapy. J Urol 128:931, 1982

64. Flamm J, Grof F: Adjuvant local immunotherapy with *bacillus Calmette-Guerin* (BCG) in treatment of urothelial carcinoma of the urinary bladder. Wein Med Wochenschr 131:501, 1981

65. Brosman SA: Experience with *bacillus Calmette-Guerin* in patients with superficial bladder carcinoma. J Urol 128:27, 1982

66. Morales A: Treatment of carcinoma in situ of the bladder with BCG: A phase II trial. Cancer Immunol Immunother 9:69, 1980

67. Herr HW, Pinsky CM, Whitmore WF, Jr, Oettgen HF, Melamed MR: Effect of intravesical BCG on carcinoma in situ of the bladder. Cancer 51:1323, 1983

68. Netto NR, Jr, Lemos GC: A comparison of treatment methods for the prophylaxis of recurrent superficial bladder tumors. J Urol 129:33, 1983

69. Lamm DL, Harris SC, Gittes RF: *Bacillus Calmette-Guerin* and dinitrochlorobenzene immunotherapy of chemically induced bladder tumors. Invest Urol 14:369, 1977

70. Gutterman JU, Mavligit G, McBride C, Grei E, Freireich EJ, Hersh EM: Active immunotherapy with BCG for recurrent malignant melanoma. Lancet i:1208, 1973

71. Bennett JA, Gruft H, McKneally MF, Zelterman D, Crispen RG: Differences in biological activity among batches of lyophilized Tice *Bacillus Calmette-Geurin* and their association with clinical course in stage I lung cancer. Cancer Res 43:4184, 1983

72. Hall RR, Bloom HJG, Freeman JE, Nowrocki A, Wallace DM: Methotrexate treatment for advanced bladder cancer. Br J Urol 46:431, 1974

73. Natale RB, Yagoda A, Watson RC, Whitmore WF, Jr, Bleumenreich M, Braun DW, Jr: Methotrexate: An active drug in bladder cancer. Cancer 47:1246, 1981

74. Hall RR, Herring DW, McGill AC, Gibb I: Oral methotrexate therapy for multiple superficial bladder carcinomata. Cancer Treat Rt 65 (suppl 1):175, 1981

75. England HR, Molland EA, Oliver RTD, Blandy JP: Systemic cyclophosphamide in flat carcinoma in situ of the bladder. p. 97. In Oliver RTD, Hendry WF, Bloom HJG (eds): Bladder Cancer: Principles of Combination Therapy. Butterworths, London, 1981

76. Pearson RM, Soloway MS: Does cyclophosphamide induce bladder cancer? Report of a case and review of the literature. Urology 11:437, 1978

77. Adolphs HD, Bastian HP: Chemoimmune prophylaxis of superficial bladder cancer. Presented at the American Urological Assoc. 77th Annual Meeting, Kansas City, Missouri, May 1982

78. Soloway MS: *Cis*-diamminedichloroplatinum (II) (DDP) in advanced urothelial cancer. J Urol 120:716, 1978

79. Soloway MS, Einstein A, Corder MP, Bonney W, Prout GR, Jr, Coombs J: A comparison of cis-platin and the combination of cis-platin and cyclophosphamide in advanced urothelial cancer—an NBCCGA Study. Cancer 52:767, 1983

80. Needles B, Yagoda A, Sogani P, Grabstald Y, Whitmore WF: Intravenous cisplatin for superficial bladder tumors. Cancer 50:1722, 1982

81. Bryan GT, Brown RR, Price JM: Incidence of mouse bladder tumors following implantation of paraffin pellets containing certain tryptophan metabolites. Cancer Res 24:582, 1964

82. Brown RR, Price JM, Satter EK, Wear JB: The metabolism of tryptophan in patients with bladder cancer. Cancer Res 16:299, 1960

83. Yoshida O, Brown RR, Bryan GT: Relationship between tryptophan metabolism and heterotopic recurrences of human urinary bladder tumors. Cancer 25:773, 1970

84. Sporn MB, Kunlop NM, Newton DL, Smith JM: Prevention of chemical carcinogenesis by vitamin A and its synthetic analogs (retinoids). Fed Proc 35:1332, 1976

85. Sporn MB, Squire RA, Brown CC, Smith JM, Wenk ML, Springer S: 13-*cis*-retinoic acid: inhibition of bladder carcinogenesis in the rat. Science 195:487, 1977

86. Cohen SM, Wittenberg JF, Bryan GT: Effect of hyper- and avitaminosis A on urinary bladder carcinogenicity of *N*-(4-(5-nitro-2-furyl)-2-thiazolyl)-formamide (FANFT). Fed Proc 33:602, 1974

87. Koontz WW: Intravesical chemotherapy and chemoprevention of superficial, low grade, low stage bladder carcinoma. Semin Oncol 6:217, 1979

88. Studer UE, Biddermann C, Chollet D, Karrer P, Craft R, Toggenburg H, Vonbank F: Prevention of recurrent superficial bladder tumors by oral etretinate. Presented at American Urologic Association Annual Meeting, April, 1983, Las Vegas

11 | First-Line Intravenous *Cis*-Platinum for Invasive Clinically Nonmetastatic Bladder Cancer

Derek Raghavan

Bladder cancer, with an annual prevalence of 16 per 100,000 males and 5 per 100,000 females, is a common malignancy of the older aged population. It appears to be related to smoking,[1] to some forms of industrial exposure,[1,2] and to prior analgesic abuse[3] and its incidence may be increasing.

The prognosis of this disease correlates with several factors, including the depth of penetration of the tumor through the bladder wall (stage), the level of histological differentiation (grade), and the histological subtype. There is no universally accepted system of staging of bladder cancer—two commonly used systems are summarized in Table 11-1.[4,5]

CONVENTIONAL MANAGEMENT OF INVASIVE BLADDER CANCER

The optimal therapy of invasive carcinoma of the bladder has been a controversial issue for many years. The major treatment options include cystectomy (simple or radical), radiotherapy (with a variety of dose schedules and fractionations), or

Table 11-1. Staging of Bladder Cancer[4,5]

Depth of Penetration	UICC	Marshall–Jewett–Strong
Preinvasive	T-I-S	0
Papillary noninvasive	Ta	0
Bimanually: freely mobile mass, which disappears after resection; no invasion beyond lamina propria	T1	A
Bimanually: induration of bladder wall, which disappears after resection; microscopic invasion of superficial muscle	T2	B1
Bimanually: induration or nodular mobile mass, which persists after transurethral resection; microscopic invasion of deep muscle or through bladder wall	T3	B$_2$,C
Tumor fixed or extending to neighboring structures; microscopic evidence of such involvement	T4[a]	D1

[a] T4a, tumor infiltrating prostate, uterus or vagina; T4b, tumor fixed to pelvic and/or abdominal wall.

combinations of the two modalities. Unfortunately, the conventional approaches to therapy of invasive bladder cancer, whatever modalities have been used, have yielded five-year survival rates of less than 40 to 45 percent (Tables 11-2, 11-3, and 11-4). Furthermore, it should be noted that, at five years, the survival curve for transitional cell carcinoma (TCC) of the bladder has not reached a true plateau, and deaths from cancer still occur—five-year survival does not mean "cure."[6-9]

Surgery

Radical surgery alone for deeply invasive TCC has been associated with long-term survival rates of less than 10 to 45 percent (Table 11-2), depending upon the stage and grade of the tumor, the selection criteria for inclusion into a study protocol, and the experience of the clinicians involved.[10-15] Furthermore, the results tabulated in surgical series often reflect pathological staging—thus the comparison of the treatment of pathological stage (PS) T3a versus clinical stage (CS) T3a may not be valid, as clinical staging is frequently inaccurate and usually associated

Table 11-2. Five-Year Survival with Cystectomy

Stage	Treatment[a]	Five-Year Survival (%)	Reference
T3/B2,C	RC	16	10
	RC	22	11
	RC	30	12
	SC	35	13
T4	RC	0	14
	RC	6.2	12

[a] RC, radical cystectomy; SC, simple cystectomy.

with understaging.[15] In fact, improved staging after surgery is often cited as a criterion in favor of the use of this modality of treatment rather than radiotherapy.

Radiotherapy

Notwithstanding the differences in the accuracy of staging, the survival results from radical radiotherapy are not greatly different from those reported with surgery alone (Table 11-3).[6-8,16-19] The five-year survival figures also range from less than 10 to 45 percent. In some instances, the total survival figures also reflect the use of "salvage cystectomy" at the time of first relapse.[7,9]

Some of the variability of survival statistics with radiotherapy may reflect the selection of patients, stage and grade of the tumor, and dose schedule and fractionation used.[6,10,15-17] As shown in Table 11-3, the survival of patients with T3 (B2,C) cancer is substantially greater than with stage T4 (D1). In clinically staged patients, the distinction between T2, T3a, and T3b is somewhat arbitrary, as it is often difficult to evaluate the level of penetration in biopsies obtained at cystoscopy.[20]

Similarly, the staging implications of computerized tomography are not yet completely clear (Husband and Hodson, 1981).[21]

Radiotherapy and Surgery

To date, the highest survival rates have been reported in patients treated with first line radiotherapy, followed by radical or simple cystectomy (Table 11-4).[6,8,10,17,22,23] With this combined approach, radiotherapy is usually delivered in one of two ways:

2,000 Rads over Two Weeks, Followed by Early Radical Cystectomy. In this situation, radiotherapy is delivered only to the bladder with the intention of sterilizing the primary tumor, decreasing the chances of intraoperative seeding, and "squeezing" viable cancer cells into the circulation at operation. Regional lymph nodes are not covered by the standard radiotherapy ports in this program.

4,000 Rads over Four Weeks. The concept of this approach is similar, but the radiation dose can be larger because less radiation is delivered per week,

Table 11.3. Five-Year Survival with Radiotherapy[a]

Stage	Radiation (rads)	5-Year Survival (%)	Reference
T3/B2,C	6,000	29	6
	7,000	20–35	16
	7,000	22	17
	5,000–6,000	38	7
	6,000–7,000	20	18
T4/D	7,000	8	16
	5,000–6,000	9	7
	6,000–7,000	10	18
	5,000–7,000	< 10	19

[a] ± salvage cystectomy.

Table 11-4. Five-Year Survival with Radiotherapy Plus Cystectomy

Stage	Radiation (rads) + Cystectomy[a]	5-Year Survival (%)	Reference
T3/B2,C	4,000 + RC	38	6
	5,000 + SC	46	17
	2,000 + RC	42	10
	4,000 + RC	41	10
	5,000 + SC	38	8
	4,000 + SC	45	22
T4/D	2,000 + RC	22[b]	23
	4,000 + RC	25[b]	23

[a] RC, radical cystectomy; SC, simple cystectomy.
[b] Small numbers of patients.

and tissue repair may occur. Thus, the regional lymph nodes may be partly encompassed in the field.

Few randomized comparative studies have been reported in which this approach is compared with either radiotherapy alone or cystectomy. The most detailed data have been reported from the Institute of Urology Cooperative Group.[6] In this detailed study, patients with T3 bladder cancer were randomized to receive 4,000 rads to the pelvis, followed by elective radical cystectomy, or 4,000 rads, followed by a 2,000-rad bladder boost. The five-year survival for the operative patients was 38 percent, compared to 29 percent for the patients treated with radiotherapy alone. In patients less than 60 years of age, combined treatment yielded a five-year survival rate of 49 percent, versus 25 percent in patients receiving only radiotherapy. These data are supported by the results of sequential trials at Memorial Sloan-Kettering Cancer Center[10] and at the M.D. Anderson Tumor Institute.[17]

NATURAL HISTORY OF BLADDER CANCER

Superficial (T-I-S, Ta, T1) bladder cancer can usually be cured by local means (radiotherapy, surgery, or intravesical chemotherapy); with superficial tumors, the five-year survival rates are in excess of 70 percent, although these figures decrease in the case of grade III tumors[24] or if other indices of poor prognosis are present. Adverse prognostic factors include increased grade and stage of the tumor, presence of squamous cell carcinoma, urinary obstruction, solid macroscopic appearance, multiple presentations, tumor size, and lack of expression of blood group substances on the tumor cell surface.[20,25-28]

As noted above, patients with invasive bladder cancer have a five-year survival of less than 10 to 45 percent (Tables 11-2, 11-3, and 11-4), whatever treatment they receive. One-half of the deaths occur within 18 months of initial treatment.[6,7,10,27] In about 20 percent of these patients, metastases are detected at relapse.[10,15,16,26,29] The bladder bed/pelvis is the commonest site of relapse, whatever the treatment. The pattern of spread and recurrence is bimodal—via the lymphatics to regional and distant nodes and via the bloodstream to the lungs, liver, bone, brain, and soft tissues. In addition, transmucosal spread or seeding may occur, with tumors developing at other sites in the bladder or uroepithelial tract. However, this could also reflect a multifocal origin of uroepithelial cancer.

CHEMOTHERAPY OF METASTATIC BLADDER CANCER

It is clear that metastatic bladder cancer is a relatively drug-sensitive disease; although cures from chemotherapy are rare,[29,30] between 20 to 40 percent of tumors treated with systemic chemotherapy show a measurable response (Table 11-5).[30-39] A wide range of response rates to single agents have been reported (Table 11-5), the variation correlating with such factors as the criteria of response, patient selection, dose and schedule of drugs, and histological subtypes. Similar data have been obtained for superficial bladder cancer with respect to the response rates to intravesical chemotherapy.[24]

Although in some series, higher response rates have been reported with combination chemotherapy (Table 11-6),[30,40-46] there have been no reports of response or survival data from well-conducted randomized studies comparing single-agent therapy versus multi-agent regimens; several such studies are in progress.

Despite these uncertainties, it appears that cytotoxic agents play some role in the treatment of bladder cancer. In an effort to improve the dismal survival statistics, we have investigated the use of first-line *cis*-platinum in previously untreated patients with invasive TCC of the bladder. The rationale for this approach is:

1. To control micrometastases as early as possible
2. To downstage tumors before "definitive" therapy, as it has been demonstrated that pre-cystectomy downstaging by radiotherapy is associated with a clear survival benefit[6,10,22]
3. To administer chemotherapy before radiotherapy to ensure maximum drug penetration into the tumor—drug access may be reduced if radiotherapy is administered first, due to vascular sclerosis induced by irradiation.
4. To attempt to decrease the viability of the tumor cells and thus to decrease the chances of seeding or spread at cystectomy

Table 11-5. Chemotherapy of Bladder Cancer: Single-Agent Response Rate

Drug	Response Rate (%)	References
Methotrexate	26–38	32,33
Adriamycin	10–20	34,35
Cyclophosphamide	0–50	36,37
Cis-platinum	33–43	30,38,39

Table 11-6. Combination Chemotherapy of Bladder Cancer

Regimen[a]	Response Rate (%)	References
ADR + 5-FU + CDDP	61	40
CYCLO + ADR + CDDP	38	41
CYCLO + ADR + CDDP	13	42
CYCLO + ADR + CDDP	20	43
CYCLO + ADR + CDDP	82	44
CYCLO + ADR + CDDP	41	45
ADR + CYCLO	33	30,46
CYCLO + CDDP	55	30,46
ADR + CDDP	54	30,46

[a] ADR, adriamycin; 5-FU, 5-fluorouracil; CYCLO, cyclophosphamide; CDDP, cis-diamminedichloroplatinum (II).

FIRST-LINE CHEMOTHERAPY OF INVASIVE BLADDER CANCER

Protocol

In August 1981, a pilot program was initiated in the Urological Cancer Research Unit, Royal Prince Alfred Hospital, in which patients with deeply invasive TCC were treated initially with intravenous cis-platinum, according to the schema shown in Figure 11-1.[47-49] Patients with clinical stage T3 and T4 TCC were initially eligible for entry into the study; subsequently, the entry criteria were extended to include patients with recurrent multifocal undifferentiated (grade III) T2 tumors (who had not previously received radiotherapy or chemotherapy).

Patients underwent an extensive staging protocol, the investigations including a detailed history and physical examination, complete blood cell count, biochemical profile, tumor marker estimations, computerized tomographic (CT) scan of the abdomen and pelvis, chest X-ray, cystoscopy, and biopsy and bimanual examination under anesthesia. Tumors were classified according to the system of the Union International Contre Cancer (Table 11-1).[4]

Cis-platinum (100 mg/m²) was administered with an aggressive hydration regimen to reduce nephrotoxicity.[47] In brief, the protocol required the initiation of a forced diuresis, with a large fluid load and mannitol and frusemide. This required close nursing and medical supervision to avoid serious fluid overload and its sequelae in this aged population. Antiemetics, including metoclopramide, haloperidol and lorazepam,[50] were employed liberally to reduce the gastrointestinal side effects of cis-platinum.

Assessment of Response

Response to two cycles of cis-platinum was assessed in terms of subjective and objective improvement. Subjective response was defined as the decrease of all symptoms that related to the tumor—frequency, dysuria, hematuria, bladder pain, and nocturia; these "responses" have been tabulated for completeness, but have not been considered in the analysis of the efficacy of this regimen.

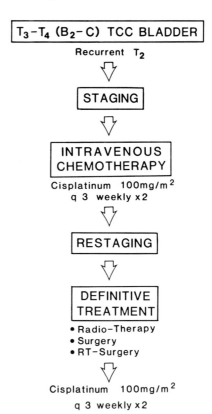

Fig. 11-1. Protocol for first-line intravenous *cis*-platinum in the management of invasive cancer.

Objective response was defined as follows:

Complete Remission. The disappearance of all symptoms and signs of disease, the return of the CT scan to normal, and the absence of viable cancer on repeat cystoscopy and biopsy.

Partial Remission. An apparent decrease of more than 50 percent in tumor diameter at cystoscopy and on CT scan, accompanied by histological evidence of tumor necrosis; no evidence of new sites of tumor.

Stable Disease. An unchanged appearance or less than 50 percent reduction in tumor diameter at cystoscopy and on CT scan; no new tumor deposits; in some instances, tumor necrosis was present upon biopsy.

Progressive Disease. An increase in observed tumor size at cystoscopy or CT scan; the presence of regions of tumor necrosis on biopsy that did not preclude evaluation as "progressive disease"; new sites of tumor.

"Definitive Treatment"

"Definitive treatment" consisted of radical radiotherapy (29 patients), radical cystectomy (4 patients), or the combination of radiotherapy and elective cystectomy (7 patients). A sole "definitive" regimen was not instituted in the pilot study for several reasons:

1. Accrual was likely to be slow initially
2. Referring clinicians were likely to have strong biases regarding "optimal definitive treatment"
3. The outcome of the study, which was designed to assess the efficacy and safety of front-line *cis*-platinum, would not be affected by differences in subsequent treatment. In view of the similarity of survival figures with the available conventional regimens, it was not likely that a major variable would be introduced with respect to overall survival by this tactic.

Patients were restaged after completion of "definitive treatment," and in some instances, received two further doses of *cis*-platinum (Fig. 11-1).

Patient Population

Forty patients have been treated between August 1981 and August 1983. All patients received chemotherapy at the Urological Cancer Research Unit and Department of Clinical Oncology, Royal Prince Alfred Hospital; 9 females and 31 males were entered into the study, with a mean age of 63.2 years (median 65 years, standard deviation 8.3, range 29 to 78 years); 29 of the patients were 60 years or older (72 percent), and 6 were 70 years or older; 31 patients were heavy smokers (>20 cigarettes/day) and 7/25 (28 percent) had abused analgesic compounds.[3] There was demonstrable renal tract obstruction on IVP or CT scan, in 20 patients and biochemical evidence of renal dysfunction was present in 14 patients (35 percent). No patients had received prior radiotherapy or chemotherapy. Of the 40 patients, 39 (98 percent) had symptoms (Table 11-7), and 32 (80 percent) of the patients were seen at their first or second presentation.

Details of Tumors

All patients had TCC, although squamous or glandular differentiation were present in some tumors. No patients had pure adenocarcinoma or squamous carcinoma. No tumors were well differentiated (grade I); 6 were grade II (15 percent), and 34 were grade III (85 percent).

Table 11.7 Presenting Symptoms of Invasive Bladder Cancer

Symptom	Patients (N)
Hematuria	31
Nocturia	23
Dysuria	21
Frequency	20
Urinary obstruction	6
Abdominal/pelvic pain	5
Incontinence	5
Backache	4
Weight loss	3
Fecal obstruction	2
Testicular pain	1
Total with symptoms	39
Total patients	40

The results of tumor staging were as follows: T2, 5 cases (12.5 percent); T3, 27 (67.5 percent); T4, 8 (20 percent), including 3 patients with prostatic infiltration (T4a).

Results

Symptomatic Improvement. A marked reduction of symptoms, particularly with respect to hematuria, frequency, and nocturia, was reported by 30 patients (75 percent). In most cases, improvement was noted within three weeks of the first dose and was sustained at least until the time of check cystoscopy and biopsy (which often caused a transient renewal of symptoms).

Objective Response. At check cystoscopy and bimanual examination under anesthesia after two doses of *cis*-platinum, 23 (58 percent) patients showed a greater than 50 percent reduction of apparent tumor diameter, with histological evidence of widespread tumor necrosis (Table 11-8). In six cases, there was no evidence, clinically or on random biopsies, of residual cancer. In two patients, a different urologist performed the initial and check cystoscopies and these cases were thus listed as "not evaluable"—however, from the initial urologists' descriptions, it appeared that there was no great change in tumor mass in either case. Two patients did not undergo check cystoscopy before "definitive treatment," although one of these patients showed a clinical partial response when examined per rectum (T4a tumor). In only one patient was there definite clinical evidence of progressive disease at check cystoscopy (although the lesion was not biopsied). In the remainder of the patients (30 percent), the tumors were either unchanged or reduced by less than 50 percent, and were classified as "stable disease."

Response to "Definitive Treatment." As previously noted, this program has been designed to evaluate the efficacy and toxicity of first-line intravenous *cis*-platinum in the treatment of bladder cancer. Thus at this stage, few significant conclusions can be drawn with respect to the superimposed effects of the specific conventional treatment programs employed—radiotherapy, surgery, etc. However, it is of interest to note that complete clinical remission was achieved in 32 patients (80 percent) after two doses of *cis*-platinum plus radiotherapy and/or surgery—the numbers of patients in each subgroup are not yet sufficiently large to permit detailed evaluation.

Table 11-8. Response at Cystoscopy to Intravenous *Cis*-Platinum: Influence of Tumor Stage

Stage	Response			
	CR/PR[a]	<PR/SD	PD	NE
T2	2	3	0	0
T3	15	8	1	3
T4	6[b]	1	0	1[b]
Totals	23[b]	12	1	4[b]

[a] CR, complete response; PR, partial response; PD, progressive disease; NE, not evaluable; SD, stable disease.

[b] One patient with T4a tumor in "remission" on rectal examination (but no check cystoscopy at that time).

Although this study is not yet mature and it is difficult to draw major conclusions with respect to patient survival, an actuarial survival curve (to October 1983) is included for completeness (Fig. 11-2).

Toxicity of First-Line Intravenous *Cis*-platinum. In general, the regimen of *cis*-platinum, 100 mg/m² three-weekly (twice) was well tolerated. As shown in Table 11-9, the major side effects were nausea and vomiting, renal toxicity, and ototoxicity. All toxicities resolved spontaneously. In one patient, serum creatinine rose from 100 mmol/liter to 970 mmol/liter (normal, < 110 mmol/liter) over a two-week period after one dose of *cis*-platinum; no other cause was found, and his renal function returned to normal within 10 days without active intervention (he was not retreated with *cis*-platinum).

The syndrome of inappropriate antidiuretic hormone production was demonstrated in one patient who became disoriented after administration of the first dose of *cis*-platinum; marginal electrolyte abnormalities consistent with this diagnosis were present in the pretreatment biochemical screen, and it is presumed that the syndrome was exacerbated by the forced diuresis. However, it is of interest to note that the patient received a second dose, with careful monitoring of electrolytes, without adverse effects.

Subsequent treatment was delivered without undue toxicity—patients receiving radiotherapy encountered the usual toxicities (dysuria and frequency, diarrhea), but did not require modification of planned radiotherapy dose. Similarly, patients who underwent cystectomy did not have unusual intra- or postoperative problems.

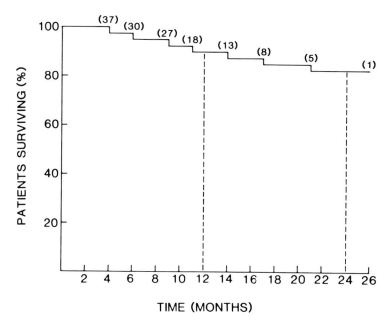

Fig. 11-2. Actuarial survival of the first 40 patients treated on protocol (October 1983); numbers in parentheses indicate patients followed to that time-point.

Table 11-9. Toxicity of Two Doses of First-Line Intravenous Cis-Platinum

Toxicity	Patients (N)
Nausea	37
Vomiting	33
Renal	7
Auditory [a]	6
Diarrhea	4
Myelosuppression	2
Infection	2
Stomatitis	2
Alopecia	2
SIADH [b]	1
Hematemesis	1
Total with toxicity	39 (98%)
Total patients	40

[a] Tinnitus or audiogram changes.
[b] Syndrome of inappropriate production of antidiuretic hormone—may have been coincidental.

To date, 10 patients have received additional doses of *cis*-platinum upon completion of radiotherapy or surgery; the spectrum of toxicity has been similar to that seen with the first doses (Table 11-9), although nausea and vomiting have been more severe, and patients have expressed greater distress and discomfort at the idea of having chemotherapy.

Discussion

It is, as yet, too early to evaluate the survival benefit that may be achieved by the use of first-line intravenous chemotherapy. In fact, a true assessment of the utility of this approach will require a randomized study, comparing this program with "standard practice" (in which a single definitive regimen is employed)—such a study is about to be launched by the Australian Bladder Cancer Group, based on the results of this pilot study.

Our data show at least a 60 percent response of primary bladder cancer to *cis*-platinum. However, an important limitation of this study is the noninvasive staging data—most of the patients have not undergone cystectomy. Nevertheless, the commonest error of clinical evaluation is understaging.[15] It is of interest to note that 16 patients have been followed for more than 12 months, and 13 remain alive between 12 and 26 months after completion of the second dose of *cis*-platinum (Figure 11-2). It should also be emphasized that we have selected a group of patients with major adverse prognostic features, including high-grade tumors (85 percent), advanced T stage (88 percent), ureteric obstruction (50 percent), and age ≥ 60 years (72 percent).

The cytotoxic regimen has been well tolerated, particularly when administered prior to radiotherapy and/or cystectomy. The National Bladder Cancer Cooperative Group A recently terminated an adjuvant chemotherapy study in which *cis*-platinum was to have been administered after radical cystectomy; the preliminary closure of the study was due to excessive toxicity. It may be that a more feasible approach is possible by the use of the drugs according to our schedule.

In a pilot study reported recently, first-line *cis*-platinum was used in the management of locally invasive bladder cancer[39]; however, it was delivered as the sole modality of treatment, and although the response rates were comparable to our own, subsequent relapse rates were high. The addition of a "definitive regimen" after chemotherapy may resolve this problem.

Finally, comment should be made regarding the choice of cytotoxic agent for this study. It appears that methotrexate and *cis*-platinum are among the most active drugs against bladder cancer (Table 11-5). A trial of methotrexate as front-line treatment, to be followed by 4,000 rads and elective cystectomy, has recently been instituted by the London and Oxford Cooperative Urological Research Group (R.T.D. Oliver, personal communication). A potential benefit of using *cis*-platinum in this context is that it may also act as a radiosensitizer,[51] thus enhancing the effect of this combined regimen.

The optimal choice and scheduling of cytotoxic drugs in the management of invasive bladder cancer will require further study. Several questions remain unanswered.

Does chemotherapy add to the effect of radiotherapy?

Can chemotherapy replace radiotherapy as a pre-cystectomy, tumor-reducing regimen?

Does such an approach confer a disease-free and total survival benefit?

Which cytotoxic drug will yield the greatest benefit in this context?

Will combination drug regimens improve the survival rates achieved with first-line chemotherapy?

Should the drugs be administered intraarterially?

How many cycles of chemotherapy are required to secure a maximum effect?

Should cytotoxic drugs be administered concurrently with radiotherapy?

Is there a role for intravenous cytotoxic chemotherapy in the treatment of superficially invasive bladder cancer?

The management of bladder cancer is undergoing a renaissance because of the increase in our knowledge of its natural history and biology and the potential applications of new treatment approaches. If the current pilot studies of front-line chemotherapy fail to yield a "quantum leap," the clear definition of its role in the management of this disease will require a series of well-designed and carefully conducted randomized clinical trials.

REFERENCES

1. Cole RP, Monson RR, Haning H, et al: Smoking and cancer of the lower urinary tract. N Engl J Med 284:129, 1971
2. Anthony HM, Thomas GM: Tumors of the urinary bladder: An analysis of the occupation of 1030 patients in Leeds, England. J Natl Cancer Inst 4:879, 1970

3. Taylor JS: Carcinoma of the urinary tract and analgesic abuse. Med J Aust 1:407, 1972
4. U.I.C.C.: Union Internationale contre le cancer, TNM Classification of Malignant Tumours, Geneva, U.I.C.C., 3rd ed., 1978
5. Marshall VF: The relation of the pre-operative estimate to the pathologic demonstration of the extent of vesical neoplasms. J Urol 68:714, 1952
6. Bloom HJG, Hendry WF, Wallace DM, Skeet RG: Treatment of T_3 bladder cancer: Controlled trial of pre-operative radiotherapy and radical cystectomy versus radical radiotherapy. Second report and review. Br J Urol 54:136, 1982
7. Blandy JP, England HR, Evans SJW, et al: T_3 bladder cancer: The case for salvage cystectomy. Br J Urol 52:506, 1980
8. Goodman GB, Hislop TG, Elwood JM, Balfour J: Conservation of bladder function in patients with invasive bladder cancer treated by definitive irradiation and selective cystectomy. Int J Rad Oncol Biol Phys 7:569, 1981
9. Vinnicombe J, Abercrombie GF: Total cystectomy—a review. Br J Urol 50:488, 1978
10. Whitmore WF, Jr: Integrated irradiation and cystectomy for bladder cancer. Br J Urol 52:1, 1980
11. Prout GR: The surgical management of bladder carcinoma. Urol Clin N Am 3:149, 1976
12. Richie JP, Skinner DG, Kaufmann JJ: Radical cystectomy for carcinoma of bladder. 16 years experience. J Urol 113:186, 1975
13. Cordonnier JJ: Simple cystectomy in the management of bladder carcinoma. Arch Surg 108:190, 1974
14. Kutscher HA, Leadbetter GW, Vinson RK: Survival after radical cystectomy for invasive transitional cell carcinoma of bladder. Urology 17:231, 1981
15. Skinner DG: Current perspectives in the management of high-grade invasive bladder cancer. Cancer 45:1866, 1980
16. Goffinet DR, Schneider MJ, Glatstein EJ: Bladder cancer: Results of radiation therapy in 384 patients. Radiology 117:149, 1975
17. Miller LS: T_3 bladder cancer: The case for higher radiation dosage. Cancer 45:1875, 1980
18. Edsmyr F: Radiotherapy in the management of bladder carcinoma. p. 139. In Oliver RTD, Hendry WF, Bloom HJG (eds): Bladder Cancer—Principles of Combination Therapy. Butterworths, London 1981
19. Hope-Stone HF, Blandy JP, Oliver RTD, England H: Radical radiotherapy and salvage cystectomy in the treatment of invasive carcinoma of the bladder. p. 127. In Oliver RTD et al (eds): Bladder Cancer—Principles of Combination Therapy. Butterworths, London, 1981
20. Chisholm GD, Hindmarsh JR, Howatson AG, et al: TNM (1978) in bladder cancer: Use and abuse. Br J Urol 52:500, 1980
21. Husband JE, Hodson NJ: Computerized axial tomography for staging and assessing response of bladder cancer to treatment. p. 17. In Oliver RTD, et al (eds): Bladder Cancer—Principles of Combination Therapy. Butterworths, London, 1981
22. Van der Werf Messing BHP: Preoperative irradiation followed by cystectomy to treatment carcinoma of the urinary bladder, category T_3 Nx, 0–4, Mo. Int J Rad Oncol Biol Phys 5:394, 1979
23. Whitmore WF, Jr, Batata MA, Ghoneim H, et al: Radical cystectomy with or without prior irradiation in the treatment of bladder cancer. J Urol 118:184, 1977
24. Soloway MS: Rationale for intensive intravesical chemotherapy for superficial bladder cancer. J Urol 123:461, 1980

25. Lange PH, Limas C, Fraley EE: Tissue blood group antigens and prognosis in low stage transitional cell carcinoma of the bladder. J Urol 119:52, 1978
26. Narayana AS, Loening SA, Slymen DJ, Culp DA: Bladder cancer: Factors affecting survival. J Urol 130:56, 1983
27. Batata M, Chu FCH, Hilaris BS, et al: Factors of prognostic and therapeutic significance in patients with bladder cancer. Int J Rad Oncol Biol Phys 7:575, 1981
28. Cummings KB: Carcinoma of the bladder: Predictors. Cancer 45:1849, 1980
29. Batata M, Whitmore WF, Chu FCH, et al: Patterns of recurrence in bladder cancer treated by irradiation and/or cystectomy. Int J Rad Oncol Biol Phys 6:155, 1980
30. Yagoda A: Chemotherapy of metastatic bladder cancer. Cancer 45:1879, 1980
31. Coates AS, Golovsky D, Freedman A: Prolonged remission in recurrent bladder carcinoma after chemotherapy with cisplatinum. Med J Aust 1:533, 1981
32. Turner AG, Hendry WF, Williams GB, Bloom HJG: The treatment of advanced bladder cancer with methotrexate. Br J Urol 49:673, 1977
33. Hall RR, Bloom HJG, Freeman JE, Nawrocki A, Wallace DM: Methotrexate treatment for advanced bladder cancer. Br J Urol 46:431, 1974
34. Yagoda A, Watson RC, Whitmore WF, Grabstald H, Middleman MP, Krakoff IH: Adriamycin in advanced urinary tract cancer. Cancer 39:279, 1977
35. O'Bryan RM, Baker LH, Gottleib JE, et al: Dose response evaluation of adriamycin in human neoplasia. Cancer 39:1940, 1977
36. Fox M: The effect of cyclophosphamide on some urinary tract tumors. Br J Urol 37:399, 1965
37. De Kernion JB: The chemotherapy of advanced bladder carcinoma. Cancer Res 37:2771, 1977
38. Herr HW: *Cis*-diamminedichloride platinum II in the treatment of advanced bladder cancer. J Urol 123:853, 1980
39. Soloway MS, Ikard M, Ford J: *Cis*-diamminedichloro platinum (II) in locally advanced and metastatic urothelial cancer. Cancer 47:476, 1981
40. Williams SD, Donohue JP, Einhorn LE: Advanced bladder cancer: Therapy with *cis*-dichlorodiammine platinum (II), adriamycin and 5-fluorouracil. Cancer Treat Rt 63:1573, 1979
41. Troner MB, Hemstreet GP, III: Cyclophosphamide, doxorubicin and cisplatinum (CAP) in the treatment of urothelial malignancy: A pilot study of the Southeastern Cancer Study Group. Cancer Treat Rt 65:29, 1981
42. Campbell M, Baker LH, Opipari M, Al-Saffaf M: Phase II trial with cisplatinum, doxorubicin and cyclophosphamide (CAP) in the treatment of urothelial transitional cell carcinoma. Cancer Treat Rt 65:897, 1981
43. Narayana AS, Loening SA, Culp DA: Chemotherapy for advanced carcinoma of the bladder. J Urol 126:594, 1981
44. Kedia KR, Gibbons C, Persky L: The management of advanced bladder carcinoma. J Urol 125:655, 1981
45. Samuels ML, Moran ME, Johnson DE, Bracken RB: CISCA combination chemotherapy for metastatic carcinoma of the bladder. p. 101. In Johnson DE, Samuels ML (eds): Cancer of the Genitourinary Tract. Raven Press, New York, 1979
46. Yagoda A: Future implications of phase II chemotherapy trials in ninety-five patients with measurable advanced bladder cancer. Cancer Res 37:2775, 1977
47. Raghavan D, Pearson B, Woods W, Green D, Tattersall M: Pilot study of "first-line" cisplatinum chemotherapy in locally invasive non-metastatic bladder cancer. Proc Am Soc Clin Oncol 2:132, 1983
48. Raghavan D, Pearson B, Wines RD, et al: Intravenous cisplatinum for invasive clinically

non-metastatic bladder cancer: Safety and feasibility of a new approach. Med J Aust 140:276, 1984

49. Raghavan D, Pearson B, Duval P, et al: Front-line intravenous cisplatinum for locally invasive (T_{3-4} N_x M_o) bladder cancer. (Submitted for publication to J Urol)

50. Friedlander ML, Kearsley JH, Sims K, et al: Lorazepam as an adjunct to antiemetic therapy with haloperidol in patients receiving cytotoxic chemotherapy. Aust NZ J Med 13:53, 1983

51. Luk KH, Ross G, Phillips T, Goldstein L: The interaction of radiation and *cis*-diamminedichloro platinum (II) in intestinal crypt cells. Int J Rad Oncol Biol Phys 5:1417, 1979

12 | Use of Etoposide (VP-16–213) in Urologic Cancers

James L. Wade III
Nicholas J. Vogelzang

VP-16-213 (etoposide) was first introduced to clinical trials in 1973, and over the last decade, it has assumed an important role in treating a wide range of cancers. This chapter will focus on the current and future use of VP-16-213 in urologic malignancies.

VP-16-213 is a semi-synthetic derivative of podophyllotoxin, a product extracted from certain plants of the genus *Podophyllum*. American Indians and natives of the Himalayan mountains first used the alcohol extract, podophyllin, for medicinal purposes hundreds of years ago.[1] American colonists used podophyllin from the dried roots and rhizomes of *Podophyllum peltatum* (known as the American mandrake or May apple) for a cathartic and an antihelminthic. It was included in the first U.S. Pharmacopoeia in 1820 as an antiemetic and was listed there until 1942, when it was removed because of its toxicity. Kaplan, in 1942, reported that podophyllin extract destroyed condylomata accuminata when applied topically[2]; the antimitotic properties of podophyllin were first demonstrated in 1947.[3] Clinical trials as an antineoplastic agent were disappointing during the 1950s because of severe toxicity and limited responses.[4] In the mid 1960s, Sandoz Laboratories synthesized various podophyllin derivatives (SPI-77 and SPG 827) that produced minimal responses in head and neck malignancies, testicular tumors, and sarcomas.[5] Further modification of podophyllotoxin led to the synthesis of VP-16-213 and VM-26 in 1973.[6]

CHEMISTRY

VP-16-213 is 4'-demethylepipodophyllotoxin-β-D-ethylidene-glucoside, with a molecular formula of C-29 H-32 O-13 and a molecular weight of 588 Daltons.[6] The structures of the parent compound podophyllotoxin, etoposide, and its congener VM-26, are shown in Figure 12-1.

Etoposide acts through several mechanisms. When added to chick fibroblasts, it initially causes metaphase arrest similar to the mitotic spindle toxin colchicine.[7]

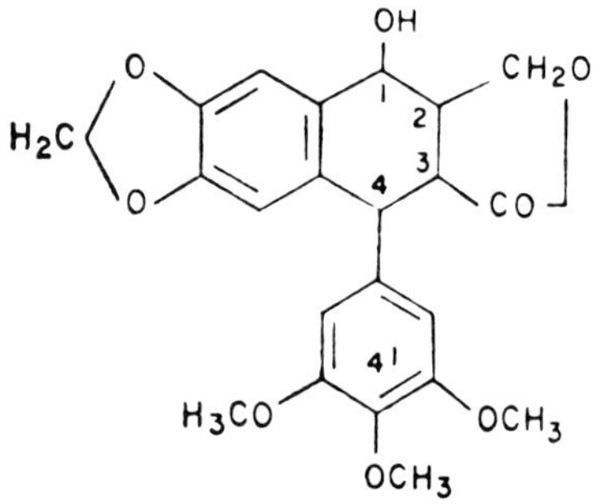

Podophyllotoxin

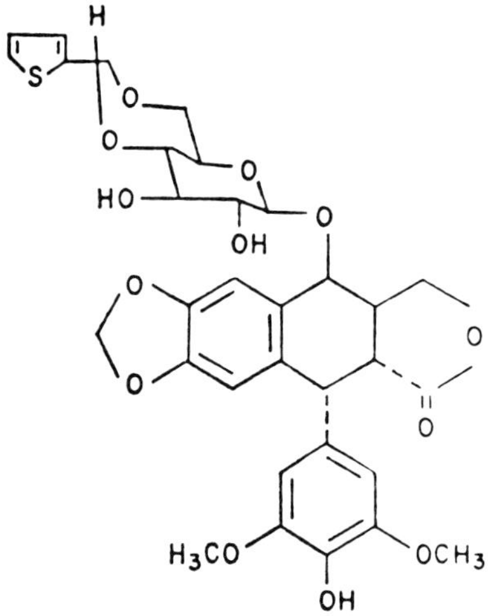

Teniposide (VM-26) 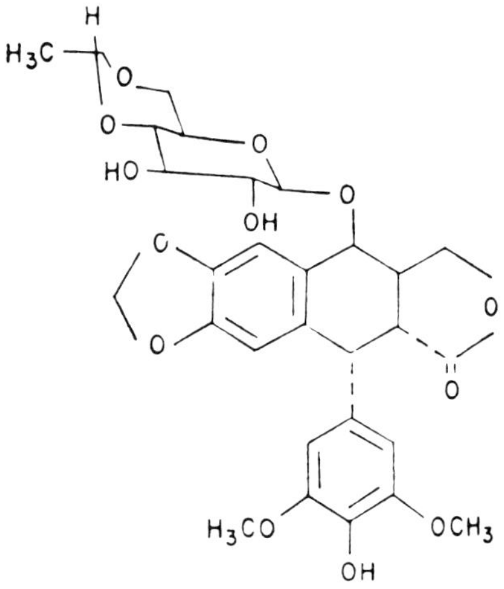   Etoposide (VP-16-213)

Fig. 12-1. Etoposide (VP-16-213). (Issell BF, Crooke ST: Etoposide (VP-16-213). Cancer Treatment Rev 6:107, 1979.)

It does not, however, bind to tubulin.[8] After a 30- to 60-minute incubation with VP-16-213, cells are prevented from entering mitosis. If cells are exposed to low concentrations of the drug (0.3 to 10 μg/ml) for two hours or more, this effect is irreversible. Cells that are exposed to higher in vitro concentrations ($>$10 μg/ml) are actually lysed when they enter mitosis.[6]

In addition to these effects on cell division, tritiated thymidine uptake by cells is inhibited. Leucine and uridine uptake are decreased also, but to a lesser degree, which implies that both DNA and RNA synthesis are inhibited.[6] Loike and Horowitz[9] also demonstrated that VP-16-213 causes single-strand breaks in DNA. Cytofluorometric studies have shown that VP-16-213 is cell cycle dependent and phase-specific, with maximum killing occurring during G_2 and S phases.[10] In summary, VP-16-213 prevents cells from entering mitosis, causes single-strand breaks in DNA, and is cell cycle-specific for G_2 and S phases.

PHARMACOLOGY

Etoposide is poorly soluble in water and will precipitate in dextrose solutions. It is supplied for clinical use in vials containing 100 mg etoposide, 400 mg Tween-80, 3.25 g of polyethylene glycol 300, 10 mg of anhydrous citric acid, and absolute alcohol to a volume of 5 ml. It should not be used if a precipitate is seen in the solution. At room temperature and shielded from light, each vial is stable for three years. Oral forms of the drug have been used, but absorption is erratic and unpredictable.[11] VP-16-213 should be diluted prior to administration with at least 20 equivalent volumes of normal saline (i.e., 100 mg in 5 cc should be diluted in 100 cc of 0.9 percent normal saline). After dilution, the drug is stable for only a short period of time, as indicated in Table 12-1.[12] The drug should be administered through a well-running IV and infused over 30 minutes; severe hypotension has been reported with more rapid infusions. The drug is apparently contraindicated for intrapleural, intraperitoneal, or intrathecal injections.[13] When administered intravenously, the drug follows a two-compartment pharmacokinetic model with a $t_{1/2} \alpha$ of 2.8 hours, a $t_{1/2} \beta$ of 15.1 hours and an overall $t_{1/2}$ of approximately 19 hours.[5,11,14] In plasma, the drug is 94 percent bound to albumin; there is also extensive tissue binding. The mean peak blood level with a 60-minute infusion of 200 mg/m² is 30 μg/ml.[14] There is poor penetration into the central nervous system with a cerebrospinal fluid concentration of approximately 4 percent that of plasma.[6] Forty percent of the drug is excreted in the urine, but 70 percent of this is not metabolized. Up to 16 percent of the drug is excreted in the feces in a metabolized form.[6,14-16] Although the metabolism of etoposide is not well under-

Table 12-1. Stability of VP-16 in Normal Saline

Concentrations (mg/ml)	Time Stable
1	30 minutes
0.4	4 hours
0.25	72 hours

stood at this time, the glucoside seems to be removed. The metabolite without the glucoside appears to be clinically active.[17]

TOXICITY

The major toxicity of VP-16-213 is dose-related bone marrow suppression. Leukopenia predominates, with a nadir at 13 to 16 days and recovery by day 22.[6] Nausea, vomiting, and occasionally diarrhea occur and are greater with the oral preparations. Alopecia occurs in most patients. Acute toxicities include hypotension with rapid infusion,[18] and rarely, fever, chills, wheezing, and bronchospasm, which respond to withdrawal of the drug and administration of antihistamines. Phlebitis will occur if the drug extravasates. Several cases of myocardial infarction have been reported during treatment with VP-16-213, but no cause–effect relationship has been shown.[19,20]

SPECTRUM OF ACTIVITY IN VITRO

VP-16-213 has been found to be active against the Walker 256 carcinosarcoma, a variety of murine leukemias, including L-1210, the Ehrlich ascites tumor, and the sarcoma 37 and 180 system.[21,22] An important schedule dependency was noted in the L-1210 system.[22] Maximum activity was demonstrated with dose intervals of 2 to 4 days, with less activity when the drug was given daily for 5 days, or weekly. Schedule dependency has also been shown in vitro with two human tumor cell lines, the RPMI myeloma 8226 and the endometrial HeLa-1A model.[23,24] The drug is also effective in vitro against human lung small cell carcinoma lines, induced bladder tumor cell lines, and nonseminoma germ cell tumor cell lines.[25-27] The drug has not been found to be effective against human prostate carcinoma grown in nude mice.[28]

DRUG SYNERGY

Therapeutic drug synergy between VP-16 and cisplatin has been observed in the P-388 murine leukemia.[29] This observation has now been used clinically, and VP-16 has been given concomantly with cisplatin (see below) in patients with refractory germ cell tumors, with moderate success. In Hodgkin's disease and non-Hodgkin lymphomas, cisplatin has been combined with VP-16 and found effective in refractory patients.[6]

DRUG RESISTANCE

The mechanisms of drug resistance to VP-16-213 are unknown at this time. Resistance can be defined either in vitro or in vivo. Growth of neoplastic cells in the presence of a specific drug is a manifestation of in vitro resistance. In vivo resistance may occur through the same mechanisms as in vitro resistance, but also through changes in drug delivery (i.e., diminished drug supply after surgery or radiation therapy) or through alteration in drug pharmacology, with accelerated metabolism to inactive products or increased excretion. Several facts are now known about in vitro resistance to VP-16-213. Using the Chinese hamster ovary tumor cell system (CHO), Gupta[30] was able to show different patterns of resistance using different microtubule inhibitors. The CHO mutant cells that become resistant to podophyllotoxin (which binds to tubulin) showed a genetic change in a microtubule-associated protein, which results in less podophyllotoxin being bound. VP-16-213, which does not bind to tubulin, is still effective in CHO cells that carry this acquired resistance. This new protein is also found in cells that manifest cross-resistance to other microtubule inhibitors, such as colchicine and vinblastine.[31] Therefore, drug resistance to microtubule inhibitors does not carry over to resistance to VP-16-213. Using the Ehrlich ascites tumor model, Seeber et al.[32] demonstrated that cells cultured for resistance to VP-16-213 are also resistant to doxorubicin, but sensitive to *cis*-platinum. Seeber[33] also observed that cell lines resistant to *cis*-platinum were sensitive to VP-16-213. Arnold and Whitehouse[34] found that inhibition of DNA repair circumvented VP-16-213 resistance. Using the TLX-5 murine ascitic tumor system, they showed that VP-16-213 alone was largely ineffective, but when given with chlorquine (a DNA repair inhibitor) the life expectancy of the mice was increased 83 percent. This implies that resistance to VP-16-213 in vitro may occur through the rapid repair of the single-strand breaks in DNA caused by VP-16-213. Further understanding of the mechanisms of VP-16-213 resistance will allow for a better drug design and more intelligent use of combination chemotherapy to circumvent resistance.

IN VIVO ACTIVITY

VP-16-213 has been found to be clinically active in a variety of neoplasms. The drug is now used in lung cancer (both small cell and non-small cell), Hodgkin's disease, histiocytic lymphoma, acute lymphocytic and non-lymphocytic leukemia, Kaposi's sarcoma, hepatoma, and genitourinary tumors.[1] This chapter will focus on the latter group.

TESTIS CANCER

Etoposide was first used in testis cancer as a single agent in the early 1970s.[1,35-38] These first reports involved phase I trials, and a cumulative response rate of 20 percent was obtained. A complete list of all trials using VP-16-213 as a single agent in refractory testis cancer is given in Table 12-2 and shows a response rate of 34 percent. In one of the largest series, Fitzharris et al. demonstrated a 46 percent response rate (12.5 percent CR and 34 percent PR) in 24 previously treated patients.[42] Interpretation of this study was hampered by the different prior therapies the patients had received (a number of patients had not received cisplatin)

Table 12-2. Studies of VP-16-213 as Single-Agent Therapy of Germ-Cell Testicular Cancer

Institution	Year	Patients (No.)	Responders (No.)
EORTC[a][35]	1973	4	0
Finsen Institute (Denmark)[36]	1972	3	0
Memorial Sloan-Kettering[37]	1973	3	0
Mayo Clinic[38]	1975	1	1
Charing Cross (England)[39]	1977	5	4
Switzerland (Berne)[40]	1977	7	4
Indiana University[41]	1980	3	3
Royal Marsden (England)[42]	1980	24	10
CALGB[b][43]	1980	5	0
Switzerland—EORTC[a][44]	1981	30	6
University of Vienna[45]	1981	9	8
W. Germany Cancer Center[46]	1982	37	4
Total		121	41 (34%)

[a] European Organization for Research on the Treatment of Cancer.
[b] Cancer and Leukemia Group B.

and by two different dosing schedules: 20 patients received 120 mg/m^2 day × 5 days, q 2 to 4 weeks, and 5 patients received 100 mg/m^2/day × 5 days, q 4 weeks. Some of the patients who responded went on to other regimens that included VP-16. In spite of its shortcomings, the study supported the evidence that etoposide is one of the most active drugs in testis cancer. The gradual increase in response rate over the decade of the 1970s probably reflects increased understanding of the optimal dose and frequency of administration of VP-16-213. Since 1981, all published reports of VP-16-213 in testis cancer have been of etoposide combined with other chemotherapeutic agents. The activity of VP-16-213 in combination with other drugs for refractory testis cancer is summarized in Table 12-3. The studies in this table are important in that these "salvage" regimens have been found to be active in spite of tumor relapse or progression with first-line cisplatin-based therapy. Several facts are now known about the behavior of testis cancer after initial chemotherapy:

1. If a patient achieves a complete remission with standard cisplatin-based therapy and later relapses, he has a significant chance (greater than 50 percent) of a second complete remission with combination cisplatin and VP-16-213-based chemotherapy.
2. If patients achieve only a partial remission on standard therapy, a complete remission with cisplatin and etoposide is highly unlikely. Although these patients have a significant chance of achieving a second partial remission, the chances of cure in this patient would be low, but has occurred.
3. The value of doxorubicin in "salvage" regimens remains unclear.
4. More potent therapy is needed for drug-resistant testis cancer.

With these points in mind, three groups began experimenting with high-dose chemotherapy, including high-dose VP-16-213, coupled with autologous bone marrow transplantation in patients with drug-resistant testis cancer (Table 12-4). The results

Table 12-3. Results of VP-16-213 as Part of Multi-Agent Chemotherapy for Previously Treated Germinal Cancer[a]

Institution	Year	Patient (No.)	Responders (No.)	Prior Therapy[b]	Drugs used with VP-16-213[b]
Indiana[41]	1980	21	18 (9 PR, 9 CR)	VLB, Bleo, DDP	ADR, DDP ± Bleo
Minnesota[47]	1981	9	8 (3 PR, 5 CR)	VLB, Bleo, DDP	ADR, DDP ± Bleo
		9	7 (4 PR, 3 CR)	VLB, Bleo, DDP	ADR/ Bleo/DDP
West Germany Cancer Treatment Center[46]	1982	36	21 (17 PR, 4 CR)	VLB, Bleo, DDP	Ifosfamide
Cleveland Clinic[48]	1982	11	11 (10 PR, 1 CR)[c]	VLB, Bleo, DDP	VLB, Bleo, DDP, ADR
MSKCC[d][49]	1983	22	7 (4 PR, 3 CR)[e]	VLB, Bleo, DDP, ADR	DDP
National Cancer Institute[50]	1983	4	4 (2 PR, 2 CR)	Not listed	VLB, Bleo, DDP
Dana-Farber[51]	1983	18	11 (6 PR, 5 CR)	VLB, Bleo, DDP	DDP, ± ADR, ± Bleo
Total		130	87 (67%)		

[a] Most series include variable numbers of patients with extragonadal tumors.
[b] VLB, velban; Bleo, bleomycin; DDP, cis-platinum; ADR, adriamycin.
[c] Four patients converted to CR after surgery.
[d] Memorial Sloan-Kettering Cancer Center.
[e] CR in patients only with prior CR.

Table 12-4. Results of VP-16-213-Based Multi-Agent Chemotherapy with Autologous Bone Marrow Transplant Support

Institution	Year	Patient (No.)	Response (No.)	Prior Chemotherapy[a]	Drug used in Addition to VP-16[a]
M.D. Anderson[52]	1981	13	7 (3 PR, 4 CR) 4 deaths	Not listed	Cytox/BCNU and others
National Cancer Institute	1982	6	4 (CR)	None	DDP/Bleo/VLB
		4	4 (2 PR, 2 CR)	Not listed	DDP/Bleo/VLB
Vanderbilt[53]	1983	4	4 (1 CR, 3 PR)	VLB/DDP/BLEO ± others	—
		6	2 (1 PR, 1 CR)	VLB/DDP/Bleo/VP-16 ± others	—
Total		33	21 (64%)		

[a] Cytox, cytoxan; DDP, cis-platinum; Bleo, bleomycin; VLB, velban.

published demonstrate some activity in previously treated patients, but significant toxicity. No patient was cured using autologous bone marrow transplantation. The most recent approach is to combine VP-16-213 with other drugs in the initial treatment of poor-prognosis testis cancer. Standard Velban–platinum–bleomycin regimens have obtained only a 30 to 50 percent CR rate in patients with poor prognostic factors.[54] Thus, the addition of VP-16-213 to front-line therapy in these patients is a natural step. The results of these studies are listed in Table 12-5. The higher response rates, particularly the CR rate, seem to imply a greater activity than that seen in historical controls. To compare the true efficacy of etoposide-containing regimens several studies are now in progress in which patients are randomized between conventional therapy, i.e., VAB-6[59] or VPB and a VP-16 based regimen.

The Memorial Sloan-Kettering Cancer Center and several associated institutions are currently categorizing patients as good risk and poor risk. These risk categories were defined by a multivariate analysis of 220 testicular cancer patients treated between 1975 and 1981.[54] Good-risk patients receive either VAB-6 or VP-16-213 (120 mg/m², IV daily × 5) plus cisplatin (20 mg/m², IV daily × 5). Currently, 51 patients have been randomized.[60] Poor-risk patients receive alternating courses of VP-16-213/cisplatin and VAB-6, for a total of six cycles. The Southeastern Cancer Study Group is randomizing all patients to either vinblastine–bleomycin and cisplatin or etoposide–bleomycin and cisplatin. The European Organization for Research in the Treatment of Cancer is studying etoposide/cisplatin versus etoposide/cisplatin/bleomycin in all metastatic testicular cancer patients. It is hoped that the results of these three randomized studies will clearly define the role of etoposide in the initial treatment of germinal malignancies. The potential elimination of vinblastine and bleomycin from "standard" regimens should reduce the risk of long-term vascular complications, such as Raynaud's phenomenon.[61] In summary, etoposide is an extremely effective drug in nonseminomatous testis cancer and is becoming part of the initial chemotherapy for many patients. Its role in salvage therapy after relapse with conventional therapy is now better appreciated. Further studies will be necessary to help clarify its role in front-line treatment.

TRANSITIONAL CELL CARCINOMA OF THE BLADDER

VP-16-213 has been tried both orally and intravenously in patients with advanced bladder cancer.[62] Falkson et al.[63] first reported the use of oral VP-16-213 200 mg/m², PO, for five days repeated every two to three weeks in a variety of tumors. Four patients with bladder cancer were treated, with two patients improving and two progressing. The newer oral preparation was used by Panduro et el.[64] and reported in 1981. All 11 patients had received prior radiation, but no prior chemotherapy, and VP-16-213 was given as drinking ampules in a dose of 130 mg/m² daily × 5 days repeated every three weeks. Three patients died early in the study and of the remaining eight, one had a complete remission lasting 9 months and one had stable disease for 18 months. The remaining six had progressive disease. Currently, VP-16 is being studied with cisplatin in patients with bladder

Table 12-5. Results of VP-16-213 in Multi-Agent Chemotherapy in Poor-Risk, Previously Untreated Patients [a]

Institution	Year	Patient (No.)	Responder (No.)	Other Drugs [b]
Charing Cross[55]	1982	64	48 (29 PR, 19 CR)	VCR/Cytox/ACT-D/Bleo MTX/DDP/HYDR/ CHLR/VLB/ADR
Cleveland Clinic[56]	1982	9	7 (2 PR, 5 CR)	VLB/Bleo/DDP/ADR
National Cancer Institute[50]	1983	6	6 (CR)	VLB/Bleo/DDP
Walter Reed Hospital[57]	1983	13	11 (2 PR, 9 CR)	VCR/Cytox/ACT-D/Bleo VLB/DDP
Royal Marsden[58] [c]	1983	19	15 (CR)	Bleo/DDP
Royal Marsden[58] [d]	1983	24	22 (CR)	Bleo/DDP
		135	109 (81%)	

[a] Some series include extragonadal germ-cell tumor patients.
[b] VCR, vincristine; Cytox, cytoxan; ACT-D, actinomycin-D; Bleo, bleomycin; MTX, methotrexate; DDP, *cis*-platinum; HYDR, hydroxyurea; CHLR, chlorambucil; VLB, velban; ADR, adriamycin.
[c] Large volume metastases ("poor risk").
[d] Small volume metastases ("good risk").

cancer at the Mayo Clinic.[65] Hahn has noted a response rate of 25 percent in 19 patients treated with this combination.

PROSTATE CANCER

In three broad-phase II studies, only seven patients with prostate cancer were treated with etoposide.[35,43,66] One had a PR, two improved, and four progressed. VP-16-213 has been tested as a continuous 5-day infusion (50 mg/m^2 daily) at the Wisconsin Clinical Cancer Center. No responses were seen in 21 patients.[67] This suggests little or no activity of VP-16-213 in this disease.

RENAL CELL CANCER

VP-16-213 also has little if any activity in cancer of the kidney. A review of 40 patients treated with VP-16-213 prior to 1979 showed no response.[68] In 1979, Hahn et al. reported 1 CR of 37 treated patients.[69] In 1980, Nissen[43] reported that twice weekly intravenous VP-16 netted 1 improved patient and 2 stable patients out of 10. There are currently no investigations studying the use of combined cisplatin with VP-16 in patients with renal adenocarcinoma.

CANCER OF THE RENAL PELVIS

There are no reports of patients with cancer of the renal pelvis or urethra being treated with VP-213. Similarly, there are no ongoing studies evaluating this drug in this tumor type. Because of similar histology, it is expected that these tumors would be as responsive, or unresponsive, as transitional cell carcinomas of the urinary bladder.

WILMS' TUMOR OF CHILDHOOD

In 1979, Chard[70] reported two of six children treated with VP-16-213 showing tumor response. That same study noted that there was a lack of cross-resistance between VP-16-213 and its cogenor VM-26. Currently, VP-16 is being used for children with recurrent solid tumors refractory to standard therapy, under the direction of the Pediatric Oncology Group in St. Louis, Missouri.

SUMMARY

VP-16-213 is a new chemotherapeutic agent with a long history. Over the next decade, its mechanism of action will be further elucidated and resistance to its effect better understood. Etoposide will be used more frequently in front-line therapy for testis cancer in combination with cisplatin and other drugs. Its role in other genitourinary malignancies remains to be elucidated.

ACKNOWLEDGMENTS

This work was supported in part by the American Cancer Society Junior Faculty Fellowship (JFCF 639) and grant CA 14599–10 from the National Institutes of Health. Dr. Vogelzang is a Gould Foundation Faculty Scholar.

REFERENCES

1. Vogelzang NJ, Raghavan D, Kennedy BJ: VP-16-213 (Etoposide): The mandrake root from Issyk-Kul. Am J Med 72:136, 1982
2. Kaplan IW: Condylomata accuminata. New Orleans Med Surg J 94:388, 1942
3. Sullivan BJ, Wechsler HI: The cytological effects of podophyllin. Science 105:433, 1947
4. Greenspan EM, Colsky J, Schoenbach ER, Shear NJ: Response of patients with advanced neoplasms to the intravenous administration of alpha-peltatin. J Natl Cancer Inst 14:1257, 1954
5. Vaitkevicius VK, Reed ML: Clinical Studies with podophyllin compounds, SPI-77 and SPG-827. Cancer Chemotherapy Rt 50:565, 1966
6. Isscll BF, Crookc ST: Etoposide (VP-16-213). Cancer Treat Rev 6.107, 1979
7. Stahelin H: Activity of a new glycoside ligand derivative VP-16-213 related to podophyllin in experimental tumors. Eur J Cancer 9:250, 1973
8. Margolis RL, Wilson L: Opposite end assembly and disassembly of microtubules in steady state in vitro. Cell 13:1, 1975
9. Loike JD, Horowitz SB: Effects of VP-16-213 on the intracellular degradation of DNA in HeLa cells. Biochemistry 15:5443, 1976
10. Krishan A, Paika K, Frei E: Cytofluorometric studies of the actions of podophyllotoxin and epidhophyllotoxins (VM-26 and VP-16-213) on the cell cycle transverse of human lymphoblasts. J Cell Biol 66:521, 1975
11. Creaven PJ: The clinical pharmacology of VM-26 and VP-16-213. Cancer Chemotherapy Pharmacol 7:133, 1982
12. Door R, Fitz WL: Cancer Chemotherapy Handbook. p. 420. Part IV, Elsevier, New York, 1980
13. Stalhelin H: Delayed toxicity of epipodophyllotoxin derivatives VM-26 and VP-16-213 due to local effects. Eur J Can 12:925, 1976
14. Allen CN, Creaven PJ: Comparison of the human pharmacokinetics of VM-26 and VP-16; two antineoplastic epipodophyllotoxin glucopyranoside derivatives. Eur J Can 11:697, 1978
15. Van Naanen JMS, VanOort WJ, Pinedo HM: Studies of the metabolism of VP-16-213 in the rat. Cancer Chemotherapy Pharmacol 7:236 (Abstract), 1982
16. Evans WE, Sinkule JA, Crom WR, Look AT, Dow LW, Rivera G: Pharmacokinetics of teniposide (VM-26) and etoposide (VP-16-213) in children with cancer. Cancer Chemotherapy Pharmacol 7:147, 1982.
17. Jardine I, Strife RJ: Is the lactone moiety of VP-16-213 necessary for activity? Synthesis and Activity of the VP-16-213 cyclic ether. Cancer Chemotherapy Pharmacol 7:235, 1982
18. Creaven PJ, Neuman FJ, Selawry OS, Cohen MH, Primack A: Phase I clinical trial

of weekly administration of (4')-demethyl-epipodophyllotoxin-9-(4,6,-0-ethylidine-β-D-glucopyranoside) (NSC-14150; VP-16-213). Cancer Chemotherapy Rep 58(6):901, 1974

19. Schector JP, Jones SE, Jackson RA: Myocardial infarction in a 27-year-old woman: Possible complication of treatment with VP-16-213 (NSC-14150), mediastinal irradiation, or both. (Letter) Cancer Chemotherapy Rt 59(5):887, 1975

20. Praga C, Beretta G, Labianca R: Cardiac toxicity from anti-tumor therapy. Oncology 37(suppl 1):51, 1980

21. Rozencweig M, Von Hoff DD, Henney JE, Muggia FM: VM-26 and VP-16-213. A comparative analysis. Cancer 40:334, 1977

22. Dombernowsky P, Nissen NI: Schedule dependancy of the anti-leukemia activity of the podophyllotoxin derivative VP-16-213 (NSC-14150) in L-1210 leukemia. Arch Pathol Mircobiol Scand 81:715, 1973

23. Loike JD: VP-16-213 and podophyllotoxin. A study of the relationship between chemical structure and biologic activity. Cancer Chemotherapy Pharmacol 7:103, 1982

24. Ludwig R, Alberts DS, Miller TP, Salmon SE, Wood DA: Scheduled dependency (SD) of anticancer drugs in the human tumor stem cell assay (HTSCA). Proc Am Assoc Cancer Res 183 (Abstract 178), 1982

25. Carney DN, Gazdar AS, Minna JD: In vitro chemosensitivity of clinical specimens and established cell lines of small cell lung cancer. Proc Am Assoc Cancer Res ASCO 22:10 (Abstract #C-37), 1981

26. Mickey DD, Neill HB, Soloway MS: Correlation of drug sensitivity of FANFT-induced mouse bladder tumors grown in syngenic mice in soft agar and microliter plates. Proc Am Assoc Cancer Res (Abstract #866), 1982

27. San Fileppo O, Silverstrini R, Zaffamoni N, Pizzocaro G: In vitro chemosensitivity of testicular tumors and its clinical perspective. p. 131. Int. Union against Cancer (Abstract #13-0152), 1982

28. Akimoto M, Tsuboi N, Kawamura N, Nakajima H, Yui Y, Yoshida K, Kanai H, Kidani Y: A study of the antitumor agents platinum complex, VP-16, and mitomycin-C (MMC) against human prostatic carcinoma in nude mice. p. 367. Proceedings of the 39th Annual Meeting of the Japanese Cancer Association, 1980

29. Schabel FM, Trader MW, Laster WR, Corbett TH, Griswold DP: *Cis*-diamminodichloroplatinum (II): Combination chemotherapy and gross resistant studies with tumors of mice. Cancer Treat Rt 63(9–10):1459, 1977

30. Gupta RS: Resistance to the microtubule inhibitor podophyllotoxin: Selection and partial characterization of mutant CHO cells. Somatic Cell Genet 7(1):59, 1981

31. Gupta RA: Podophyllootoxin resistant mutant of chinese hamster ovary cells: Gross resistant studies with various microtubule inhibitors and podophyllotoxin analogs. Cancer Res 43:505, 1983

32. Seeber S, Schmidt CG, Achterrath W, Crooke ST: In vivo resistance towards anthracyclines, etoposide and *cis*-diammine-dichloroplatinum (II). Cancer Res 42:4719, 1982

33. Seeber S: Model studies with etoposide resistance. Cancer Treat Rev 9(suppl A):18, 1982; 18, 1981

34. Arnold AM, Whitehouse JFM: Interaction of VP-16-213 with the DNA repair antagonist chloroquine. Cancer Chemotherapy Pharmacol 7:123, 1982

35. European Organization for Research on the Treatment of Cancer, Clinical Screening Group: Epipodophyllotoxin VP-16-213 in the treatment of acute leukemias, haematosarcomas and solid tumors. Br Med J 3:199, 1973

36. Nissen NI, Larson V, Pederson H, Thomsen K: Phase I clinical trials of a new antitumor agent 4'-demethylepipodophyllotoxin 9-(4,6,-0-ethylidene-β-D-glucopyranoside) (NSC-141540; VP-16-213). Cancer Chemotherapy Rt. 56 (I), 769, 1972

37. Young CW, Ihde DL, Von Stubble W: Prelimnary clinical trial of 4'-demethylepipodo-phyllotoxin-β-D-ethylidene-glucopyranoside) (VP-16-213). Proc Am Assoc Cancer Res 14:60, 1973

38. Eagen RT, Ahmann DL, Hahn RG, O'Connell MJ: Pilot study to determine an intermit-tent dose schedule for VP-16-213. Proc Am Assoc Cancer Res ASCO. 16:55, 1975

39. Newlands ES, Bagshawe KD: Epipodophyllotoxin derivative VP-16-213 in malignant teratomas and choriocarcinomas (Letter). Lancet ii:87, 1977

40. Cavalli F, Sontag RW, Brunner KW: Epipodophyllin derivative (VP-16-213) in the treatment of solid tumors. Lancet ii:322, 1977

41. Williams SD, Einhorn LD, Greco FA, Oldham R, Fletcher R: VP-16-213 salvage therapy for refractory germinal neoplasm. Cancer 2154, 1980

42. Fitzharris BM, Kaye SE, Saverymuttu S, Newlands ES, Barrett A, Peckham MJ, McEl-wain TJ: VP-16-213 as a single agent in advanced testicular tumors. Eur J Cancer 16:1193, 1980

43. Nissen NI, Pajak TF, Leone LA, et al: Clinical trial of VP-16-213 (NSC 141540) I.V. twice weekly in advanced neoplastic disease: A study of the Cancer and Leukemia Group B. Cancer 45:232, 1980

44. Cavalli F, Klepp O, Renard J, Röhrt M, Alberto P, EORTC: A phase II study of oral VP-16-213 in non-seminomatous testicular cancer. Eur J Cancer 17:245, 1981

45. Aiginger E, Kuhboch J, Kuzmits R, Schwartz HP: VP-16 therapy in *cis*-platinum resistant testicular tumors. 12th Intl. Congr. Chemotherapy (Abstract #1149), 1981

46. Bremer K, Niederle N, Krischke W, Higi M, Scheulen ME, Schmidt CG, Seeber S: Etoposide and etoposide-ifosfamide therapy for refractory testicular tumors. Cancer Treat Rev 9(Supply A):79, 1982

47. Vogelzang NJ, Kennedy BJ: Salvage chemotherapy for refractory germ cell tumors. Proc Am Soc Clin Oncol 22:471, 1981 (Abstract #546)

48. Mortimer J, Bukowski RM, Montie J, Hewlett JS, Livingston RB: VP-16-213 cis-plati-num and adriamycin salvage therapy of refractory and/or recurrent nonseminomatous germ cell neoplasms. Cancer Chemotherapy Pharmacol 7:215, 1982

49. Bosl GJ, Yagoda A, Whitmore WF, Sogani P, Herr H, Vugrin D, Dukemar M, Golbey R: VP-16-213 and cisplatin in the treatment of refractory germ cell tumors. Am J Clin Oncol (In press).

50. Ozols RF, Deisseroth AB, Javadpour N, Barlock A, Messerschmidt GL, Young RT: Treatment of poor prognosis non-seminomatous testicular cancer with a "high dose" platinum combination chemotherapy regimen. Cancer 51:1803, 1983

51. Lederman GS, Garnick MB, Richie JP, Canellos GP: Chemotherapy of refractory germ cell cancer with etoposide. J Clin Oncol 1:706, 1983

52. Blijham G, Spitzer G, Litam J, Zander A, Verma ES, Bellekoop L, Samuels M, McCredie KB, Dicke KR: The treatment of advanced testicular carcinoma with high dose chemo-therapy and autologous bone marrow support. Eur J Cancer 17:433, 1981

53. Wolfe SN, Johnson DH, Hainsworth JD, Greco FA: High dose VP-16-213 monotherapy for refractory germinal malignancies—a phase II study. J Clin Oncol 2:271, 1984

54. Bosl GJ, Geller NC, Cirricione C, Vogelzang NJ, Kennedy BJ, Whitmore WF, Vugrin P, Scher H, Nisselbaum J, Golbey RB: Multivariate analysis of prognostic variables in patients with metastatic testicular cancer. Cancer Res 43:3403, 1983

55. Begent RHJ, Newlands ES, Rustin GJS, Bagshaw EK: Combination chemotherapy for advanced malignant teratoma. Cancer Chemotherapy Pharmacol 7(43):243, 1982

56. Bukowski RM, Montie J, Livingston RB, Weick JK, Groppe CW, Hewlett JS, Purvis

J: Combination chemotherapy including VP-16 in poor prognosis germ cell tumors. Proc Am Assoc Cancer Res 23:163, 1982 (Abstract #604)

57. Taylor G, Knight R, Major W, Boyd J, Perry D, Skoog S, McLeod D, Stutzman R: Improved outcome in bulky stage III germ cell tumors treated with cyclophosphamide, actinomycin, vinblastine, cisplatinum alternating with VP-16, vincristine. Proc Am Soc Clin Oncol 1:137, 1983 (Abstract #538)

58. Barrett A, Peckham MJ, Liew KH, McElwain TJ, Horwich A, Robinson B, Dobbs MJ, Hendry WF: The treatment of metastatic germ cell testicular tumors with bleomycin, etoposide, and cisplatin (BEP). Br J Cancer 47:613, 1983

59. Vugrin D, Whitmore WF, Golbey RB: VAB-6 combination chemotherapy without maintenance in treatment of disseminated cancer of the testis. Cancer 51:211, 1983

60. Bosl G: Personal communication. November 1983

61. Vogelzang NJ, Bosl GJ, Johnson K, Kennedy BJ: Raynaud's phenomenon: A common toxicity after vinblastine, bleomycin, and cisplatin therapy of testicular cancer. Ann Int Med 95:288, 1981

62. Yagoda A: Chemotherapy of metastatic bladder cancer. Cancer 45(7):(suppl):1879, 1980

63. Falkson G, Van Dyk JJ, von Eden EB, van Dermerwe AM, van den Berghe JA, Falkson HC: A clinical trial of the oral form of 4'-dimethylepipodophyllotoxin-β-D-ethylidene-glucose (NSC-141540) VP-16. Cancer 35:1141, 1975

64. Panduro J, Hansen M, Hansen HH: Oral VP-16-213 in transitional cell carcinoma of the bladder: A phase II study. Cancer Treat Rt 65(7–8):703, 1981

65. Hahn RG: Personal communication. November 1983

66. Jungi WF, Senn HT: Clinical study of the new podophyllotoxin derivative 4'-dimethyl-epipodophyllotoxin 9-4,6,-0-ethylidene-β-D-glucopyranoside (NSC-141540; VP-16-213) in solid tumors in man. Cancer Chemotherapy Rt 59(4):737, 1975

67. Trump DL, Loprinzi MD: Phase II trial of Etoposide (VP-16-213) in advanced prostate cancer. In press

68. Arnold AM: Podophyllotoxin derivative VP-16-213. Cancer Chemotherapy Pharmacol 3:71, 1979

69. Hahn RG, Bauer M, Wolter J, Creech R, Bennett JM, Wampler G: A phase II study of single agent therapy with megestrol acetate, Vp-16-213, cyclophosphamide, and dian-hydrogalactitol in advanced renal cell cancer. Cancer Treat Rt 63:1755, 1979

70. Chard RL, Krivit W, Bleyer WA, Hammond D: Phase II study of VP-16-213 in child-hood malignant disease: A children's cancer study group report. Cancer Treat Rt 63:1755, 1979

13 | Interferon in Urologic Malignancies

John M. Kirkwood
Marc S. Ernstoff

The interferons (IFN) comprise a complex group of several different families and an undetermined number of subfamilies of hormonelike proteins. They are relatively species-specific, with some cross-reactivity apparent between IFN of higher and lower vertebrates. The methods for production of IFN in vivo and in vitro will be reviewed, as well as assays required for typing and quantification of IFN as these are pertinent to treatment programs for cancer. The preclinical and clinical basis for the application of IFN alpha and IFN beta to renal cell carcinoma and bladder carcinoma will be discussed, with an examination of the results of studies reported to date.

Interferons were first described by Isaacs and Lindenmann[1] as substances produced by cultured cells, in response to noninfectious viruses, which induced cellular resistance to subsequent lytic virus infection. This antiviral activity has been a basis for the bioassay of all IFNs, despite the wide range of other biological effects that have been recognized. The production of IFN by virtually all types of eukaryotic cells is now recognized, following induction by live virus, derived natural and synthetic nucleic acids, and other substances. The IFN were initially categorized according to their cell of origin, inductive stimuli, or crude physicochemical properties, such as acid lability. Table 13-1 reviews the recognized families of IFN, designated alpha, beta, and gamma according to their cell of origin. The manner of induction of virus-induced (alpha, beta) and immune (gamma) IFN provides an additional differentiation between the IFN and has been the basis for classification of human and murine IFN into types I and II, respectively.

Interferon alpha comprises a number of subfamilies coded on human chromosomes 2, 5, and 9. Genes for more than 14 distinct IFN alpha proteins are now

Table 13-1. Interferons

Type	Cell Source	Classical Stimulus	Acid Stability	Molecular Size	Recognized Subspecies
Alpha	Leukocyte	Virus	$+(-)$	15–21,000	≥ 16 with $>80\%$ homology
Beta	Fibroblast	Virus dsRNA	$+$	20,000	29–45% homology with alpha
Gamma	T Lymphocyte	Mitogen	$-$	17–46,000	1% with Introns, distinct from alpha or beta

documented among the alpha family, with homology from 80 to >95 percent. The chromosomal location of genes that specify IFN alpha was first suggested by somatic cell genetic analysis,[2] and has been amplified in more recent studies by recombinant DNA technology. Interferon production by appropriately stimulated cells ensues rapidly, following the appearance of new messenger RNA. Production may be manipulated by inhibitors of protein synthesis or even by the addition of small quantities of interferon. Intact blood buffy-coat leukocytes or cultured fibroblasts have been used as the classical source of alpha and beta IFN, respectively. The methods of Cantell,[3] which have been the standard for production of human leukocyte IFN alpha for clinical trials over much of the past decade, are outlined in Figure 13-1. Buffy-coat leukocytes have been freshly purified from units of whole blood and stimulated by means of Sendai virus in vitro for 18 hours. Interferon produced in the crude supernatant culture fluid has been purified by ethanol precipitation and adjustment of the pH 2.5.[3] The Cantell-type IFN alpha obtained from buffy-coat leukocytes used in most large trials in Scandinavia and the United States during the past decade have been approximately 1 percent pure (1×10^6 antiviral units per milligrams protein, as defined below).

Production of IFN alpha has recently been refined by purification using monoclonal antibody affinity columns,[4] achieving up to 1.0×10^8 μ/mg protein, in more limited quantities. The Burroughs Wellcome Corp. has produced IFN alpha from a lymphoblast line (Namalva) on a large scale, using methods capable of achieving specific activities up to 2×10^8 μ/mg, with only modest pyrogen (0.4 ng/ml Limulus lysate endotoxin equivalents).

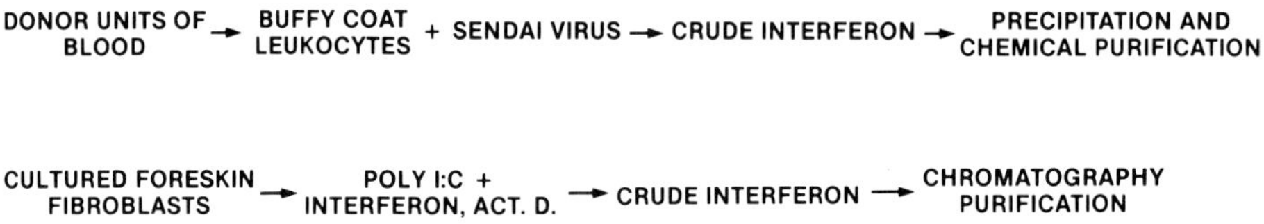

DONOR UNITS OF BLOOD → BUFFY COAT LEUKOCYTES + SENDAI VIRUS → CRUDE INTERFERON → PRECIPITATION AND CHEMICAL PURIFICATION

CULTURED FORESKIN FIBROBLASTS → POLY I:C + INTERFERON, ACT. D. → CRUDE INTERFERON → CHROMATOGRAPHY PURIFICATION

Fig. 13-1. Classical purification of cellular interferon.

Interferon beta has been classically produced from fetal foreskin fibroblasts after induction by synthetic polynucleotides. Production of IFN beta from cultured fibroblasts has been enhanced by the addition of interferon in small quantities, with inhibitors of protein synthesis.[5] These methods of "superinduction" have yielded IFN of a purity comparable to that of whole-leukocyte IFN, in sufficient quantities to allow limited national trials similar to those carried out with Cantell-type IFN alpha. Methods have recently been described for production of even larger quantities of IFN beta from fibroblasts at 60 percent or greater purity, with a specific activity of $>1.5 \times 10^8$ μ/mg protein and homogeneity in polyacrylamide gel electrophoresis.[6]

Interferon gamma has been shown to be produced by T lymphocytes, prototypically, in response to antigenic or mitogenic stimuli. The instability of IFN gamma at an acid pH has been a defining characteristic of this species, and its general instability has complicated production and purification of quantities required for clinical studies. Although production of limited amounts of IFN gamma is possible, using potent antigens or mitogens such as staphylococcal protein A and phytohemagglutinin in combination with phorbol esters, purification of IFN gamma from these inducers, or other contaminating cellular lymphokines such as interleukin-2, has been difficult.

Production of IFN alpha, IFN beta, and IFN gamma have now all been achieved by recombinant DNA techniques in bacteria. The feat of isolation and cloning of cDNA in one of several plasmid vectors with high-level expression, and purification by means of crystallization (rIFN alpha-2) or monoclonal immunosorbent antibody (rIFN alpha-A) has allowed a quantum leap in the design of clinical trials. Methods used for the production of IFN by genetic engineering are schematically portrayed in Figure 13-2. These techniques are likely to be the source of individual subspecies of IFN for most future clinical applications, as well as other lymphokines (such as interleukins), and even larger hormones, and proteins for which natural biological sources are lacking or undesirable. Commercial-scale production of the most common subspecies of IFN alpha, by Schering-Plough Corp. (rIFN alpha-2) amd the Hoffman La-Roche Corp. (rIFN alpha-A) has allowed the first phase I and phase II clinical experience with highly purified

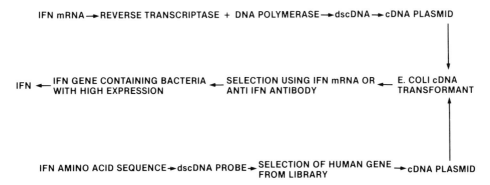

Fig. 13-2. Production of interferon by recombinant DNA technology.

IFN, unfettered by limited supply. The purified drug itself has proven to be among the most potent biological agents ever administered to human beings, with an unprecedented range of effects in vitro and in vivo, many of which remain to be fully detailed in man.

Interferons are as pleiotropic in basic biological systems as they are in the clinic. The basic biology of IFN may help to explain its clinical effects, but the molecular biology of IFN action in antiviral, anticellular, and immunomodulatory applications is beyond the scope of the present review. The reader is referred to recent reviews.[2,7] Here, we will note the assay methods for quantification of all IFN, some of which depend upon antiviral actions. Antiproliferative effects of IFN itself provide a direct explanation for at least some antitumor results with IFN and may, in the future, prove to be a more rational basis for its bioassay. It is already clear that IFN alpha, IFN beta, and IFN gamma have different antiproliferative potency per unit of antiviral activity. It is also apparent that IFN alpha and IFN beta interact with one cell surface receptor and IFN gamma interacts with a different receptor. This must be borne in mind when unit cases of the different species are compared in the clinic.

Viral infection in tissue-cultured cells produces a cytopathic effect that may be quantitated and that is highly reproducible for given combinations of virus and target cells. Inhibition of cytopathic effect is the simplest and crudest of bioassays for the IFN. Interferon is then quantitated in reference to a standard and expressed in units of antiviral activity. This assay may be carried out with or without vital staining with eosin, using an end point of 50 or 100 percent lytic destruction of the monolayer. The assay has an intrinsically variable sensitivity for the different species of human IFN, depending upon the virus, as well as the target cell, used. Reduction of virus yield by IFN affords a means to more precise and sensitive measurements of IFN action than inhibition of cytopathic effect. Assays for reduction of virus yield require a second step, with titration of virus from infected cells and are more lengthy and tedious.[7]

Anti-IFN antibodies are the most rapid and precise means for assay of the IFN, and allow a dissection of the relative effects of different species and subspecies of IFN when quantitation of a complex mixture by measurement of antiviral effects is attempted.[4] However, immunoassay of interferons by radioisotopic or enzyme-linked methods in the serum of patients or induced in vitro is problematic. Because we have already noted the existence of multiple subspecies of IFN alpha, and a potential complexity of IFN beta and IFN gamma, it is obvious that antibodies to all active subspecies must be employed for definitive immunoassay. Moreover, it is probable that inactivated (denatured or biologically defective) species may retain full immunoreactivity. The most appropriate use for immunoassay will thus be the measurement of homogeneous, genetically engineered subspecies of IFN in vivo during clinical trials or for purification in the laboratory. The potential detection of immunoreactive, but nonfunctional molecules is a problem that precludes complete reliance on immunoassay. It is thus desirable to quantitate IFN species both by bioassay and immunoassay.

Effects of the IFN, whether antiviral, antiproliferative, or immunological, appear to follow a rapid binding of IFN to a cell-surface receptor. It has long been recognized that the IFN sensitivity of cells varies with the complement of chromosome-21, being increased in trisomy 21. Analysis of mouse–human hybrid cells lacking various human chromosomes has corroborated the evidence that chromosome-21 codes for a cell-surface structure associated with IFN response.[8] Antibody to a cell-surface structure coded by chromosome-21 inhibits interferon activation of human cells.[9] The receptors for IFN alpha and IFN beta appear to be similar, as determined using isotopically labeled species in cross-competition experiments. The receptor for IFN gamma is believed to differ from the receptors for IFN alpha and IFN beta, suggesting that a potential for combination of alpha and beta and gamma species, with synergy, may be realized. However, it is clear that exposure of a cell to IFN affects the expression of IFN receptors, with down-regulation analogous to observations with other smaller polypeptide hormones, such as insulin. Interactions between the IFN alpha/beta and gamma subspecies are now also reported, but full examination of these effects awaits the availability of labeled homogeneous preparations of both IFN alpha and IFN gamma.[10]

Intracellular molecular mechanisms of the IFN have largely been worked out in murine systems, in which early induction of several enzymes appear to be related to the antiviral, if not antiproliferative and immunological effects observed with purified IFN alpha. An oligoadenylate synthetase is induced, which is capable of producing a novel 2'5' oligoadenylate in the presence of double-stranded RNA and other co-factors.[11] This enzyme is activated by double-stranded RNA and converts ATP to oligo 2'5' adenylate (2'5'A) in lengths ranging from 2 to 15. Oligo 2'-5' adenylate, in turn, activates an endoribonuclease capable of cleaving single-stranded RNA in both murine and human cells. Interferon has recognized inhibitory effects upon transcription as well as translation of a number of RNA and DNA viruses, which may be related to oligo 2'5'A synthetase induction and activation of an endoribonuclease, which is preferentially able to degrade *m* RNA linked to double-stranded RNA (such as the replicative intermediate of RNA viruses). Oligo 2'5' adenylate introduced into normal and neoplastic cells appears to inhibit both protein and DNA synthesis.[12] Most recently, it has been recognized that separate nuclear and cytoplasmic oligo 2'5' A synthestases of differing molecular size and with corresponding *m* RNA may be induced by IFN.[13] Additional molecular mechanisms of relevance to antiviral and antiproliferative action are known to be induced by IFN. A kinase is induced that is able to phosphorylate and thereby inactivate peptide elongation initiation factor (eIF-2), thus inhibiting ribosomal protein synthesis. A phosphodiesterase that removes the CCA terminus of *t* RNA also contributes to the inhibition of protein synthesis in IFN-treated cells. The role of these enzymatic mechanisms of IFN action in cancer therapy remains to be determined.

Immunomodulatory activities are recognized, distinct from other cellular antiproliferative, surface membrane, and antiviral functions of the IFN. These are especially relevant for the T-cell lymphokine, IFN gamma. Humoral and cellular immunity have been shown to be altered in both animals and man. Primary humoral responses to both T-cell–dependent and T-cell–independent antigens are inhibited in vitro. Both primary and secondary responses to sheep red blood cells have been modified upward as well as downward, depending upon the time sequence of exposure to antigen and IFN in mice. Immune response is diminished when IFN is administered before, or together with antigen. Response is augmented when IFN administration follows antigenic challenge.[14]

The most widely accepted effects of IFN upon the cellular immune system occur in the natural killer cell and the monocyte–macrophage. The macrophage is a recognized participant in tumor rejection, and responds to IFN with activation by augmented surface Fc receptor expression and Fc-dependent phagocytosis, superoxide production, and peroxide release. These responses have been partially documented, in vivo in mice and in vitro, but not in vivo in man.[15-17] The effects of IFN upon immunity are dose dependent, beyond their time dependence, in man and in mice.[18-21]

The natural killer lymphocyte is a lymphocyte without the phenotypic markers of the mature T- or B-lymphocyte series. It is lytic to certain lymphoid and solid tumor cells in vitro without the sensitization required for cytotoxic T cells.[22] The ultimate role of this cell in vivo is uncertain, but it may have to do with inhibition of metastasis and/or primary tumor development. It is highly responsive to IFN in vitro and in vivo, in a dose-dependent and time-dependent fashion.[18,19,21] In vivo, the natural killer cell activity of peripheral blood wanes despite continued repetitive daily administrations of IFN. This may be due to regulation by adherent macrophage–monocyte elements or to appropriate peripheral tissue disposition and the natural killer cell.[22,23] Interferon has major effects upon the cell surface, which may augment or alter the susceptability of tumor cells to recognition and destruction by the immune system. Augmentation of certain domains in the histocompatibility locus, but not others, argues for selective or specific action of IFN upon cell-surface antigens.[24-26]

Cell growth inhibition in normal and neoplastic tissues is recognized as a direct effect of the IFN.[27] Inhibition of liver regeneration in partially hepatectomized mice, as well as neonatal liver development in unoperated mice, has been thoroughly documented.[28] Reversible cytostatic, rather than cytotoxic effects have been observed in general, upon both virally and nonvirally induced tumors.[29-31] Growth inhibition in some, but not other in vitro studies has appeared to be greater in certain phases of the cell cycle (e.g., G_0-G_1).[31,32] The differentiative effects of IFN in hemopoietic systems appear to be dose dependent, in keeping with their immunomodulatory functions.[33] Further study will be required to elucidate the importance and mechanism of antiproliferative, surface membrane, and genetic effects upon human tumor cells and the host.

CLINICAL EXPERIENCE

The IFN were first applied to the treatment of human cancer in far-reaching trials commenced more than a generation ago in France.[34] The choice of leukemia, and subsequently of osteosarcoma, for the first clinical trials of IFN was based, in part, upon the suspected viral etiology of these neoplasms. Partial antitumor effects in 1/11 leukemia patients and a suggested improvement in disease-free survival of children with osteosarcoma, spurred national investigations of the efficacy of IFN alpha in breast cancer, lymphoma, multiple myeloma, and melanoma, as well as renal cell carcinoma under the auspices of American Cancer Society in the United States. Toxicity of the whole-cell alpha IFN have been fairly consistent in published trials of Cantell-type IFN alpha and lymphoblastoid IFN alpha, showing a similar range of toxicities for whole-cell and recombinant DNA-produced IFN. The dosages attained in trials with lymphoblastoid and recombinant DNA products have been higher as a consequence of the availability of virtually unlimited drug.[21,39,43]

TOXICITY AND PHARMACOKINETIC STUDIES

Acute toxicity reported with IFN alpha has fallen into two large categories, the acute and the subacute/chronic. Acute toxicity of IFN, in general, has included fever, chills, and an influenza-like syndrome of myalgia, arthralgia, headache, and malaise, commencing approximately 30 to 120 minutes posttreatment and enduring for hours.[20,36-38] A blunting or tachyphylaxis of the acute constitutional flu-like toxicities has been noted in patients treated repetitively on a daily or thrice-weekly schedule.[21,37,38] Maximum tolerated daily dosages have been shown to depend upon the schedule and route and, potentially, may differ among the species as well as subspecies of IFN. Tolerance has been improved by intravenous as compared with intramuscular or subcutaneous routes of administration.[39] Acute toxicity is minimized by continuous or frequent (daily) IFN administration, and is most pronounced in intermittent dosing schedules, when an interval of two days between doses is exceeded and the tolerance to the acute toxicity wanes.[38] Acute toxicities may also be lessened by escalation from low to high doses over several days to induce tolerance.

Subacute/chronic constitutional, hematological, hepatic/gastrointestinal, and neurological toxicity are known with the IFN and is seen in a period of days to weeks with repetitive dosing. Hematological toxicity has been observed with neutropenia, the most common objective basis for discontinuation of IFN therapy in reported studies.[19,36-41] Neutropenia or occasional thrombocytopenia have been the dose-limiting toxicities of whole leukocyte, lymphoblastoid, and recombinant DNA-produced IFN alpha subspecies at dosages of from 10 to 200 $\times$ 10^6 u/day, depending upon route and schedule.[21,38,42-44] Neutropenia with IFN appears to be due to a reversible inhibition of myeloid maturation, with an element of sequestration.[45] Hepatotoxicity, manifested as elevations of SGOT and SGPT, have been dose-related and noted in a smaller proportion of patients, chiefly at the higher doses of 30 to 100 $\times$ 10^6 u/day.[35-38,42,43] This toxicity is rapidly reversible upon withdrawal of the drug and unassociated with functional hepatic abnormalities. No systematic biopsy studies have been carried out to evaluate the liver pathology associated with abnormal liver enzymes during IFN treatment, except in individuals under treatment with lower doses of IFN alpha (HuLe) for hepatitis.

Neurological toxicity has proved to be an unexpected and occasionally dose-limiting side effect of IFN. This toxicity has merged from the somnolence, lethargy, and malaise commonly observed in the acute setting to a progressive syndrome of debilitation and decreased ability to perform the activities of daily life.[41,42] The occasional occurrence of stupor and psychosis has been noted during phase I investigations of IFN. Electroencephalographic manifestations of IFN neurotoxicity may be much more common than previously thought, with characteristic, diffuse slowing observed in the gamma waves. Peripheral neuropathy, characterized by paraesthesia in the hands and feet, with changes in nerve conduction velocities has been reported.[36-38] The most dramatic of these manifestations of neurological toxicity have been observed after protracted exposure at dosages $\geq 10 \times 10^6$ μ/day, with lymphoblastoid- or recombinant DNA-produced IFN alpha subspecies.[43,46]

Gastrointestinal toxicity observed with IFN has been mild, in general, with anorexia commonly observed, but nausea, vomiting, and occasional diarrhea have been noted. Stomatitis and conjunctivitis have been observed at higher doses in phase I trials, especially with repetitive daily schecules of treatment.[38,45,46] Activation of labial Herpes simplex, associated with febrile acute toxicity, has been a problem in 7 to 10 percent of treated individuals.[37,38]

Cardiac toxicity has been noted infrequently and is dominated by sinus tachyarrhythmias at doses $\geq 30 \times 10^6$ u/day, chiefly in elderly ($>$70 years) patients who have had a prior history of arrythmia, heart failure, ischemia, or cardiotoxic drugs.[38,47]

Metabolic abnormalities associated with IFN have been noted only at very high and sustained IFN doses (200×10^6 u/m^2 daily, $\times$ 3–5 days of lymphoblastoid IFN alpha). Hypocalcemia, hyperkalemia, and transiently elevated creatinine and urea nitrogen in such cases could not be ascribed to tumor lysis. These dose-limiting toxicities, in conjunction with neurotoxicity, may be associated with continuous exposure to serum levels of IFN in excess of 1,000 u/ml for periods of more than several days. Neutralizing antibody against IFN beta has been reported in an individual treated with IFN beta for nasopharyngeal carcinoma.[48] Subsequently, naturally occurring antibodies reactive with IFN alpha had been noted, with an especially high incidence of neutralizing antibody to one preparation of recombinant IFN alpha in a cohort of patients with renal cell carcinoma.[36,49,50] These antibodies against rIFN alpha-A have shown broad specificity among recombinant subspecies of IFN alpha, suggesting that subtle differences in native IFN alpha (HuLe) may have induced an autoimmune response that is generalized against a broader range of IFN alphas. Physiological consequences of such antibodies, other than nullification of toxic and therapeutic effects of exogeneous IFN therapy, have not been observed.[49,50] No abnormality could be found in beta IFN produced by fibroblasts of one individual who developed anti-IFN beta antibody during therapy with homologous whole-cell IFN beta.[51]

Pharmacokinetic studies in man are well documented for IFN alpha, with peak serum levels following IM injection attained in four to six hours, and an initial half-life of six to eight hours is reported.[36] Pharmacokinetic studies during repetitive daily IM dosing trials explain the rapidly progressive dose-limiting toxicity observed at dosages of 30×10^6 u or greater, when accumulation of the drug can be demonstrated in serum.[38,46]

CLINICAL TRIALS

A range of human tumors have now been treated with IFN alpha of leukocyte and lymphoblastoid cell origin; trials of fibroblast-derived IFN beta have been more limited. Trials with recombinant DNA-produced IFN alpha of the major subspecies (alpha-2 or alpha-A) are now as extensive as those with the native cellular product, and are soon to be followed by rIFN beta and gamma. The species, derivation, dosage, schedule, and route of IFN administration in clinical trials are important in analyzing the results of any treatment programs for cancer.

UROLOGICAL CANCER

Bladder Carcinoma

The early recorded benefits of IFN alpha (HuLe) in children with laryngeal papillomatosis, treated in Sweden, were the basis for studies of bladder papilloma and early-stage invasive bladder carcinoma.[52] Recurrent superficial bladder carcinoma is often refractory to topical/intravesical chemotherapy (see Chapter 10). Local intravesical therapy with *bacille Calmette Guerin* (BCG) has been effective and has been taken to support the hypothesis that bladder carcinoma might be responsive to immunomodulators of a variety of types.[53] Bladder carcinoma appears likely to be carcinogen-induced, in general, and evidence for the presence of cell-surface antigens recognized by the host exists in bladder carcinoma, as in experimental carcinogen-induced neoplasms of mice.[54] BCG is known to induce production of IFN (IFN alpha and IFN gamma), and it was therefore reasonable to examine the role of exogenous IFN as a treatment in bladder carcinoma.

Before HuLeIFN alpha or rIFN alpha became available for large-scale clinical trials, the IFN inducer poly I:C was administered systemically (25 μg/kg, IV, every two weeks) to patients with low-stage bladder carcinoma at Memorial Hospital. This phase II trial demonstrated a modest reduction of recurrences at three months, of borderline statistical significance (5/18 receiving poly I:C and 0/14 controls free of disease). At year one, 4/14 treated and 1/12 untreated patients remained free of disease. The trial was closed to further accession after 32 patients, on the basis of this early analysis. No difference in recurrence rate, thereafter, nor any difference in the rate of salvage cystectomy or pathology findings at operation have been noted in the two groups. The median survival of treated individuals was 170 months, compared to 76 months for controls. Among the low-grade or in situ tumors of controls, four were fatal; none in the treated group were fatal.[55]

This trial of poly I:C involved doses sufficient to cause fever in 90 percent and chills in 70 percent of the patients, but there were no other hematological or hepatic toxicities, and in the absence of any reported absolute levels of IFN measured over time, the question of optimal/maximal dosing may be raised. The rationale for the use of a systemic IFN-inducing treatment, instead of local therapy, may also be questioned. It is of interest that the short-term benefit of this system was taken as evidence of an effect against mature implanted tumor; late effects upon the frequency of recurrence were interpreted as evidence of activity against premalignant and evolving lesions. The true meaning of IFN effects in bladder carcinoma (as well as in other tumors) treated in vivo is impossible to assess now. The limited numbers and admixture of cases of papilloma and transitional carcinoma in situ (stage 0, grades 1,2) in the reported literature makes further evaluation of IFN and/or poly I:C necessary before any definitive conclusions can be drawn.

Early European trials examined the antitumor effects of the available crude IFN alpha preparations in small series of patients with several types of tumor.[56-58] Intralesional or perilesional, cystoscopically directed inoculation of IFN alpha was reported in eight patients with "malignant papillomatosis" of the bladder, using HuLe IFN alpha of only 3×10^4 u/mg specific activity (0.01 percent purity), given daily $\times 21$ days.[56] Patients had experienced 2 to 11 recurrences of papilloma at intervals of one to six months, all grade II, except one case. In addition to this protocol, tumors were resected transurethrally in two of eight patients following the first cycle, and systemic treatment, in addition to intravesical/intralesional treatment was given to two patients (2×10^6 u/day, IM). Monthly cycles of treatment were given until remission. The authors report complete regression in all patients, enduring for 4 to 46 months (median, 25 months). Tumor regression was complete by the third cycle of therapy in all patients except for the two who required resection; treatment was for 14 to 16 months to remit disease completely. Relapse in one patient in this study failed to respond to retreatment with IFN alpha, using the same protocol. This is in contrast to the experience in lymphoma patients, in whom reinduction of remission has been noted on retreatment of relapse.[59]

Scorticatti et al.[60] have carried out a trial with systemic intramuscular administration of higher doses of IFN alpha (HuLe 1×10^6 u qod) in eight patients for six months; the patients have been followed for over 2 years. Similar antitumor activity of IFN alpha in bladder carcinoma was reported, and retreatment was effective in patients who relapsed following response. Unfortunately, neither this nor Ikic's[56] trials were controlled. The regression of transitional carcinoma of the ureter (grade 2, stage 3) has been anecdotally reported in Japan with crude HuLe IFN alpha (1×10^5 u/mg of protein). Three intralesional inoculations were followed by systemic treatment with 10×10^4 u/week, IM, achieving complete response of 27 months as documented, histologically.[61]

RENAL CELL CARCINOMA

Renal cell carcinoma is among the most unresponsive tumors known to medicine and there is no standard effective therapy, once unresectable metastatic disease has occurred. The predominance of renal cell carcinoma among spontaneously regressing neoplasms documented in the literature has provided fuel for speculation that the immune response might hold a key to better control of metastatic disease.[62] There has been no compelling evidence of antitumor efficacy of any standard drug or hormone regimen at a response rate of over 20 percent.[63-67] Many of the modalities previously reported to be of some limited efficacy in small series, such as immune RNA, BCG, and tumor vaccines, have had a strong likelihood of inducing interferon (alpha, beta, or gamma) as well. It would be of interest to have documented IFN levels in patients treated by these modalities.

Early studies with HuLe IFN alpha at the M.D. Anderson Hospital first suggested the potential of systemic treatment with a modest dosage of IFN alpha (HuLe, 3×10^6 u/day, IM) to induce regression in metastatic renal cell carcinoma.[68] Of 19 patients, 7 (36 percent) gave some evidence of response, 5 (26 percent) of these with partial regression fulfilling standard criteria of 50 percent reduction in the product of greatest perpendicular diameters of measureable disease. An additional three patients showed mixed evidence of contemporaneous response in some, and progression in other, lesions. Toxicity observed in this trial was minimal, and response was of four to nine months duration (median four months), equally in minimal and objective partial responders. Responses were observed in lung metastases, in general, and all were noted at 30 to 90 days of treatment. Responders had a significantly higher performance status (median Karnofsky score, 97 percent) and a longer disease-free interval (with 4/7 at > 24 months) compared with performance status of 80 percent and a disease-free interval of less than 24 months in 9/12 nonresponders. Nadir granulocyte count was 1,400/mm^3 in responders, and 1,700 in nonresponders (median weekly neutrophils). These data suggest a greater biological effect of IFN alpha in responsive patients than nonresponsive patients. The dose–response question was otherwise tangentially addressed in selected patients during this trial; these patients were given up to 18 to 36×10^6 u/day without apparent benefit, but also without a strict protocol.

The American Cancer Society initiated plans to investigate the question of dose–response relationships in the treatment of renal cell carcinoma with IFN alpha in 1980, choosing dosages of 1×10^6 and 10×10^6 u/day, which, by chance, bracketed those of the M.D. Anderson group. These doses were the minimum effective and maximum tolerable daily dosages suggested from scattered European and American data up to that time. A collaborative trial between the Yale Comprehensive Cancer Center and the Illinois Cancer Council was activated in 1981, with 30 patients with biopsy-proven, measurable, metastatic renal cell carcinoma, not involving the brain. Patients were randomly allocated to 1 or 10×10^6 u/day IFN, IM, for 28 days. Patients treated at the lower dosage who were stable at the time of the first (28-day) evaluation were randomized again to receive an additional 28 days of therapy, with reevaluation for response at day 56 (see Table 13-2). Of 30 patients, 16 were treated at 10×10^6 u/day ×28 days yielding five responses, including one partial (PR) and one complete response (CR), as well as three minimal responses. Of 14 patients treated at 1×10^6 u/day ×28 days, only 1 minimal response was obtained. The responses in the high-dose group were of 8 ± 15 months duration and were observed in predominantly pulmonary metastatic sites. Minimal responses were of median 4½ months duration (a 2½- to 7-month range). Extended treatment for a second month in nine eligible patients gave 1/5 PR at high dosage, lasting four months; none of four patients responded to a second month at low dosage. Responses were observed in this trial from 28

Table 13-2. Renal Cell Carcinoma: Trials of Intramuscular Interferon Alpha

Author	IFN Species	Dose (× 10⁶u)	Duration	Patients (Evaluable)	Response	Duration	Characteristics
Quesada et al.[50]	Alpha HuLe	3/day	4–14 mos	19[a]	5 PR 2 MR	4–14 mos	Little toxicity; predominantly pulmonary responses
	Alpha HuLe	3/day	4–14 mos	36[a]	2 CR 9 PR 4 MR		
Kirkwood et al.[46]	Alpha HuLe	1/day 10/day	4–8 wks 4–8 wks	30 (30)	1 MR 1 CR 2 PR 3 MR	2½ mos 15 mos 4–12 mos 2–7 mos	Little toxicity at 1 or 10/day; predominantly pulmonary responses
Quesada et al.[68]	Alpha REC A	2/m²/day 20/m²/day	8 wks	30 (8) (8)			Toxicity ↓ dose ½ @ 20/m²
Krown et al.[49]	Alpha REC A	50/m²		27 (19)	2 PR 4 MR	4–7⁺ mos 2½–4½ mos	Toxicity ↓ dose in 11/19; 4 with Ab, predominantly pulmonary responses

[a] Same trial

to 120 days following initiation of treatment. One late responder experienced complete regression of pulmonary disease nearly three months after his last treatment, in the initial 28-day IFN treatment period. A trend toward improved antitumor activity at this higher dosage is apparent, with the most durable responses being those that were complete, and achieved at the higher dosage. This trend is not statistically significant for the aggregate of patient treatment–courses at high dosage compared to those at low dosage.[38] No relationship of response to performance status or total granulocyte or nadir granulocyte counts has been identified in this collaborative trial carried out by Yale and the Illinois Cancer Council. Indeed, the median disease-free interval of responders (9 months) was only one-half that of nonresponders (19 months) in this trial. This trial clearly corroborates the responsiveness of metastatic renal cell carcinoma to interferon, despite the lack of correlation of disease-free interval to response.

A similar response rate has been reported by Krown et al.[49] using rIFN alpha-A in 27 renal adenocarcinoma patients, at a dose of 50×10^6 u/m^2, IM, TIW. Of 19 evaluable patients, 6 had documented responses (2 PR and 4 minimal responses). Responses lasted from 20 to 32+ weeks, and were associated with antibody formation to IFN as in the M.D. Anderson experience previously noted.[50]

SUMMARY

In summary, research into the use of IFN in therapy for urologic cancers has only just begun. A number of newer protocols are examining the efficacy of higher doses of IFN given for extended periods of time (up to three months) in renal adenocarcinoma or at direct intravesical installation of IFN in patients with bladder cancer.

Although the IFN have not proved to be as innocuous as they were once held to be, toxicities remain mild, reversible, and well tolerated, in general. Toxic effects involve a constitutional symptom complex similar to a viral illness and are noted in the hematological, hepatic, neurological, and cardiac systems. The prime cause of dose-limiting toxicity has been leukopenia, which is transient and normalizes rapidly once IFN is discontinued. These effects are dose related, for the most part, and have not caused any irreversible damage to date. Anti-IFN antibodies pose theoretical, but unsubstantiated worries that lasting consequences of anti-IFN immunity will develop.

The efficacy of IFN in treatment of renal adenocarcinoma was shown by a reproducible finding at a number of independent institutions, using both whole human leukocyte- and recombinant DNA-produced IFN. Although the true response rate to IFN has yet to be determined in head-on comparisons, the early data point to a level of activity that is above that noted with either standard chemotherapy or hormonotherapy.

Future work must center upon determination of (1) optimum schedule, route of administration, and species of IFN, (2) the utility of IFN in more appropriate adjuvant settings of microscopic residual disease, and (3) design of rational programs of combination therapy with IFN. The use of IFN alpha/beta and gamma is suggested by their separate receptor mechanisms. The use of IFN and more conventional chemotherapy, hormonal therapy, or radiotherapy is an obvious sequel to the current phase II studies. The most interesting combinations of biological agents will be those of IFN and the more specific immunological agents, such as antibody. Interferon plus antitumor–antibody combinations would afford the opportunity to prime the whole Fc-dependent cellular immune system, and follow-up with an antibody capable of directing the nonspecific mechanisms set into motion by IFN.

REFERENCES

1. Isaacs A, Lindemann JJ: Virus interference: The interferon. Proc Roy Lond Soc (Biol) 147:258, 1957
2. Sehgal PB: The interferon gene. Biochem Biophys Acta 695:17, 1982
3. Cantell K, Hervonen S, Mogensen KE: Human leukocyte interferon production, purification, and animal experimental. p. 35. In Waymouth C (ed): In Vitro Baltimore Tissue Culture Assoc, 1975
4. Secher DS, Burke DC: A monoclonal antibody for large-scale production of human leukocyte interferon. Nature 285:446, 1980
5. Horoszewicz JS, Leong SS, Ito M, et al: Human fibroblast interferon in human neoplasia: Clinical and laboratory study. Cancer Treat Rt 62:1899, 1978
6. Dembinski W, O'Malley JA, Sulkowski E: Large scale purification procedure for human fibroblast interferon. Proc. AACR 778:69, 1983
7. Stewart WE III (ed): The Interferon System. Academic Press, New York, 1979
8. Tan YH, Tisdefield J, Ruddle FH: Linkage of genes for the human interferon induced antiviral protein and indophenol oxidase-B to chromosome G21. J Exp Med 137:317, 1973
9. Revel M, Bash D, Ruddle FH: Antibodies to a cell-surface component coded by human chromosome 21 inhibit action of interferon. Nature 260:139, 1976
10. Williams Bryan RG, personal communication, 1983
11. Lengyel P: Biochemistry of interferons and their actions. Ann Rev Biochem 51:251, 1982
12. Revel M, Kimchi A, Shulman L, et al: Role of interferon induced enzymes in the antiviral and antimitogenic effects of interferon. Ann NY Acad Sci 350:459, 1980
13. St. Laurent G, Yoshie U, Floyd-Smith G, et al: Interferon action: Two (2'5') (A)n synthetases specified by distinct mRNAs in Ehrlich ascites tumor cells treated with interferon. Cell 33:95, 1983
14. Sonnenfeld G, Mandel AD, Merigan TC: Time and dosage dependence of immunoenhancement by murine type II interferon preparations. Cell Immunol 40:285, 1978
15. Hamburg SI, Cassell GH, Rabinovitch M: Relationship between enhanced macrophage phagocytic activity and the induction of interferon by New/Castle disease virus in mice. J Immunol 124:1360, 1980
16. Coleman DC, Ernstoff MS, Kirkwood JM, Ryan JL: Macrophage Fc dependent phagocytosis in man during treatment with interferon alpha-2. J Interferon Res 1984
17. Nathan CF, Murray HW, Wiebe ME, Rubin BY: Identification of IFN gamma as the lymphokine that activates human macrophage oxidative metabolism and antimicrobial activity. J Exp Med 158:670, 1983

18. Ernstoff MS, Fusi S, Kirkwood JM: Parameters of interferon action I. Immunological effects of whole cell leukocyte interferon in phase I-II trials. J Biol Resp Mod 2(6): December 1983

19. Ernstoff MS, Fusi S., Rudnick S, and Kirkwood JM: Parameters of interferon action II. Immunological effects of recombinant leukocyte interferon in phase I-II trials. J Biol Resp Mod 2(6): December 1983

20. Horning SJ, Levine JF, Miller RA, Rosenberg SA, Merigan TC: Clinical and immunologic effects of recombinant leukocyte A interferon in eight patients with advanced cancer. JAMA 247:1718, 1982

21. Laszlo J, Huang AT, Brenckman WD, et al: Phase I Study of pharmacological and immunological effects of human lymphoblastoid interferon given to patients with cancer. Cancer Res 43:4458, 1983

22. Herberman R (ed): Natural Cell-Mediated Immunity against Tumors. Academic Press, New York 1980

23. Miehlke K: Regulation of NK activity by macrophages. Proc. XIII Int. Congress of Chemotherapy. In press

24. Lindahl P, Leary P, Gresser I: Enhancement by interferon of the expression of surface antigens on murine leukemia L1210 cells. Proc Nat Acad Sci USA 70:2785, 1973

25. Gresser I, DeMaeyer E, Guignard J, Tovey MG, DeMaeyer E: Electrophorectically pure mouse interferon exerts multiple biological effects. Proc Nat Acad Sci USA 76(10):5308, 1979

26. Sonnenfeld G, Meruelo D, McDevitt, HO: Effect of type I and type II interferons on murine thymocyte surface antigen expression induction for selection. Cell Immunol 57:427, 1981

27. Paucker K, Cantell K, Hurler W: Quantitative studies on viral interference in suspended L-cells. III. Effect of interfering viruses and interferon on the growth of cells. Virology 17:325, 1962

28. Gresser F, Tovey M, Maury C, et al: Lethality of interferon preparations for newborn mice. Nature 258:76, 1975

29. Gresser I: On the varied biologic effects of interferon. Cell Immunol 34:406, 1977

30. Stewart WE, II: The Interferon System. p. 134. Springer-Verlag, New York, 1979

31. Ratner L, Nordlund JJ, Lengyel P: Interferon as an inhibitor of cell growth: Studies with mouse melanoma cells (40760). Proc Soc Exp Biol Med 163:267, 1980

32. Creasey AA, Bartholomew JC, Merigan TC: Role of G_0G_1 arrest in the inhibition of tumor cell growth by interferon. Proc Nat Acad Aci USA 77:1471, 1980

33. Rossi GB, Dolei A, Capubianchi MR, et al: Interactions of interferon with *in vitro* model systems involved with hemopoietic cell differentiation. Ann NY Acad Sci 350:279, 1980

34. Falcoff E, Falcoff R, Fournier F, Chany C: Production en masse, purification partille et characterization d'un interferon destive a des essais therapeutiques humans. Ann Inst Pasteur 3:562, 1966

35. Gutterman JU, Blumenschein GR, Alexanian R, et al: Leukocyte interferon-induced tumor regression in human metastatic breast cancer, multiple myeloma, and malignant lymphoma. Ann Int Med 93:399, 1980

36. Gutterman JU, Fine S, Quesada J, et al: Recombinant leukocyte A interferon: Pharmacokinetics, single-dose tolerance, and biologic effects in cancer patients. Ann Int Med 96(5):549, 1982

37. Sherwin SA, Knost JA, Fein S, et al: A multiple-dose phase I trial of recombinant leukocyte A interferon in cancer patients. JAMA 248(19):2461, 1982

38. Vera R, Kirkwood JM, Harris J, et al: Randomized trial of low and high dose interferon

14 | Is There a Role for Pulmonary Nodulectomy in Urologic Cancers?

Daniel F. Hayes

INTRODUCTION

Most physicians would consider the appearance of metastases distant from the primary site of malignancy to be an indication of failure in their attempts to effect a cure for that patient. This pessimistic attitude has been particularly prevalent among doctors caring for patients who develop multiple lung metastases. Nonetheless, data now exist to refute this once hopeless outlook toward patients with pulmonary metastases.[1-6] In the late 1920s, Divis published a case report concerning the resection of metastases to the lung.[7] A decade later, Barney and Churchill reported the five-year survival of a patient from whom metachronous lung metastases had been resected 15 months after a nephrectomy for a renal adenocarcinoma. The patient went on to survive for 29 years and ultimately died from coronary artery disease, free of cancer.[8] That report forms the basis for the widely held notion that patients with renal cell cancer from whom pulmonary metastases are resected tend to fare better than those patients with other metastatic cancers. However, ample precedent exists for long-term survival after pulmonary metastatic nodulectomy in patients with other primary nonurologic and urologic cancers. In this chapter, the indications for an aggressive approach toward these patients will be discussed, and an attempt will be made to relate the success gained to the knowledge about the biological behavior of metastases. In addition, a separate section has been devoted to the treatment of patients with pulmonary metastases from nonseminomatous testicular carcinomas, in order to relate several issues which are unique to that disease adequately.

GENERAL BACKGROUND OF PULMONARY METASTASECTOMY

In the 45 years since the report of Barney and Churchill, more than 30 papers have been published documenting experiences from a variety of institutions regarding metastatic pulmonary nodulectomies.[9-37] Most of these papers have included a wide variety of tumor types, indications for surgery, patient profiles, and operative approaches. It is clear that the absolute number of patients cured by resection of pulmonary nodules is small. It has been estimated that 30 percent of all cancers metastasize to the lung.[10] Approximately one-half of these will occur in conjunction with widespread systemic disease, obviating a surgical cure. Of the remaining patients who have metastases only in the lungs, about 50 percent will be surgically rendered "disease-free." Thus, of all patients with malignancies, only 5 to 6 percent can be considered as candidates for surgical resection. As will be discussed below, the percentage of those who remain disease-free for three to five years is about 20 to 30 percent. Consequently, the overall salvage rate of all patients with malignancies is a meager 2 to 3 percent. Although cure is the major indication for nodulectomy, successful palliation from pain, bronchial obstruction, hemorrhage, and pulmonary osteoarthropathy can be obtained in highly selected patients for whom no other effective noninvasive therapy is available.

DIAGNOSIS

Because metastatic lesions tend to be peripheral, the overwhelming majority of patients with pulmonary metastases will be asymptomatic until very late in their course. Only 15 to 40 percent will present with cough, hemoptysis, wheezing, or pain[3,14-16,30,32,34,36,37] (Table 14-1). This is quite different from what is commonly seen with primary bronchogenic tumors of the lung, from which patients tend to present with these classic symptoms.[38]

These data suggest that the physician's efforts to discover potentially resectable metastases will be successful only with very compulsive follow-up of patients whose primary tumor has been eradicated. In light of recent concerns about the rising expense of routine medical care, the cost-effectiveness of this approach has been questioned. If recurrent disease is usually asymptomatic, then the physician must rely on either serological markers or radiographic studies to monitor the patient. The clinical utility of markers is limited, at present, in most solid neoplasms other than germ cell cancer, although several potentially valuable serological tests are currently under investigation.[39] However, serological markers have been shown to be invaluable in the care of patients with testicular carcinoma and will be discussed below.

Table 14-1. Presenting Signs and Symptoms
of Pulmonary Metastases in Order of
Relative Frequency

Signs and Symptoms	Frequency (%)
Cough	30–40
Hemoptysis	15–30
Wheezing	15–30
Pain	<15
Fever	
Weight loss	
Dyspnea	<10
Sputum production	
Osteoarthropathy	

The appropriate utilization of radiological tests for routine follow-up is not well defined.[40] Although many of the earlier studies relied solely on plain chest radiography (CXR) for the detection of recurrent pulmonary metastases, it is clear that whole lung tomography (WLT), and more recently, computerized tomography (CT) offer greater sensitivity and perhaps specificity to the clinician. These are, unfortunately, gained at the expense of cost, overuse of already limited facilities, and increased radiation exposure to the patient.[40] Several authors have addressed these issues, but each investigation suffers from lack of suitable controls, insufficient numbers of patients, heterogeneity of tumor types and patient characteristics, and/ or a retrospective experimental design. In addition, rapid technological advances in radiology alter the validity of the data from many studies soon after they are published.[40,41]

In 1976, Polga and Watnick reviewed 100 patients with extrapulmonary primary neoplasms who had had both CXR and WLT[42] (Table 14-2). They found that of those patients with normal CXR, 97 percent had normal WLT. They also found that of those patients with positive CXR, 71 percent would have positive WLT, which confirmed the results of the CXR. Importantly, they also reported two patients with negative CXR and positive WLT, and eight patients with nodules seen on plain films, but who had a higher number of lesions present on WLT. Thus, chest radiography was felt to be falsely negative in 10 percent of their patients.[42]

In 1977, Neifeld et al. reported their retrospective analysis of 152 patients with extrathoracic cancers who underwent thoracotomies for evaluation of pulmonary nodules at the National Institutes of Health[43] (Table 14-2). They found 25 patients with normal CXR who were shown to have nodules by WLT. Sixteen (64 percent) of these patients were found at thoracotomy to have metastatic lesions. Of 64 patients who were felt to have unilateral nodules on CXR 14 were found to have bilateral nodules by WLT. The sensitivity of WLT in detecting metastatic lesions was also questioned. Twenty-four patients were found to have more nodules at thoracotomy than were suggested by WLT preoperatively. They concluded that WLT influenced the clinical management in 35 of 152 patients (23 percent) and is thus justified in routine serial evaluation of appropriate patients following treat-

Table 14-2. Role of Plain Chest Radiography, Whole Lung Tomography, and Computerized Tomography in Pulmonary Metastases Diagnosis

Author	Conclusions[a]
Polga[42]	WLT more sensitive than CXR
Neifeld[43]	WLT versus CXR changed the clinical course in 23% of patients—suggest routine WLT
Sindelar[44]	88% accuracy for abnormal WLT; 64.3% accuracy for abnormal CXR; 3 patients with normal CXR and abnormal WLT cured by resection
Chang[45]	CT more sensitive than CXR or WLT with size limit of 4.5 mm, but decreased specificity precludes routine use of CT.
Curtis[47,48]	CT too nonspecific to add new or unsuspected information in patients with breast cancer[47] or melanoma[48]
Cohen[49]	WLT justified only if CXR abnormal or questionable in children
Bergman[50]	WLT positive when CXR normal in 17% of patients with testicular cancer and 10% of patients with renal cell cancer
Jochelson[51]	Only 1 of 120 patients required alteration of treatment based on findings on WLT not discernible on CXR

[a] WLT, whole lung tomography; CXR, plain chest radiography; CT, computerized tomography.

ment of the primary malignancy. They came to this conclusion, even though the false positive rate for WLT was between 5 and 10 percent.

In a later paper from the same institution, Sindelar et al. reviewed the records of 415 patients who had localized extrapulmonary primary malignancies and later had CXR and WLT[44] (Table 14-2). Of the 54 patients who ultimately had metastatic disease confirmed, 36 (67 percent) were detected by routine CXR, whereas 51 (94.4 percent) were identified by WLT. Of particular note, 15 patients (3.6 percent) with normal plain CXR were found to have pulmonary metastases by WLT, while the same number had false positive plain radiographs. They suggested predictive values (defined as the index of clinical confidence that the radiographic results truly reflect the actual situation) for normal CXR and WLT to be 94.9 and 99.2 percent, respectively, and for abnormal films, 64.3 and 87.9 percent, respectively. Three patients with normal CXR and metastases by WLT ultimately survived longer than two years after resection of their metastases.

More recently, the use of CT has been reviewed. Chang et al. from the National Cancer Institute attempted to prospectively correlate operative findings with preoperative CXR, WLT, and CT from 25 patients who underwent thoracotomy for resection of pulmonary metastases[45] (Table 14-2). They found CT to be more sensitive than either CXR or WLT. Computerized tomography identified 58 percent of those nodules found at thoracotomy, as opposed to 47 and 36 percent for WLT and CXR, respectively. The limits of size of the nodules visible by CT were smaller than with either of the other modalities (median size 4.5 mm with CT versus 7.0 mm for WLT). However, the greater sensitivity of CT was gained at the expense of loss of specificity. Although 90 percent of the nodules seen by plain CXR were truly malignant, only 66 percent of those seen by WLT, and an unacceptable

45 percent of those found with CT were. More than one-half of the nodules seen by CT were not found at thoracotomy. Of those found, 42 percent were not malignant. They concluded that until technology allowed better specificity, the routine use of CT to screen for pulmonary metastases could not be justified. These data were consistent with an earlier paper by these authors, in which they had suggested that CT scanning offered little when compared to CXR or WLT in the routine follow-up of patients with prior extrathoracic malignancies.[46]

Curtis et al. from Yale–New Haven Hospital have published two consecutive prospective studies in which they compared the utility of CT with WLT and CXR for routine follow-up of patients who had breast cancer[47] and melanoma[48] (Table 14-2). These patients were without measurable disease at the time of these studies. In both reports, the authors found that CT added new or unsuspected information in only 2 of 144 patients with breast cancer and 3 of 62 patients with melanoma, with six false positives in the latter group.

Children with prior cancer have also been evaluated radiologically. Cohen et al. (Table 14-2) have reviewed the WLT and CT in 120 children with variety of neoplasms.[49] They reported that if the CXR was normal, only 5 of 190 tomographic studies (2 percent) were different, and two of these were benign or false positives. If the CXR was abnormal, WLT confirmed this routinely and added new information in 15 of 47 cases (28 percent). Six of these WLT scans showed new lesions, although therapy was changed only once. Importantly, the other nine studies were all negative, refuting the abnormal CXR. These negatives were all substantiated with long-term clinical follow-up.

More germane to this discussion, at least two recent papers have analyzed these questions in patients with urologic carcinomas.[50,51] Bergman, Lippert, and Javadpour reviewed 36 patients with renal cell or Wilms' carcinoma and 83 patients with germ cell carcinoma of the testis on whom WLT had been performed[50] (Table 14-2). They found that 17 percent of the patients with testicular carcinoma had falsely negative CXR, although it is not clear how many of these patients were treated differently with the knowledge gained by WLT. Of 21 patients with renal cell carcinoma, 2 (10 percent) also had falsely negative CXR. They found a 37 and 40 percent false positive rate for CXR in patients with renal cell carcinoma and testicular carcinoma, respectively. The authors concluded that WLT offered a more sensitive and specific tool for routine follow-up than CXR, but that clearly neither test was optimal.

Jochelson et al. have recently published a prospective study of 120 patients with germ cell tumors treated and followed at the Brigham and Women's Hospital and Dana-Farber Cancer Institute[51] (Table 14-2). All patients had initial and post-treatment CXR and WLT. Stage II patients who achieved a complete remission were followed by CXR and WLT bimonthly. They found four patients (3 percent) with normal CXR and positive WLT. However, only one of these had his treatment course altered; the other three had simultaneous visceral and/or other extrathoracic disease, which obviated any change in treatment. These authors concluded that, in testicular carcinoma, the routine use of WLT is not warranted in initial staging or subsequent management and should be reserved for cases in which questionable lesions on CXR need clarification.

These investigations are summarized in Table 14-2. The role for WLT and CT in following patients who have been cured of a primary, extrathoracic malignancy is not well defined. A reasonable policy is that routine CXR is satisfactory in the majority of patients, and that WLT and CT should be reserved for those cases in which there is a question regarding the plain chest films and for those patients in whom a nodule has been found and further delineation of the size, number, and location of other lesions is required. However, some physicians may feel more comfortable with serial WLT, especially in those patients that they would otherwise consider excellent candidates for nodulectomy. Some authors suggest routine CT in highly selected patients.[52] At present, interpretation of CT is too nonspecific to justify its use for routine follow-up, but the obvious potential in diagnosing early lesions should certainly be studied and exploited. As technology and experience become more advanced, CT may prove particularly useful in detecting peripheral pleural-based lesions and distinguishing benign from malignant lesions and primary from metastatic nodules.[40] Nuclear magnetic resonance (NMR) is a new modality with an exciting potential, but it has yet to be tested in extensive clinical trials.[53]

As discussed, one cannot rely on the radiographic appearance of a new pulmonary lesion to provide a definitive diagnosis. The incidence of false positive radiographic studies ranges from 5 to 15 percent.[40-53] The differential diagnosis of a pulmonary nodule found radiographically in a patient with a history of an extrathoracic neoplasm includes a new bronchogenic primary, a metastatic lesion, or a benign process. The incidence of a secondary primary carcinoma is particularly high if the patient has a history of tobacco abuse. For example, the risk of an occurrence of a second aerodigestive primary neoplasm in patients with prior head and neck cancer has been well documented to be in the range of 30 percent.[54] Cahan has reviewed 60 patients with a prior history of colon cancer, who had pulmonary nodules resected, and found that in 29 patients the nodules were pathologically consistent with new primaries.[55] Of interest, it has been suggested that patients who have complete resection of pulmonary metastases do as well as those who have had thoracotomies for primary bronchogenic carcinoma.[26] Nonetheless, the most common diagnostic dilemma is distinguishing metastases from granulomas and vessels.[40,44,45]

Other preoperative diagnostic modalities, such as sputa cytology and fiberoptic bronchoscopy, have been shown to be diagnostic in less than 15 percent of cases studied.[2,24,56,57] Recently, Patterson et al. reported a 75 to 80 percent diagnostic rate utilizing percutaneous needle aspirations of the tumor.[34] This technique requires further investigation and experience before it gains widespread clinical acceptance. Thus, once a nodule is identified in a patient with a history of prior malignancy, thoracotomy is usually indicated for diagnosis if otherwise appropriate.

PREOPERATIVE CLINICAL CONSIDERATIONS

Most authors agree that the basic criteria for operating on a patient who has had a previous non-germ cell malignancy and later develops a pulmonary nodule or nodules include complete eradication of the primary tumor and no evi-

Table 14-3. Minimum Criteria for Consideration
of Pulmonary Metastases Resection

Primary tumor eradicated
No extrapulmonary metastases
Low surgical risk

dence of extrapulmonary metastases. Additionally, the patient must otherwise be considered to be at low operative risk (Table 14-3). A review of the literature suggests that if at least these three criteria are fulfilled, approximately 30 percent of all patients will survive five years or more without recurrence of disease if the operation completely resects all pulmonary metastases.[9-37]

Authors do not agree on what preoperative factors are important prognostically (Table 14-4). Somewhat surprisingly, neither the *age* nor the *sex* of the patient seems to influence the ultimate outcome. Many reports in the pediatric literature confirm the efficacy of pulmonary nodulectomy in children with malignancies,[49,58,59,60] especially in patients with osteogenic sarcoma.[61-70] This topic has been extensively reviewed elsewhere and will only be mentioned briefly here. Similarly, advanced age is not a contraindication to nodulectomy if the medical condition of the patient is sufficiently stable to allow a major operation. The overall survival results in this selected group are equal to those in younger patients.[13,15,16,18,21,28,29]

The *pathology* of both the primary and resected tissue is of great interest. Most authors have reported their experiences with patients with different tumor types. Notably, overall five-year survival rates of patients who have soft tissue sarcoma are similar to those patients who have carcinomas.[10-12,14,18,21,25,28,29,37] A higher percentage of patients with a previously treated sarcoma do become candidates for pulmonary resection because of the unique biology of that pathological entity. Sarcomas tend to have a specific predilection for metastasizing to the lungs, without spreading elsewhere.[71] Thus, failure in patients with soft tissue sarcomas is usually either at the site of the primary or in the lungs, as opposed to the tendency toward more widespread dissemination in patients with carcinomas.[71]

There is a broad range of reported survival rates of patients with different carcinomatous primaries.[2-34] These results are summarized in Table 14-5. The survival for any given tumor type depends heavily on the particular series chosen, probably as a result of patient selection, surgical technique, and postoperative follow-up. Surprisingly, patients with both melanoma and breast cancer manifest relatively high, long-term survival rates after pulmonary metastectomy. In fact, Ehrenhaft et al. originally suggested that a patient with a history of previous

Table 14-4. Potential Factors in the Prediction
of Prognosis for Pulmonary Nodulectomy
Candidates

Age, sex (of less importance)
Histology of primary
Number, size, and location of nodules
Presence or absence of metastases to hilar or mediastinal lymph nodes
Disease-free interval
Tumor doubling time

Table 14-5. Summary of Five-Year Survival Based on Histology of Primary Tumor after Pulmonary Metastases Resection

Primary Tumor	No. of Patients	Five-Year Survival (%)	Range Reported (%)
Head and neck	62	37	30–100
Melanoma	56	21	14–100
Breast	101	26	7–43
Colon	190	25	9–51
Cervix uterus	39	20	0–66
Corpus uterus	29	75	50–100
Miscellaneous (thyroid, adrenal, mandible, ovary)	9	55	0–100

breast cancer should be excluded from consideration from resection because of the very poor results obtained.[12] In a later paper, however, they reported a 20 percent five-year survival in this same population.[29] Previously, a report from Memorial Hospital in New York City documented a 30 percent, five-year survival in women who had resection of pulmonary metastases from breast cancer.[28] These data prompted the former authors to revise their earlier guidelines to consider such women as operative candidates.[29]

Considerable controversy exists regarding the significance of other preoperative factors in predicting which patients will enjoy long-term survival after nodulectomy. The presence of *multiple pulmonary metastases,* especially if bilateral, was initially considered to contraindicate aggressive surgical treatment.[10] Many surgeons still feel that the presence of multiple metastases worsens the patient's prognosis, especially if the tumors are bilateral.[15,18,65,67,72] Nonetheless, later authors documented that patients with more than one, and even bilateral, lesions could achieve satisfactory, long-term, disease-free remissions.[11] Several investigators have subsequently reported that the incidence of five-year, disease-free survival in patients with multiple nodules may be as high as in those with solitary metastases, ranging from 18 to 62 percent.[13,14,19,27,31,34,62,66,73]

There is also disagreement over the *size* of potentially resectable lesions. Klein and Young reported that only 2 of 16 patients (12 percent) with lesions greater than 5 cm survived more than five years, whereas 5 of 14 patients (35 percent) with smaller lesions had a five-year disease-free survival.[19] On the other hand, several series have suggested that size was of no prognostic importance.[15,18,32,74] In fact, Edlich reported that the patient with the largest tumor resected in his series was alive and disease-free at seven years.[15]

Most authors agree that the presence of metastatic tumor in *hilar* or *mediastinal nodes* in a resected sample predicts a dismal outcome.[13-16,72] However, recently, Wilkins et al. have reported that patients with nodal involvement survived as long as those with negative nodes after lobectomy or pneumonectomy for metastatic lesions (22 versus 25 percent, respectively).[26] Those who had no lymph nodes examined fared even better (40 percent survival).[26] These data are difficult to interpret, since most surgeons attempt to resect as little tissue as possible, relying on wedge resections rather than lobectomies or pneumonectomies in order to avoid a postoperative compromise of pulmonary function. Thus, the failure of the surgeon to perform a lymph node dissection may reflect the necessity of a less extensive procedure to achieve total resection of malignancy. Nodal tissue is not often available for careful review. However, many reports of apparent cures after more extensive procedures have been published.[18,19,21,26]

The *disease-free interval* (DFI), defined as the elapsed time from control of the primary lesion until appearance of recurrent disease, may or not predict ultimate outcome. One might logically deduce that a short DFI would indicate that the patient has a more aggressive tumor. However, the literature contains at least 11 studies claiming that survival may be as good or better in patients whose disease recurs within 3 to 12 months, than in those with a longer DFI.[10-12,25,27,29,32,61,62,65,75] At least as many studies have been published that have reported that a DFI of less than 12 to 24 months significantly worsens the prognosis.[13-16,19,21,31,34,66,67,73, 74,76] This disparity almost certainly arises from multiple differences between studies, including patient selection, tumor types, presence or absence of other predictive factors, and adequacy of patient follow-up.

In the early 1970s, two separate groups suggested that the *tumor doubling time* (TDT), a concept similar to, yet quite distinct from the DFI, was predictive of ultimate success or failure of a metastectomy.[20,63] They hoped that this would help in a more careful selection of patients for resection of pulmonary metastases, while avoiding operations in those destined to fail. This concept was based on studies of the measurements of tumor growth rates done in the preceding two decades by Collins.[77,78] He suggested that tumor growth appeared to be exponential, and that the TDT could be determined from knowledge of change in tumor volume over a given interval of time. When plotted on a semi-logarithmic graph, a straight line is produced. This slope is a function of rate of tumor growth, whereas the horizontal distance between the vertical lines drawn from the two measuring points is a close approximation of the TDT.[20,63,77,78] Examples of three hypothetical patients with TDT of 9, 24, and 48 days are illustrated in Figure 14-1.

From these calculations, Morton and Joseph attempted to retrospectively calculate and correlate the DFI and the TDT in several patients with a variety of tumors, but predominantly patients with sarcomas.[20,24] They compared survival of patients according to their preoperative TDT (Fig. 14-2). They found a significant survival advantage for those patients who manifested a preoperative TDT of greater than 40 days, as compared with those whose TDT were 20 to 40 days and those with TDT of less than 20 days. They also compared a group of patients who had similar TDT, but who were not resected, and suggested that the survival in this group was worse than in those patients on whom an operation was performed. In summary, they suggested that the TDT and DFI were proportional and reflected the biological aggressiveness of the respective neoplasms in patients with short (less than 40 days) and long (greater than 40 days) TDT (Fig. 14-2). Their data led them to propose that a preoperative TDT of less than 40 days might contraindicate resection of pulmonary metastases, and that a delay of one to two months to calculate the TDT was justified.

Although intriguing, a number of faults exists in this retrospective study. The criteria used to choose the control patients is not clear, and one must assume

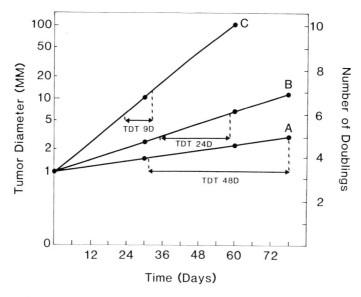

Fig. 14-1. Calculation of tumor doubling times (TDT) of three hypothetical patients based on changes in tumor diameter during a specific time period. Tumor diameter given as logarithmic scale (see text)· Patient A, TDT, 48 days; patient B, TDT, 24 days; patient C, TDT, 9 days.

that there were contraindications to operative intervention, which would have worsened the prognosis anyway. The number of patients studied was small, and there is great heterogeneity among tumor type, location, size, and number of lesions, making intergroup comparisons difficult. Finally, follow-up was relatively brief, although all patients with shorter TDT were dead of disease within three years. Reflecting on these ambiguities, subsequent authors have differed widely in their support of the use of TDT as a prognostic and selective preoperative factor.[21,25,63,75,79] In association with Morton, Huth et al. have described similar preoperative selection techniques in a group of patients with sarcomas.[73] They

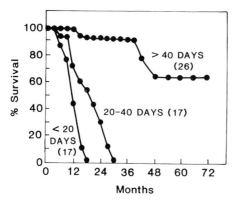

Fig. 14-2. Percent survival after resection of pulmonary metastases. Three groups of patients based on preoperative TDT (Morton DL, Joseph WL, Ketcham AS, Geelhoed GW, Adkins PC: Surgical resection and adjunctive immunotherapy for selected patients with multiple pulmonary metastases. Ann Surg 178:360, 1973.)

suggested that the two survival curves representing shorter and longer TDT separated early, but may converge after three or four years.[73] In addition, the Roswell Park experience has been similar to that of Morton and Joseph.[21,25,75] They did, however, report that DFI and TDT did not necessarily correlate.[75]

Other authors have argued that a delay of one to two months in therapy to calculate the TDT might allow metastatic spread to the hilar or mediastinal lymph nodes.[74] Also, it has been shown that a new pulmonary lesion might represent a primary bronchogenic carcinoma, as discussed earlier.[26,80]

In summary, one can conclude that both the DFI and TDT may be important in determining the advisability of an aggressive operative approach for the treatment of pulmonary metastases. However, a short DFI and/or TDT are certainly not absolute contraindications to surgery for any individual patient. Several reports of survivors who have one or both are in the literature.[10-12,25,27,29,32,61-63,65,75] Also of interest is a recent preliminary report from UCLA suggesting that if the TDT is altered preoperatively by the use of effective chemotherapy, the prognosis after metastatic resection changes appropriately.[73] These data require confirmation.

TUMOR BIOLOGY

The discussion of these clinical prognostic factors raises several interesting issues regarding the natural biology of neoplasms and metastases. Recent investigators have emphasized the importance of tumor heterogeneity and the differences in metastatic potentials. These subjects have been thoroughly reviewed.[81-83] Metastasis to a particular organ has been shown to occur through various specific, though as yet unidentified recognition systems. Fidler et al. have demonstrated that tumors implanted and consecutively passed in nude mice will eventually show a propensity for a specific organ, if the material passed is serially harvested from that organ only.[84] Nicholson et al. have described the presence of phenotypic cell-surface variations within malignant cell lines that are characteristic for each subclone, which has a specific predilection for colonizing a particular organ.[81,85] In addition, they have shown that simple anatomical placement of tumor cells in the pulmonary system will not select for lung-specific clones.[86] These cell-surface recognition factors, presumably proteins or glycoproteins, may be critical in determining which tumors will metastasize only to the lungs and be amenable to curative resective approaches. Other tumors with presumably different phenotypes tend to metastasize widely to other organs. One might speculate that the ability to define these determinants in an in vitro study of resected material might even predict the ultimate clinical course, allowing more accurate preoperative patient selection. On the other hand, Talmadge and Fidler have shown that metastases can be either organ-specific or can occur randomly in their growth patterns, depending on the parent tumor population.[87] These studies offer great potential clinical applicability for the future.

The concept of inter- and intra-tumor heterogeneity has been of great interest.[82,83,85,88-90] Most malignancies contain several subpopulations of cells with different microscopic, biochemical, biological, and clinical characteristics.[89,90] This heterogeneity has significance for the clinical investigator trying to define empiric prognostic factors that allow appropriate selection of patients as candidates for nodulectomy. For example, the TDT, which is determined for a given tumor based on measurement of one or more lesions seen on chest radiographs, may not accurately reflect all the tumor nodules present. Determination of TDT may become even more difficult after chemotherapeutic intervention. Preoperative chemotherapy might eliminate sensitive cell populations, thus selecting for insensitive subclones. These subclones may, in fact, be slower or faster growing, but their malignant and metastatic potential would be difficult to predict.[90] The resultant TDT would be similarly ambiguous. The Gompertzian growth-curve model, which predicts that cell growth slows exponentially with increasing tumor mass,[91] would predict a shorter doubling time for those cells remaining in a tumor nodule. The clinical implications of these possibilities are unclear. Huth's suggestion that a preoperative response to chemotherapy might improve the results of a nodulectomy[73] must be substantiated in more extensive trials. However, as more effective adjuvant treatment programs become available, these considerations will be foremost in coordinating operative and systemic treatment programs for metastases.

The latency period between treatment of the primary and appearance of the metastatic lesion is also perplexing. It is not known whether the host immune system plays a surveillance role in tumor inhibition and whether failure of that system allows the growth of neoplasms. Alternatively, it has been postulated that an immune response might, in fact, stimulate tumor growth.[92] Obviously, the metastatic clones must have been present, but undetectable when the primary lesion was treated. The appearance of the lesions at a later date might simply represent linear growth of the clones to a size visible by current techniques, but this does not explain the considerable variation in size and weight often seen between metastatic nodules. Alternatively, subclone heterogeneity with variable antigenic expressions and, thus, different responses to either stability or changes in the immune system might exist.[92] Another hypothesis is the suggestion that staggered release of metastases from the primary neoplasm occurs prior to definitive treatment. One might also speculate that metastases arise from metastases, rather than from the original malignancy.[93] The testing of these hypotheses will directly affect the approach to pulmonary nodulectomy. The possibilities of metastatic spread from metastases and of changing immunogenicity of the tumor with growth might argue against conservative preoperative observation of metastatic nodules for one or two months if the patient is an otherwise excellent operative candidate. Additionally, effective adjuvant therapy after treatment of the primary is necessary to eliminate micrometastatic subclones.[94] The reader is referred to more extensive discussions of metastatic potential, tumor heterogeneity, and adjuvant chemotherapy for further insight into these fascinating areas.[81-95]

PULMONARY NODULECTOMY IN UROLOGIC CANCER

Is there a role for pulmonary nodulectomy in nongynecological urologic cancer? Although most authors of larger series include case reports of metastases arising from non-testicular primaries, their results in this particular subset is infrequently mentioned.[5,11-19,21-23,26-29] Table 14-6 summarizes the renal cell cancer data. In spite of the original report by Barney and Churchill[8] patients with metastases from renal cell carcinoma do no better than other patients.[23,27,29] Several investigators have published series describing resection of pulmonary metastases from urothelial and renal primaries.[8,96-104] As mentioned, the classic case of Barney and Churchill concerned a woman with renal cell carcinoma.[8] Subsequent isolated case reports suggested that five-year, disease-free survival following resection of pulmonary metastases originating from renal cell carcinoma is possible.[96] The tendency of renal cell carcinoma to follow an unusual and unpredictable clinical course has complicated interpretation of the available data.[105] Although long latency periods from the time of resection of the primary to the time of tumor recurrence are not necessarily characteristic of renal cell carcinomas, several authors have reported disease-free intervals in excess of 6 to 10 years.[96,102,106] Consequently, any series requires long follow-up to assess the success of the therapeutic intervention adequately. In addition, renal cell carcinoma has been shown to manifest great intra- and inter-tumor heterogeneity (vida supra). Although many patients with renal cell carcinomas have rapidly progressing disease, it is not uncommon to see patients survive several years, even with widespread incurable metastases.[100,102,107] In the absence of concurrent, matched controls, the influence of metastasectomy in prolonging survival may be more apparent than real.

A great deal of attention has been directed toward the issue of spontaneous regression of metastases from renal cell carcinoma.[99,100,102,108-113] Although certainly well documented, spontaneous regression occurs in less than 1 percent of all patients with metastatic renal cell carcinoma.[112] Classically thought to occur after nephrectomy, spontaneous regression is now believed to occur randomly.[113] Again, unpredictable behaviors make evaluation of surgical results difficult. They also reflect a very complex and as yet poorly understood interaction between tumor biology and host defense mechanisms.

Table 14-6. Reported Five-Year Survivals of Patients Who Have Undergone Resection of Pulmonary Metastases from Primary Renal Cell Cancer

Author	No. of Patients	Five-Year Survival (%)
Alexander[10]	6	50
Gliedman[11]	7	29
Ehrenhaft[12]	4	25
Wilkins[13]	16	31
Edlich[15]	9	11
Johnson[16]	8	25
Turney[18]	7	14
Cline[19]	4	25
Chokski[21]	6	40
Turnbull[22]	1	0
Hutchinson[23]	2	100
Wilkins[26]	28	44
Mountain[27]	16	50
McCormack[28]	22	28
Wright[29]	14	5
Marks[32]	7	43
Patterson[34]	16	25

Finally, the histological identification of resected pulmonary nodules can be ambiguous. Renal cell carcinomas can appear microscopically as several cell types, including clear, granular, spindle, and small cell carcinomas.[114] Confusion can arise between spindle cell tumors and sarcomas, small cell tumors and oat cell carcinomas of the lung, or clear cell tumors and the so-called "sugar" tumor arising in the lung.[72,115-117] The latter are, fortunately, quite rare.[115-117]

Preoperative diagnosis of renal cell carcinoma metastases does not differ significantly from that for other cell types. This has been discussed above. The production of serological markers by renal cell carcinomas, some of which are functional hormones and peptides, has been well documented.[118] These markers are present in only a few patients. Their clinical utility as a measure of disease activity has not been satisfactorily established. Consequently, one cannot rely on the clinical use of these markers to detect metastatic disease or follow response to treatment.

Review of the literature suggests that of those patients with renal cell carcinoma, 2 to 8 percent have solitary metastases to a single organ, and approximately 30 percent of those are found in the lung.[99,100,102,104,119] In 1978, Katzenstein et al. reviewed a series of 44 patients with renal cell carcinoma metastatic to the lung.[72] Nineteen patients had synchronous metastases or discovery of their metastases prior to diagnosis of a primary renal cell carcinoma. The remaining 25 patients had disease-free intervals, ranging from 1 to 120 months. In contrast to the larger general series, 90 percent of these patients had pulmonary symptoms manifesting metastatic disease. In this retrospective study, most patients selected for resection of their metastases had unilateral nodules, which appeared metachronously in relation to the primary neoplasm. Those with bilateral lesions were biopsied only, without aggressive attempts at curative operations. Of 17 patients who underwent resection, 2 (12 percent) were alive and free of disease at 16 and 148 months postoperatively. Both these patients had solitary lesions. One had a DFI of less than two years; the other a DFI of more than two years. These authors concluded that, in selected patients, pulmonary nodulectomy was justified, especially if the patients had a solitary nodule or a minimal number of unilateral nodules.[72] They also reviewed 19 patients who presented with pulmonary nodules shown to be metastases from subsequently diagnosed renal cell carcinoma primaries. Of 17 patients, 4 (23 percent) were long-term survivors but only three of these were free of cancer at 21 months to 6 years from initial diagnosis. All four had unilateral lung lesions completely excised and all underwent nephrectomies after the primaries were discovered. Thus, it can be concluded that the presence of metastatic lesions at the time of diagnosis of the primary does not exclude long-term disease-free survival.[72]

Several series evaluating the results of treating and following patients with solitary metastases from renal cell cancer to a variety of single organs have been published.[99,100,102] Tolia and Whitmore found that 35 percent of those patients who had aggressive therapy, including surgery, irradiation, or cryosurgery, survived for five years, although only 24 percent were disease-free.[99] Three patients had a single pulmonary nodule. Two of these were resected, and one patient lived at least five years without recurrence. O'Dea et al. obtained similar results at the Mayo Clinic in patients with solitary renal cell carcinoma metastases.[100] They reported seven patients with lung nodules, six of whom were treated with surgery. Two of these patients were alive and disease-free 6.5 and 8.5 years after the operation, although the latter required resection of a brain metastasis 16 months after his thoracotomy. Although one patient died of widespread disease within two years of his operation, three others who ultimately died of metastases were disease-free for 9, 8, and 8 years after their thoracotomies. These data again emphasize the unpredictable nature of this neoplasm and the need for long-term follow-up.

Finally, Kjaer and Engelholm have reviewed the experience at the Finsen Institute with patients with renal cell carcinoma who exhibited solitary metastases.[102] Of six patients with solitary pulmonary nodules, three underwent resection and three were treated with aggressive radiotherapy. At five years, one of the surgically treated patients was alive without disease, and two of the latter group had survived without recurrence. The successful use of aggressive radiotherapy in this situation is intriguing. Radiation therapy might prove to be an alternative therapy for those patients whose medical condition obviates major surgery. The use of radiotherapy for treatment of gross metastases or sterilization of micrometastases has been investigated in patients with Wilms' tumor[22,120,121] and osteogenic sarcoma.[120,122] Although both of these tumors are relatively radiosensitive, whole lung radiation at the dose required to produce cytotoxicity of uroepithelial tumor cells is quite toxic.[22] This modality would have to be reserved for isolated metastases.[120]

All the above reports deal primarily with patients with solitary metastatic lesions. Mayo et al. have recently reported the resection of multiple metastatic renal carcinoma metastases requiring a bilobectomy from a 51-year-old woman who had had a nephrectomy for clear cell carcinoma of the kidney four years previously.[101] At the time of their report, she had survived 8.5 years without evidence of disease. These data are summarized in Table 14-7.

Thirty-three patients who have undergone resection of pulmonary metastases from transitional cell carcinoma of the bladder have been reported in the literature.[11,12,15,17,18,21,32,97,98,103] Of these, eight (27 percent) survived at least one year without disease recurrence. In the only series specifically addressing this issue,

Table 14-7. Summary of Papers on Resection of Pulmonary Metastases from Primary Renal Cell Carcinoma

Author	Patients (N)	Five-Year Survival (%)	Comments
Katzenstein[12]	17	12	All solitary, metachronous
Tolia[99]	3	33	All solitary
O'Dea[100]	7	28	One survivor also had brain metastases. Several patients relapsed after more than five disease-free years
Kjaer[102]	3	33	Three patients successfully palliated with radiation therapy
Mayo[101]	1	100	Multiple, bilateral metastases resected

Table 14-8. Patient Survival after Resection of Pulmonary Metastases Originating from Transitional Cell Carcinoma of the Urothelium

Author	No. of Patients	Survival (%)
Gliedman[11]	1	0
Ehrenhaft[12]	1	0
Edlich[15]	2	0
Fallon[17]	14	11
Turney[18]	2	50
Chokski[21]	3	0
Marks[32]	4	25
Cowles[103]	6	83

four of six patients survived five years or more.[103] All patients in this series had isolated pulmonary metastases (Table 14-8).

Only 13 patients with prostatic carcinoma who have undergone pulmonary metastectomy have been reported in the world literature, and there is only one long-term survivor.[12,17,29] The sparsity of reports of resection of metastases from prostate cancer undoubtedly reflects the tendency exhibited of this particular primary to metastasize widely (Table 14-9).

In summary, renal and uroepithelial neoplasms present enigmatic problems to the clinician. On the one hand, the unique biology of these malignancies separates them from other types of tumors on the basis of their relative tendencies to metastasize solely to the lungs. Renal cell carcinoma has a proportionately higher propensity to do so; uroepithelial and prostatic cancers do not.[99,100-102,104,119] Of those patients whose metastases are solely in the pulmonary system, the preoperative criteria for selection are the same as for those patients with other neoplasms, and the expected five-year disease-free survival is also probably about 20 to 35 percent.

RESECTION OF PULMONARY METASTASES FROM TESTICULAR CARCINOMA

The biology and natural history of nonseminomatous testicular carcinomas are so different than those of other solid tumors that a separate discussion of resection of metastases arising from these tumors is justified. Prior to the advent of consistently curative chemotherapy, several authors published scattered case reports of patients who enjoyed long-term disease-free survivals after having isolated and recurrent pulmonary metastases excised.[12-14,123-126] These results are surprising in light of the characteristically rapid growth rate and short TDT of testicular

Table 14-9. Patient Survival after Resection of Pulmonary Metastases Originating from Adenocarcinoma of the Prostate

Author	No. of Patients	Survival (%)
Ehrenhaft[12]	1	100
Fallon[17]	9	0
Wright[29]	3	0

carcinoma.[20,77,127] It has been estimated that the mean TDT of testicular metastases to the lung is 39 days, considerably less than the mean value of approximately 100 days calculated for breast and colorectal tumors.[127] Tumor heterogeneity is further emphasized by the broad range of TDT within the same histological groupings.[127] If other sites of metastases, particularly the retroperitoneum, could also be sterilized surgically, an aggressive surgical approach seemed justified in this predominantly young population prior to the availability of effective chemotherapy.[124,126] Unfortunately, cures remained the exception rather than the rule in stage III patients.[123-126]

These anecdotal survival data shed some insight into the metastatic characteristics of testicular carcinoma. Most authorities agree that testicular cancer manifests a predictable stepwise pattern of metastatic spread. The tumor usually first invades the regional lymphatics and ascends the lymphatic channels accompanying the spermatic vein to the retroperitoneal lymph nodes. Although hematogenous access may be gained by infiltration of the spermatic veins, more commonly, pulmonary metastases appear to arise through the lymphatic distribution via the lymphatic duct with bloodborne metastases occurring late in the clinical course.[128] Consequently, the manifestation of pulmonary metastases can be correlated with the presence of retroperitoneal disease.[129] Unlike the situation with non-germ cell cancers, in which extrapulmonary metastases contraindicate an operative approach, one cannot discuss the surgical management of testicular metastases to the lung without considering the retroperitoneum. This is reflected in the literature. More than 20 papers have reported the results of resection of metastases from nonseminomatous testicular cancer, yet only a few primarily discuss pulmonary nodulectomies.[123-126,128,130-147]

The advent of curative combination chemotherapy with *cis*-diamminedichloroplatinum, has drastically altered the clinical course of testicular carcinoma.[145,148] Complete response (CR) rates as high as 60 to 80 percent for patients with widespread metastases have been reported with chemotherapy and chemotherapy followed by surgery.[145,148,149] These remarkable results have dramatically changed the role of surgery in the physician's approach toward the patient with metastatic disease. Whereas surgery was previously used only as a last effort to salvage a failing patient, it has now become an integral part of the comprehensive, curative treatment program of the patient with metastatic disease.[123-126,128-149]

There is some confusion concerning the staging of testicular cancer, and a plea has been made for better standardization, to allow more accurate comparisons of different treatment programs.[140] For the purposes of this discussion, the category of stage III disease (or stage C) will be subdivided into two classes: one group includes those patients with minimal pulmonary disease, defined as five or less metastases per lung field with each nodule less than 2 cm; the other group includes patients with advanced disease with any mediastinal or hilar mass, any intrapulmonary nodule greater than 2 cm, more than five pulmonary nodules, or pleural effusion.[150] Using these designations, up to or more than 90 percent of patients with minimal stage III disease can expect to achieve complete remission with chemotherapy.[140,142,151] However, 40 to 50 percent of those with advanced pulmonary metastases are left with residual masses after chemotherapy.[140,142,151] It is this group of patients who are left with residual masses after aggressive effective chemotherapy for whom surgery now plays an integral part. As noted by Vugrin et al.,[142] "when the tremendous potential of combination chemotherapy for curative germ cell tumors was first appreciated, it seemed probable that the role of the surgeons would be dramatically curtailed. Contrary to this prediction, modern chemotherapy has increased the role of the surgeons."

The timing of curative resection of metastases has been thoroughly investigated. Merrin and Takita have reported that, initially, they performed pre-chemotherapy "debulking" procedures, based on theoretical suggestions that resistance to chemotherapy is less likely to develop if the overall tumor burden is small.[128,132,134] However, they found that the time required for recovery from surgery delayed the initiation of systemic treatment and permitted rapid dissemination of metastases. In addition, they found that preoperative chemotherapy facilitated the technical aspects of the procedure by decreasing tumor size and vascularity and altering the basic histology of the resected mass (see below). Finally, as discussed above, a large proportion of patients will achieve complete remission with chemotherapy alone, obviating the need for surgery.[134,147] The early experience at Indiana University was consistent with these findings.[124] Recently, investigators at the National Cancer Institute published a well-conceived, prospective trial in which 39 patients with stage III nonseminomatous testicular cancer were randomized for either a cisplatin-containing chemotherapeutic regimen, followed by resection of any residual masses, or up-front debulking surgery, with postoperative chemotherapy.[150] Extent of disease at presentation was similar for the two groups. Although surgical cytoreduction was feasible, they found no difference between the two groups in overall response rates, CR rates, or survival. Their conclusion, in agreement with the above authors, was that cytoreductive surgery prior to chemotherapy has no role in the treatment of stage III testicular patients.[150] Although exact timing varies from surgeon to surgeon, Mandelbaum et al. have suggested waiting four to eight weeks from the end of chemotherapy to the time of surgery.[147]

Detection of resectable metastases and selection of patients for nodulectomy have been recently evaluated. Several authors have reported that of all patients who are found to have stage III disease at presentation, between 10 and 40 percent will be left after effective chemotherapy with a residual mass either in the retroperitoneum, the lungs, or both.[132,133,138,139,142,145,147] The investigators at Indiana University have reported that about 10 percent of their patients have only residual pulmonary masses.[138,147] Since most, if not all, of these patients are asymptomatic,[145] the clinician must rely on either radiological detection of residual or recurrent metastatic disease. It should be noted that considerable controversy exists over the adequacy of routine CXR to evaluate the lung and mediastinum. Many authors suggest that routine WLT after chemotherapy, supplemented by CT, is indicated.[40,42-50,52,147] However, a recent study by Jochelson et al. disputes this approach and suggests that the latter two modalities are not required unless the chest X-ray is abnormal or equivocal.[51]

The clinician may have difficulty distinguishing true neoplastic disease from bleomycin-induced nodules.[152] Although elevated serological markers suggest active cancer, normal markers do not suggest the reverse. The radiological characteristics of the nodules may have some diagnostic significance.[40,51,52,152,153] Observation over time to assess any change in size may also be helpful. Frequently, however, the diagnosis ultimately requires thoracotomy and resection of the nodules for pathological review.[146,147,152]

The use of serological markers, especially beta human chorionic gonadotropin (hCG), alphafetroprotein (AFP), and lactic dehydrogenase (LDH) has been of more value in nonseminomatous testicular carcinoma than perhaps in any other tumor to date.[154] The level of these markers after chemotherapy and prior to surgery in patients who have residual masses may be of value. Several authors have reported that if preoperative markers are elevated, the residual mass will almost always contain carcinomatous elements.[133,136,139,142] Interestingly, both Garnick et al.[145] and Mandelbaum et al.[138,147] have reported patients whose preoperative markers were elevated, but whose masses were found to be only fibrotic. These patients subsequently suffered a carcinomatous relapse. In addition, two patients with elevated markers from whom only mature teratoma was resected have been reported, but both have since relapsed and died.[145]

The Indiana University Group excludes patients with rising markers after cisplatin-containing chemotherapy from surgical consideration because of their poor prognosis.[147] Conversely, negative markers do not assure that residual tissue masses will be benign. Although all patients who ultimately had only fibrosis and/or teratoma resected and have not relapsed have had normal markers, many authors have reported several patients whose preoperative markers were normal, but whose resected masses contained carcinomatous elements.[133,136,138,139,141,142,145-147] Thus, elevated serum markers, preoperatively imply residual cancer, but normal serum markers do not exclude the presence of cancer in the residual mass.

The appropriate operative approach depends on the individual surgeon. Although some authors suggest bilateral or staged thoracotomies for the resection of pulmonary nodules,[126,133,139,140,144] others claim superior results with a midline median sternotomy.[128,132,143] The group at Indiana University makes their decisions on a case-by-case basis.[138,139,147] Most investigators feel that a single operation, whether done via a sternal to pubic midline incision[128,132,143] or a thoracoabdominal incision,[131,133,138,139,144,147] is preferred for patients for resection of retroperitoneal and pulmonary masses. Postoperative mortality is low, ranging from 0 to 2 percent.[132-134,138-141,143-145,147] Unlike patients with non-germ cell cancer, who tend to be in an older age group and who have a higher incidence of significant coronary artery disease, patients with testicular cancer are commonly younger and are better surgical risks. However, bleomycin administration can produce pulmonary fibrosis, which may make postoperative care extremely difficult. Several authors have published cases in which severe morbidity and mortality has occurred, presumably due to pulmonary fibrosis.[132,145,153,155,156] Concern over this toxicity has led some institutions to initiate special protocols using low inspired oxygen tensions and careful fluid replacement during anesthesia. These precautions have allegedly reduced or eliminated this problem.[143,153,155,156]

The masses that remain after chemotherapy in patients who have had nonseminomatous testicular carcinoma, are of three histological types; fibrosis, teratoma, or residual carcinoma. Mixtures of these have also been found within lesions from a single patient.[126,130,134,136,138-145,147] These pathological entities are distributed evenly, with roughly one-third of surgical patients having each kind.[134,136,138,139,141,145,146]

Teratoma are infrequently found after chemotherapy,[134,135,139,141,143,146,157-159] and only in patients who initially had embryonal cell carcinoma or teratocarcinoma.[134,143,157,158] Some investigators have suggested that these lesions are the result of a cytotoxic elimination of surrounding malignant elements, with retention of the chemotherapy-resistant mature teratoma. A second theory is that chemotherapy, in some way, stimulates differentiation of embryonal elements.[134,135] The latter seems more plausible, in that mature elements are not always seen histologically in the original, prechemotherapy biopsy specimen in patients who ultimately develop mature teratoma.[134] Additionally, spontaneous maturation has been reported in the absence of chemotherapy.[157] That a drug may be responsible for differentiation is pure conjecture, although differentiation was observed before the advent of cisplatin therapy.[155,157] The theory of chemotherapy-induced tumor differentiation has precedence in in vivo animal studies[160] and other recently reported tumor-chemotherapeutic agent systems.[146,161]

A recent paper from Indiana University has described non-germ cell malignant elements in pathological specimens from 11 male patients with primary germ cell tumors.[159] They reported a variety of different sarcomas and an occasional carcinoma. The authors proposed that these non-germ cell elements arose within teratomatous foci and were "unmasked" by the destruction of more sensitive germ cell fractions during chemotherapy.[159]

The prognostic implications of the surgical findings are dramatic. Mandelbaum et al. have recently reported that only 4 of 22 patients from whom carcinomatous pulmonary nodules were resected after chemotherapy are alive and well.[147] This corroborates their earlier reports,[138] as well as those of others, who report that 30 to 100 percent of those patients with residual cancer ultimately relapse and die.[133,134,136,142-145] Conversely, a pure mature teratoma is predictive of an excellent long-term outcome.[133,134,136,141-145,147] More than 90 percent of these patients are alive and free of disease. Those who are not had such extenuating circumstances as operative-associated mortality,[142] a very high-grade primary,[144] a second testicular malignancy,[141] or late bleomycin-induced pulmonary toxicity.[147] Discovery of the third histological component fibrosis also indicates a good prognosis, although it does not ensure a cure. As noted, there have been cases of patients with elevated preoperative serum markers who had only fibrotic masses and who ultimately relapsed.[138,145,147] In addition, recurrence of cancer in patients in whom only fibrosis was resected, even though preoperative markers were normal, has been reported.[138,142,145] The finding of rhabdomyosarcomatous malignant elements in germ cell foci is particularly ominous, with only one of six patients having survived in the largest series.[159] Conversely, other forms of sarcoma that develop within germ cell tumors do not appear to affect the prognosis adversely. If patients with teratoma could be distinguished from those with cancer preoperatively, one wonders if an operation could be avoided in the former. Merrin et al. have reported two locally invasive, but histologically mature teratomas,[134] and metastases from histologically benign teratomas have also been reported.[157] In 1984, the clinician is forced to recommend resection of any remaining masses after aggressive standard chemotherapy for patients who have had a nonseminomatous testicular neoplasm.

Almost all authors concur that postoperative chemotherapy is necessary for those patients in whom residual carcinoma is found, although agents and schedules differ widely.[132,133,136,139-141,143,145-147] Even with postoperative chemotherapy, long-term, disease-free survival is significantly less than in those patients who obtain complete remission, either with chemotherapy alone or with chemotherapy plus surgery.[132,133,136,139-141,143,145,147] Encouragingly, Einhorn et al. have recently reported that 8 of 10 patients who had residual cancer after lymphadenectomy and/ or pulmonary nodulectomy, and received two additional courses of cisplatin, bleomycin, and vinblastine, have remained in a continuous, disease-free remission for more than two years.[139] When only fibrosis or teratoma is found, most authors do not recommend the use of adjuvant chemotherapy,[138,145-147] or if chemotherapy is given, cisplatin is usually deleted to avoid further toxicity[140,143,144] (Fig. 14-3).

Retrospectively, it is difficult to define other preoperative clinical factors that predict success or failure of metastectomy in patients with nonseminomatous testicular carcinoma. The initial extent of pulmonary disease may determine whether chemotherapy alone will result in complete remission. However, assuming that postoperative pulmonary function is adequate and that all nodules can be resected, the number or size of the resected nodules may have no prognostic significance.[128,138,143,147] A recent report by Callery et al. refutes this.[144] They found that 90 percent of patients with a single metastatic nodule resected had a sustained, disease-free survival. Only 40 percent of those with more than one nodule, and 14 percent of those who required bilateral thoracotomies had a durable complete remission.[144] Unfortunately, patient selection is biased in many of these studies.

Callery et al. also suggested that cancer in the retroperitoneal lymph nodes worsens the prognosis.[144] Mandelbaum et al. have recently reported three patients

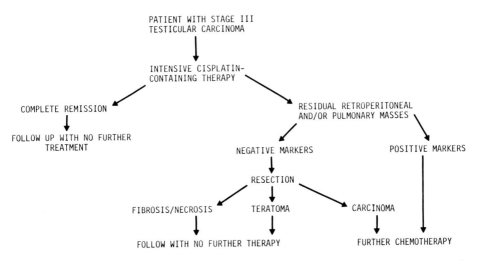

Fig. 14-3. Suggested treatment schema for patients with Stage III nonseminomatous carcinoma of the testicle.

with concurrently resected retroperitoneal and pulmonary carcinoma who are long-term, disease-free survivors.[147] No difference was noted between those whose retroperitoneal disease was resected prior to or simultaneously with the pulmonary lesions.[144] Garnick et al. have suggested that patients with extragonadal primary tumors do less well in all categories, including patients who had metastatic resections.[145] There has been no systematic evaluation of preoperative TDT in metastatic testicular carcinoma and the importance of the disease-free interval from the time of treatment of the primary to the time of nodulectomy is also difficult to assess.[137,138,147] Thus, the histology of the resected specimen remains the single most important prognostic factor. Experience from resection of metastases from patients who have primary testicular seminomas is limited, but success has been reported.[142]

In conclusion, 20 to 30 percent of *selected* patients who have had a primary non-testicular urologic cancer completely excised and who have no evidence of extrathoracic metastases can expect to enjoy a long-term, disease-free survival after resection of metastatic pulmonary nodules. The preoperative diagnosis and prognostic factors are similar to those of patients with non-urologic carcinomas. Patients with metastatic testicular cancer are in an entirely different category, and the decision to operate will depend on the initial response of the metastases to chemotherapy and the presence (or absence), and histology, of residual masses. A treatment schema suggesting a stepwise approach to the patient with stage III nonseminomatous texticular carcinoma is presented in Figure 14-3.

REFERENCES

1. Temple WJ, Ketcham AS: Surgical management of isolated systemic metastases. Semin Oncol 7:468, 1980
2. Holmes EC, Ramming KP, Eilber FR, Morton DL: The surgical management of pulmonary metastases. Semin Oncol 4:65, 1977
3. van Dongen JA, van Slooten EA: The surgical treatment of pulmonary metastases. Cancer Treat Rev 5:29, 1978
4. Mountain CF: The basis for surgical resection of pulmonary metastases. Int J Rad Oncol Biol Phys 1:749, 1976
5. Wilkins EW Jr: Solitary metastases in the lung. Int J Rad Oncol Biol Phys 1:735, 1976
6. Weinlechner V: Tumoren an der brustwand und deren behandlung (resektion der rippen, eroffnung der brusthohle, partielle enffernung der lunge). Weiner Med Woch 20:21, 1882
7. Divis G: Ein Beitrag zur operativen behandlung der lungeneschwulste. Arch Chir Scand 62:329, 1927
8. Barney JD, Churchill EJ: Adenocarcinoma of the kidney with metastasis to the lung. J Urol 42:269, 1939
9. Torek F: Removal of metastatic carcinoma of the lung and mediastinum. Arch Surg 21:1416, 1930
10. Alexander J, Haight C: Pulmonary resection for solitary metastatic sarcomas and carcinomas. Surg Gynecol Obstetr 85:129, 1947

11. Gliedman ML, Horowitz S, Lewis JF: Lung resection for metastatic cancer. Surgery 42:521, 1957
12. Ehrenhaft JL, Lawrence MS, Sensenig DM: Pulmonary resections for metastatic lesions. Arch Surg 77:606, 1958
13. Wilkins EW, Burke JF, Head JM: The surgical management of metastatic neoplasms in the lung. J Thorac Cardiovasc Surg 42:298, 1961
14. Thomford NR, Woolner LB, Clagett OT: The surgical treatment of metastatic tumors in the lings. J Thorac Cardiovasc Surg 49:357, 1965
15. Edlich RF, Shea MA, Foker JE, Grondin C, Castaneda AR, Varco RL: A review of 26 years' experience with pulmonary resection for metastatic cancer. Dis Chest 49:587, 1966
16. Johnson RM, Lindskog G: 100 cases of tumor metastatic to lung and mediastinum: treatment and results. JAMA 202:94, 1967
17. Fallon RH, Roper CL: Operative treatment of metastatic pulmonary cancer. Ann Surg 166:263, 1967
18. Turney SZ, Haight C: Pulmonary resection for metastatic neoplasms. J Thorac Cardiovasc Surg 61:784, 1971
19. Cline RE, Young CW: Long-term results following surgical treatment of metastatic pulmonary tumors. Am Surgeon 36:61, 1970
20. Joseph WL, Morton DL, Adkins PC: Prognostic significance of tumor doubling time in evaluating operability in pulmonary metastatic disease. J Thorac Cardiovasc Surg 61:23, 1971
21. Choksi SB, Takita H, Vincent RG: The surgical management of solitary pulmonary metastasis. Surg Gynecol Obstet 134:479, 1972
22. Turnbull AD, Pool JL, Arthur K, Golbey R: The role of radiotherapy and chemotherapy in the surgical management of pulmonary metastases. Am J Roentgenol 114:99, 1972
23. Hutchinson DE, Deaner RM: Resection of pulmonary secondary tumors. Am J Surg 124:732, 1972
24. Morton DL, Joseph WL, Ketcham AS, Geelhoed GW, Adkins PC: Surgical resection and adjunctive immunotherapy for selected patients with multiple pulmonary metastases. Ann Surg 178:360, 1973
25. Takita H, Merrin C, Didolkar M, Douglas HO, Edgerton F: The surgical management of multiple lung metastases. Ann Thorac Surg 24:359, 1977
26. Wilkins EW, Head JM, Burke JF: Pulmonary resection for metastatic neoplasms in the lung. Am J Surg 135:480, 1978
27. Mountain CF, Khalil KG, Hermes KE, Frazier OH: The contribution of surgery to the management of carcinomatous pulmonary metastases. Cancer 41:833, 1978
28. McCormack PM, Martini N: The changing role of surgery for pulmonary metastases. Ann Thorac Surg 28:139, 1979
29. Wright JO, Brandt B, Ehrenhaft JL: Results of pulmonary resection for metastatic lesions. J Thorac Cardiovasc Surg 83:94, 1982
30. Vyas JJ, Shaparia CL, Desai PB: The changing role of surgery for pulmonary metastasis. Ind J Chest Dis Allied Sci 23:179, 1981
31. Blondet R, Zlatoff P, Frieh JPH, Brunat-Mentigny M, Pasini E, Bobin JY, Mayer M: Results of combined chemosurgical therapy for pulmonary metastases. J Surg Oncol 18:105, 1981
32. Marks P, Ferrag MZ, Ashraf H: Rationale for the surgical treatment of pulmonary metastases. Thorax 36:679, 1981

33. Johnson H Jr, Fantone J, Flye MW: Histologic evaluation of the nodules resected in the treatment of pulmonary metastatic disease. J Surg Oncol 21:1, 1982

34. Patterson GA, Todd TRJ, Ilves R, Pearson FG, Cooper JD: Surgical management of pulmonary metastases. Canad J Surg 25:102, 1982

35. Johnston MR: Median sternotomy for resection of pulmonary metastases. J Thorac Cardiovasc Surg 85:1515, 1983

36. Farrell JT: Pulmonary metastasis: A pathologic, clinical, roentgenologic study based on 78 cases seen at necropsy. Radiology 24:444, 1935

37. Martini N, Bains MS, Huvos AG, Beattie EJ: Surgical treatment of metastatic sarcoma to the lung. Surg Clin N Am 54:841, 1974

38. Cohen M: Signs and symptoms of bronchogenic cancer. In Straus MA (ed): Lung Cancer: Clinical Diagnosis and Treatment. 2nd ed. Grune & Stratton, New York, 1983

39. Waldmann TA, Herberman RB. Tumor markers in diagnosis and in monitoring therapy. In Holland JF, Frei E III (eds): Cancer Medicine. 2nd ed. Lea & Febiger, Philadelphia, 1982

40. Libshitz HI, North LB: Pulmonary metastases. Radiol Clin N Am 20:437, 1982

41. Mintzer RA, Malave SR, Neiman HL, Michaelis LL, Vanecko RM, Sanders JH: Computed vs. conventional tomography in evaluation of primary and secondary neoplasms. Radiology 132:653, 1979

42. Polga JP, Watnick M: Whole lung tomography in metastatic disease. Clin Radiol 27:53, 1976

43. Neifeld JP, Michaelis LL, Doppman JL: Suspected pulmonary metastases. Cancer 39:383, 1977

44. Sindelar WF, Bagley DH, Felix EL, Doppman JL, Ketcham AS: Lung tomography in cancer patients. JAMA 240:2060, 1978

45. Chang AE, Schaner EG, Conkle DM, Flye MW, Doppman JL, Rosenberg SA: Evaluation of computed tomography in the detection of pulmonary metastases: A prospective study. Cancer 43:913, 1979

46. Schaner EG, Chang AE, Doppman JL, Conkle DM, Flye MW, Rosenberg SA: Comparison of computed and conventional whole lung tomography in detecting pulmonary nodules: A prospective radiologic-pathologic study. Am J Roentgenol 131:51, 1978

47. Curtis AM, Ravin CE, Collier PE, Putnam CE, McCloud T, Greenspan RH: Detection of metastatic disease from carcinoma of the breast: Limited value of full lung tomography. Am J Roentgenol 134:253, 1980

48. Curtis AM, Ravin CE, Deering TF, Putnam CE, McCloud TC, Greenspan RH: The efficacy of full-lung tomography in the detection of early metastatic disease from melanoma. Radiology 144:27, 1982

49. Cohen M, Provisor A, Smith W, Weetman R: Efficacy of whole lung tomography in diagnosing metastases from solid tumors in children. Radiology 141:375, 1981

50. Bergman SM, Lippert M, Javadpour N: Value of WLT in early detection of metastatic disease in patients with renal cell carcinoma and testicular tumors. J Urol 124:860, 1980

51. Jochelson M, Garnick MB, Balikian JP, Richie JP: Efficacy of routine whole lung tomography in germ cell tumors. Cancer (In press)

52. Muhm JR, Brown LR, Crowe JK, Sheedy PF, Hattery RR, Stephens DH: Comparison of whole lung tomography and computed tomography for detecting pulmonary nodules: Am J Roentgenol 131:981, 1978

53. Kaufman L, Crooks LE, Margulis AR (eds): NMR imaging in medicine. Igaka Shoin, New York, 1981

54. Tepperman BS, Fitzpatrick PJ: Second respiratory and upper digestive tract malignancies after oral cancer. Lancet i:547, 1981

55. Cahan WG, Castro EB, Hadju SI: Therapeutic pulmonary resection of colonic carcinoma metastatic to the lung. Dis Col Rect 17:302, 1974

56. Sherwin RP: The differentiation of primary lung cancer from metastatic disease. In Weiss L, Gilbert HA (eds): Pulmonary Metastasis. Vol. 1. G.K. Hall, Boston, 1978

57. Vincent RG, Choksi LB, Takita H, Gutierrez AC: Surgical resection of the solitary pulmonary metastasis. In Weiss L, Gilbert HA (eds): Pulmonary Metastasis. Vol. 1. G.K. Hall & Co, Boston, 1978

58. Cliffton EE, Pool JL: Treatment of lung metastases in children with combined therapy. J Thorac Cardiovasc Surg 54:403, 1967

59. Kilman JW, Kronenberg MW, O'Neill JA, Klassen KP: Surgical resection for pulmonary metastases in children. Arch Surg 99:158, 1969

60. Goorin AM, Delorey MJ, Williamson KR, Levy R, Tapper D, Link M, Abelson HT: Outcome of patients who develop pulmonary metastatic disease after adjuvant chemotherapy for osteosarcoma. Proc Am Soc Clin Oncol p. 184 (C-717), 1982 (Abstract)

61. Sweetnam R, Ross K: Surgical treatment of pulmonary metastases from primary tumours of bone. J Bone Joint Surg 49B:74, 1967

62. Martini N, Huvos A, Mike V, Marcove RC, Beattie EJ: Multiple pulmonary resections in the treatment of osteogenic sarcoma. Ann Thorac Surg 12:271, 1971

63. Ishihara T, Ikeda T, Yamazaki S, Shibata H: Treatment for pulmonary metastasis arising from osteogenic sarcoma. Keio J Med 20:195, 1971

64. Beattie EJ, Martini N, Rosen G: The management of pulmonary metastases in children with osteogenic sarcoma with surgical resection combined with chemotherapy. Cancer 35:618, 1975

65. Spanos PK, Payne WS, Ivins JC, Pritchard DJ: Pulmonary resection for metastatic osteogenic sarcoma. J Bone Joint Surg 58A:624, 1976

66. Dunn D, Dehner LP: Metastatic osteosarcoma to lung. Cancer 40:3054, 1977

67. Telander RL, Pairolero PC, Pritchard DJ, Sim FH, Gilchrist GS: Resection of pulmonary metastatic osteogenic sarcoma in children. Surgery 84:335, 1978

68. Rosen GR, Huvos AG, Mosende C, Beattie EJ, Exelby PR, Capparos B, Marcove RC: Chemotherapy and thoracotomy for metastatic osteogenic sarcoma: A model for adjuvant chemotherapy and the rationale for the timing of thoracic surgery. Cancer 41:841, 1978

69. Burgers JMV, Breur K, van Dobbenburgh OA, Hazebroek F, Vos A, Voute PA: Role of metastatectomy without chemotherapy in the management of osteosarcoma in children. Cancer 45:1664, 1980

70. Levine AS, Appelbaum FR, Echelberger C, Wesley R, Johnston M, Rosenberg S: Metastatectomy followed by multi-agent intensive chemotherapy (CT) in osteosarcoma. Proc Am Soc Clin Oncol p. 184 1982 (Abstract C-716)

71. Morton DL, Eilber FR. Soft tissue sarcomas. In Holland JF, Frei E III (eds): Cancer Medicine. 2nd ed. Lea & Febiger, Philadelphia, 1982

72. Katzenstein AL, Purvis R, Gmelich J, Askin F: Pulmonary resection for metastatic renal adenocarcinoma. Cancer 41:712, 1978

73. Huth JF, Holmes EC, Vernon SE, Callery CD, Ramming KP, Morton DL: Pulmonary resection for metastatic sarcoma. Am J Surg 140:9, 1980

74. Feldman PS, Kyriakos M: Pulmonary resection for metastatic sarcoma. J Thorac Cardiovasc Surg 64:784, 1972

75. Huang MN, Edgerton F, Takita H, Douglas HO, Karakousis C: Lung resection for metastatic sarcoma. Am J Surg 135:804, 1978

76. Creagan ET, Fleming TR, Edmonson JH, Pairolero PC: Pulmonary resection for metastatic nonosteogenic sarcoma. Cancer 44:1908, 1979

77. Collins VP, Loeffler RK, Tivey H: Observations on growth rates of human tumors. Amer J Roentgenol 76:988, 1956

78. Collins VP: Time of occurrence of pulmonary metastases from carcinoma of colon and rectum. Cancer 15:387, 1962

79. Hegemann G, Muhe E: Exstirpation von Metasten. Langenbecks Arch Chir 342:261, 1976

80. Adkins PC, Wesselholft CW, Newman W, Blades B: Thoracotomy on the patient with previous malignancy: metastases or new primary? J Thorac Cardiovasc Surg 56:351, 1968

81. Nicolson GL: Cell surfaces and cancer metastasis. Hosp Practice 17:75, 1982

82. Fidler IJ, Poste G: The biologic diversity of cancer metastases. Hosp Practice 17:57, 1982

83. Spremulli EN, Dexter DL: Human tumor cell heterogeneity and metastasis. J Clin Oncol 1:496, 1983

84. Fidler IJ: Selection of successive tumor lines for metastasis. Nature New Biol 242:148, 1973

85. Nicolson GL: Cell surface antigen heterogeneity and blood borne tumor metastasis. In Owens AH, Coffey DS, Baylin S (eds): Tumor Cell Heterogeneity: Origins and Implications. Academic Press, New York, 1982

86. Nicolson GL, Custead SE: Tumor metastasis is not due to adaptation of cells to a new organ environment. Science 215:176, 1982

87. Talmadge JE, Fidler IJ: Cancer metastasis is selective or random depending on the parent population. Nature 297:593, 1982

88. Poste G, Tzeng J, Doll J, Greig R, Rieman D, Zeidman I: Evaluation of tumor cell heterogeneity during progressive growth of individual lung metastases. Proc Natl Acad Sci 79:6574, 1982

89. Fidler IJ, Hart IR: The origin of metastatic heterogeneity in tumors. Eur J Cancer 17:487, 1981

90. Fidler IJ, Poste G: The heterogeneity of metastatic properties in malignant tumor cells and regulation of the metastatic phenotype. In Owens AH, Coffey DS, Baylin S (eds): Tumor Cell Heterogeneity: Origins and Implications. Academic Press, New York, 1982

91. McCredie JA, Inch WR, Kruuv J, Watson TA: The rate of tumor growth in animals. Growth 29:331, 1965

92. Prehn RT: Antigenic heterogeneity: A possible basis for progression. In Owens AH, Coffey DS, Baylin S (eds): Tumor Cell Heterogeneity: Origins and Implications. Academic Press, New York, 1982

93. Viadana E, Bross IDJ, Pickren JW: Cascade spread of blood-borne metastases in solid and nonsolid cancers of humans. In Weiss L, Gilbert HA (eds): Pulmonary Metastasis. Vol 1. G.K. Hall, Boston, 1978

94. Salmon SE, Jones SE (eds): Adjuvant Therapy of Cancer. II. Grune & Stratton, New York, 1979

95. Weiss L, Gilbert HA (eds): Pulmonary Metastasis. Vol. 1. G.K. Hall, Boston, 1978

96. Kradjian RM, Bennington JL: Renal carcinoma recurrent 31 years after nephrectomy. Arch Surg 90:192, 1965
97. Orteza AM, Kandzari SJ, Milam DF: Transitional cell carcinoma of the bladder with pulmonary metastasis: Case report on 5 year survival following resection of metastasis. J Urol 105:232, 1971
98. Seymour JE, Malin JM, Pierce JM: Late metastasis of a superficial transitional cell carcinoma of the bladder. J Urol 108:277, 1972
99. Tolia BM, Whitmore WF, Jr: Solitary metastasis from renal cell cancer. J Urol 114:836, 1975
100. O'Dea MJ, Zincke H, Utz, DC, Bernatz PE: The treatment of renal cell cancer with solitary metastasis. J Urol 120:540, 1978
101. Mayo P, Saha SP, McElvein RB: Long-term survival after resection of multiple pulmonary metastases from adenocarcinoma of the kidney. South Med J 74:1161, 1981
102. Kjaer M, Engelholm SA: The clinical course and prognosis of patients with renal adenocarcinoma with solitary metastasis. Br J Rad Oncol Biol Phys 8:1691, 1982
103. Cowles RS, Johnson DE, McMurtrey MJ: Long-term results following thoracotomy for metastatic bladder cancer. Urology 20:390, 1982
104. Saitoh H, Hida M, Nakamura K, Shimbo T, Shiramizu T, Satoh T: Metastatic processes and a potential indication of treatment for metastatic lesions of renal adenocarcinoma. J Urol 128:916, 1982
105. Middleton RG: Surgery for metastatic renal cell carcinoma. J Urol 97:973, 1967
106. Dunnick NR, Wixson D, Dopmann JL, Bakins KG, Javadpour N: Metastatic renal cell carcinoma to the remaining kidney 14 years after nephrectomy, Cardiovasc Radiol 2:127, 1979
107. Walter CW, Gillespie DR: Metastatic renal cell carcinoma of 50 years duration. Minn Med 43:123, 1960
108. Snow RM, Schellhammer PF: Spontaneous regression of metastatic renal cell carcinoma. Urology 20:177, 1982
109. Braren V, Taylor JN, Pace W: Regression of metastatic renal carcinoma following nephrectomy. Urology 3:777, 1974
110. Bartley O, Hultquist GT: Spontaneous regression of renal cell carcinoma. Acta Pathol Microbiol Scand 27:448, 1963
111. Degiorgi S: Regression of pulmonary metastasis during radiation to a renal cell carcinoma. Cancer 30:895, 1972
112. Freed SZ, Halperin JP, Gordon M: Idiopathic regression of metastases from renal cell carcinoma. J Urol 118:538, 1977
113. Middleton HW: Indications for and results of nephrectomy for metastatic renal cell carcinoma. Urol Clin N Am 7:711, 1980
114. Mostofi FK: Pathology and spread of renal cell carcinoma. In King JS (ed): Renal Neoplasia. Little Brown, Boston, 1967
115. Becker NH, Soifer I: Benign clear cell tumor of the lung. Cancer 27:712, 1971
116. Leibow AA, Castleman B: Benign clear cell tumor of the lung. Yale J Biol Med 43:213, 1971
117. Morgan AD, MacKenzie DH: Clear cell carcinoma of the lung. J Pathol and Bacteriol (London) 87:25, 1964
118. Altaffer LF: Paraneoplastic endocrinopathies associated with renal tumors. J Urol 122:573, 1979
119. Saitoh H, Nakayama M, Nakamura K, Satoh T: Distant metastases of renal adenocarcinoma in nephrectomized cases. J Urol 127:1092, 1982

120. Kagan AR, Rao AR, Nussbaum H, Gilbert HA, Chan PYM: Radiation therapy of pulmonary metastasis. In Weiss L, Gilbert HA (eds): Pulmonary Metastasis. Vol. 1. G.K. Hall & Co., Boston, 1978

121. Phillips T: The radiotherapeutic management of pulmonary metastases. Int J Rad Oncol Biol Phys 1:743, 1976

122. Breur K, Cohen P, Schweisgirth O, Hart AAM: Irradiation of the lungs as adjuvant therapy in the treatment of osteosarcoma of the limbs. Eur J Cancer 145:461, 1978

123. Thompson HT, Goldstein AM: Resection in the treatment of pulmonary metastases from testicular tumors and its influence on overall survival rate. Br J Surg 56:349, 1969

124. Rees GM, Cleland WP: Surgical treatment of pulmonary metastases from testicular tumors. Br Med J 3:467, 1971

125. Skinner DG, Leadbetter WF, Wilkins EW: The surgical management of testis tumors metastatic to the lung: A report of 10 cases with subsequent resection of from one to seven pulmonary nodules. J Urol 105:275, 1971

126. Wettlaufer JN: Stage III germinal testis tumors: aggressive approach. J Urol 116:593, 1976

127. Straus MJ: The growth characteristics of lung cancer and its application to treatment design. Sem Oncol 1:167, 1974

128. Merrin CE: Combined surgical and chemotherapeutic approach to metastases and testicular tumors. In Weiss L, Gilbert HA (eds): Pulmonary Metastasis. Vol. 1. G.K. Hall & Co, Boston, 1978

129. Peckham MJ: The investigation and management of testicular tumors. In Carter SK, Glatstein E, Livingston RS (eds): Principles of Cancer Treatment. McGraw-Hill, New York, 1982

130. Staubitz WJ, Early KS, Magoss IV, Murphy GP: Surgical treatment of nonseminomatous germinal testes tumors. Cancer 32:1206, 1973

131. Merrill DC: Modified thoracoabdominal approach to the kidney and retroperitoneal tissue. J Urol 117:15, 1977

132. Merrin CE, Takita H: Cancer reductive surgery. Report on the simultaneous excision of abdominal and thoracic metastases from widespread testicular tumors. Cancer 42:495, 1978

133. Scardino PT, Skinner DG: Germ-cell tumors of the testis: Improved results in a prospective study using combined modality therapy and biochemical tumor markers. Surgery 86:86, 1979

134. Merrin C: Combination of chemotherapy and debulking surgery. In van Oosterom AT et al (eds): Therapeutic Progress in Ovarian Cancer. Martinus Nijhoff, Boston, 1980

135. Merrin C, Baumgartner G, Wajsman Z: Benign transformation of testicular carcinoma by chemotherapy. Letter. Lancet i:43, 1975

136. Donohue JP, Einhorn LH, Williams SD: Cytoreductive surgery for metastatic testis cancer: Considerations of timing and extent. J Urol 123:876, 1980

137. Hendry WF, Barrett A, McElwain TJ, Wallace DM, Peckham MJ: The role of surgery in the combined management of metastases from malignant teratomas of testis. Br J Urol 52:38, 1980

138. Mandelbaum I, Williams SD, Einhorn LH: Aggressive surgical management of testicular carcinoma metastatic to lungs and mediastinum. Ann Thorac Surg 30:224, 1980

139. Einhorn LH, Williams SD, Mandelbaum I, Donohue JP: Surgical resection in disseminated testicular cancer following chemotherapeutic cytoreduction. Cancer 48:904, 1981

140. Skinner DG: Advanced metastatic testicular cancer: The need for reporting results according to initial extent of disease. J Urol 128:312, 1981

141. Stahel RA, Von Hochstetter AR, Largiader F, Schmucki O, Honegger HP: Surgical resection of residual tumor after chemotherapy in nonseminomatous testicular cancer. Eur J Cancer Clin Oncol 18:1259, 1982

142. Vugrin D, Whitmore WF Jr., Sogani PC, Bains M, Herr HW, Golbey RB: Combined chemotherapy and surgery in treatment of advanced germ-cell tumors. Cancer 47:2228, 1981

143. Vugrin D, Whitmore WF Jr., Bains M, Golbey RB: Role of chemotherapy and surgery in the treatment of thoracic metastases from nonseminomatous germ cell testis tumor. Cancer 50:1057, 1982

144. Callery CD, Holmes EC, Vernon S, Huth J, Coulson WF, Skinner DG: Resection of pulmonary metastases from nonseminomatous testicular tumors. Cancer 51:1152, 1983

145. Garnick MB, Canellos GP, Richie JP: Treatment and surgical staging of testicular and primary extragonadal germ cell cancer. JAMA 250:1733, 1983

146. Vogelzang NJ, Stenlund R: Residual pulmonary nodules after combination chemotherapy of testicular cancer. Radiology 146:195, 1983

147. Mandelbaum I, Yaw PB, Einhorn LH, Williams SD, Rowland RG, Donohue JP: The importance of one-state median sternotomy and retroperitoneal node dissection in disseminated testicular cancer. Ann Thorac Surg 36:524, 1983

148. Einhorn LH, Donohue JP: *Cis*-diamminedichloroplatinum, vinblastine and bleomycin combination chemotherapy in disseminated testicular cancer. Ann Int Med 87:293, 1977

149. Vugrin D, Herr H, Whitmore W, Sogani P, Golbey RB: VAB-6 combination chemotherapy in disseminated cancer of the testes. Ann Int Med 95:59, 1981

150. Javadpour N, Ozols RF, Anderson T, Barlock AB, Wesley R, Young RC: A randomized trial of cytoreductive surgery followed by chemotherapy versus chemotherapy alone in bulky stage III testicular cancer with poor prognostic features. Cancer 50:2004, 1982

151. Einhorn LH, Williams SD: The management of disseminated testicular cancer. In Carter SK, Glatstein E, Livingston RB (eds): Principles of Cancer Treatment. McGraw-Hill, New York, 1982

152. McCrea ES, Diaconis JN, Wade JC, Johnston CA: Bleomycin toxicity simulating metastatic nodules to the lungs. Cancer 48:1096, 1981

153. Bauer KA, Skarin AT, Balikian JP, Garnick MB, Rosenthal DS, Canellos GP: Pulmonary complications associated with combination chemotherapy programs containing bleomycin. Am J Med 74:557, 1983

154. Bosl GJ, Geller NL, Cirrincione C, Nisselbaum J, Vugrin D, Whitmore W, Golbey RB: Serum tumor markers in patients with metastatic germ cell tumors of the testes: a ten year experience. Am J Med 75:29, 1983

155. Ginsberg SJ, Comis RL: The pulmonary toxicity of antineoplastic agents. Sem Oncol 9:34, 1982

156. Goldiner PL, Carlon GC, Cvitovic E, Schweizer O, Howland WS: Factors influencing postoperative morbidity and mortality in patients treated with bleomycin. Br Med J 1:1664, 1978

157. Willis GW, Hajdu SI: Histologically benign teratoid metastases of testicular carcinoma. Report of five cases. Am J Clin Pathol 59:338, 1973

158. Hong WK, Wittes RE, Hajdu ST, Cvitovic E, Whitmore WF, Golbey RB: The evolution of mature teratoma from malignant testicular tumors. Cancer 40:2987, 1977

159. Ulbright TM, Loehrer PJ, Roth LM, Einhorn LH, Williams SD, Clark SA: The development of non-germ cell malignancies within germ cell tumors: A clinicopathologic study of eleven cases. Cancer (In press)
160. Martin JR: Teratocarcinomas and mammalian embryogenesis. Science 209:768, 1980
161. Griffin JD, Major PP, Munroe D, Kufe D: Induction of differentiation of human myeloid leukemia cells by inhibitors of DNA synthesis. Exp Hematol 10:774, 1982

Index

Page numbers followed by t represent tables; those followed by f represent figures.